MUSCULOSKELETAL
PRIMARY CARE

D1440739

MUSCULOSKELETAL
PRIMARY CARE

Sharon J. Gates, RN, MSN, ANPC

Nurse Practitioner, Musculoskeletal Medicine Unit
Beth Israel Deaconess Medical Center
Adjunct Assistant Professor of Nursing
Northeastern University
Boston, Massachusetts

Pekka A. Mooar, MD

Assistant Professor
Medical College of Pennsylvania/Hahnemann University School of Medicine
Chief of Orthopaedics
Medical College of Pennsylvania Hospital
Philadelphia, Pennsylvania

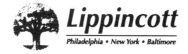

Lippincott

Philadelphia • New York • Baltimore

Acquisitions Editor: Lisa Stead
Editor: Claudia Vaughn
Project Editor: Tom Gibbons
Senior Production Manager: Helen Ewan
Senior Production Coordinator: Nannette Winski
Assistant Art Director: Doug Smock
Index: Lynne Mahan
Compositor: The PRD Group
Printer: RR Donnelley, Crawfordsville

This book is published as a re-titled, revised edition of *Orthopaedics and Sports Medicine for Nurses,* © 1989 Williams & Wilkins.

Library of Congress Cataloging in Publication Data

Musculoskeletal primary care / [edited by] Sharon Gates, Pekka Mooar.
    p.   cm.
Includes bibliographical references and index.
ISBN 0-7817-1430-3 (alk. paper)
    1. Musculoskeletal system—Diseases—Treatment.   2. Primary care
(Medical care)   3. Musculoskeletal system—Diseases—Prevention.
4. Orthopedics.   5. Orthopedic nursing.   I. Gates, Sharon J.
II. Mooar, Pekka A.
    [DNLM: 1. Musculoskeletal Diseases—therapy.   2. Musculoskeletal
Diseases—diagnosis.   3. Primary Health Care.   WE 140M9862 1999]
RC925.M856   1999
616.7—dc21
DNLM/DLC
for Library of Congress   98-38544
                                                                        CIP

Care has been taken to confirm the accuracy of the information presented and to describe generally accepted practices. However, the authors, editors, and publisher are not responsible for errors or omissions or for any consequences from application of the information in this book and make no warranty, express or implied, with respect to the contents of the publication.

The authors, editors and publisher have exerted every effort to ensure that drug selection and dosage set forth in this text are in accordance with current recommendations and practice at the time of publication. However, in view of ongoing research, changes in government regulations, and the constant flow of information relating to drug therapy and drug reactions, the reader is urged to check the package insert for each drug for any change in indications and dosage and for added warnings and precautions. This is particularly important when the recommended agent is a new or infrequently employed drug.

Some drugs and medical devices presented in this publication have Food and Drug Administration (FDA) clearance for limited use in restricted research settings. It is the responsibility of the health care provider to ascertain the FDA status of each drug or device planned for use in their clinical practice.

9   8   7   6   5   4   3   2   1

To our families
Irving, Robert and Glenn
and
Sally, Ethan, Rebecca and Sarah

Contributors

Harris Gellman, MD
Professor, Orthopaedic and Plastic
  Surgery
Director, Center for Hand and Upper
  Extremity Surgery
Department of Orthopaedic Surgery
University of Arkansas
Little Rock, Arkansas

Paul A. Glazer, MD
Instructor in Orthopaedic Surgery
Harvard Medical School
Beth Israel Deaconess Medical Center
Boston, Massachusetts

Katherine S. Lyman, RN-C, MSN
Geriatric Nurse Practioner
Division of Gerontology
Beth Israel Deaconess Medical Center
Boston, Massachusetts

**Frances Lynn McCullough,
  MNSc, RNP**
Arkansas Spine Center
Little Rock, Arkansas

James E. Nixon, MD
Emeritus Clinical Professor of
  Orthopaedics
University of Pennsylvania
Philadelphia, Pennsylvania

Sally Pullman-Mooar, MD
Clinical Assistant Professor
Thomas Jefferson University
Philadelphia, Pennsylvania

William H. Simon, MD, FACS
Clinical Associate Professor
Department of Orthopaedic Surgery
University of Pennsylvania School of
  Medicine
Philadelphia, Pennsylvania

Katherine Taft, RN-C, MSN
Orthopaedic Nurse Practioner
Department of Nursing
Beth Israel Deaconess Medical Center
Boston, Massachusetts

Jeffery L. Zilberfarb, MD
Instructor in Orthopaedic Surgery
Harvard Medical School
Beth Israel Deaconess Medical Center
Boston, Massachusetts

Reviewers

Katherine Brew Barbee, MSN,
  ARNP
Nurse Practitioner
Primary Care Center
Adjunct Faculty, Nurse Practitioner
  Program
George Washington University
Washington, DC

Patricia C. Birchfield, RN, DSN
Associate Professor
College of Nursing
University of Kentucky
Lexington, Kentucky

Michael H. Cox, PhD
Corporate Vice President for
  Occupational Health
Center for Preventative Medicine and
  Human Performance and the
  Urgent Care Business
Crozer-Keystone Health System
Crozer, Pennsylvania

Eileen M. Crutchlow, EdD, FNP,
  APRN
Associate Professor
Department of Nursing
Southern Connecticut State University
New Haven, Connecticut

Catherine Foster, BSN, MSN,
  CNP
Graduate Faculty in Women's Health
  and Community Health
Family Nurse Practitioner Program
College of Nursing and Health
  Sciences
Women's Health Nurse Practitioner
Student Health Center
The University of Texas at El Paso
El Paso, Texas
Women's Health Nurse Practitioner
Mesilla Valley Health Care Associates
Las Cruces, New Mexico

Delwin Jacoby, MSN, CFNP
Family Nurse Practitioner
Anderson Family Health Center
Adjunct Faculty
Family Nurse Practitioner Program
Spalding University
Louisville, Kentucky

James P. Ressler, PA-C
Associate Faculty Senior Physician
  Assistant
Department of Orthopaedic Surgery
University of California, San
  Francisco Medical Center
San Francisco, California

Benita Walton-Moss
Assistant Professor
Coordinator, Nurse Practitioner Program
School of Nursing
The Catholic University of America
Washington, DC

Forewords

The 1990s have brought about a dramatic change in health care. The introduction of managed care with its emphasis on cost saving has placed a spotlight on both outpatient and primary health care. The challenge for health care providers is to continue to provide comprehensive and high quality care while containing costs. Patients with musculoskeletal problems make up a large percentage of those now seen in the primary care setting. Individuals in all stages of the lifespan come to the office with concerns related to musculoskeletal pain and various degrees of immobility. This book, devoted to the common musculoskeletal and orthopaedic problems encountered by these individuals—from young children to seniors—offers the convenience of one-stop shopping for the primary care provider searching for tips on how to evaluate and manage these individuals of diverse age groups.

Musculoskeletal Primary Care is unique in several respects. The first chapter offers the reader the opportunity to understand the psychosocial, physiologic, and developmental changes and concerns across the lifespan by discussing children, adolescents, adults, and older adults with musculoskeletal problems. The following chapters on specific, regional conditions provide the reader with focused guidelines for evaluating and treating specific age-related disorders. As more physicians and advanced practice nurses join forces to provide primary care to patients, it is especially helpful to find a text that incorporates an interdisciplinary approach using the expertise of both nurses and physicians to provide care.

Another unique characteristic of this book is its emphasis on prevention and patient education. The information about exercise prescriptions, laboratory studies, and diagnostic procedures greatly enhances the primary care provider's ability to build and maintain the patient–provider partnership in care. It is through this kind of solid and mutual partnership with the patient that the primary care provider is able to offer and oversee both continuity and quality of care. Nurses and physicians will find this book to be a valuable and much-utilized addition to their professional libraries.

Suzanne R. Langner, PhD, CRNP, FAAN
Associate Professor
Department of Nursing
Thomas Jefferson University College of Health Professionals
Philadelphia, Pennsylvania

This book is designed to elaborate the musculoskeletal problems occurring at all ages and create an interdisciplinary approach in caring for patients with common musculoskeletal problems.

The aging population brings new challenges to all areas of medicine. The task for health care at the beginning of the 21st century is to provide adequate care for an increasingly older population and to deliver that care so that it promotes a sense of well-being and independence. A focus on function should be a major characteristic of good health care for the elderly. That level of quality health care will require an interdisciplinary approach to patient assessment and a more holistic consideration of patients and their quality of life.

Traditional medicine and its systems are in the process of change, as consumers become more informed of their choices of available health care and what they can expect for their health care dollars. Providers are currently required to uphold and perform to a standard of excellence that customers are expecting. Patients are more empowered as to the choice of their health care providers; This includes a choice of physicians and nurses. Wellness and healing are hallmarks of these moves. These changes require an emphasis on prevention and patient education. This book helps to seek an interdisciplinary approach among physicians and advanced practice nurses in the evaluation and care of patients with common musculoskeletal problems.

Stephen J. Lipson, MD
Chairman
Department of Orthopaedic Surgery
Beth Israel Deaconess Medical Center
Harvard Medical School
Boston, Massachusetts

William P. Docken, MD
Department of Medicine
Beth Israel Deaconess Medical Center
Harvard Medical School
Boston, Massachusetts

Preface

I
n 1983 we began to work together to develop a concept of collaborative practice in orthopaedics. We discovered that collaborative practice between a nurse practitioner and an orthopaedic surgeon enhanced patient care, through the merging of nursing and medical philosophies of care.

Our commitment to patient care through a collaborative practice model became the driving force behind the writing of this text. It is our hope that the reader will find as we have, that practicing in a collaborative, complementary manner allows the patient to experience the uniqueness of both nursing and medicine. It is this collaboration that ultimately helps the patient to obtain the best possible outcome.

Our motivation for this edition focused on the expanding role of primary care providers in the diagnosis and medical management of patients with regional musculoskeletal disease. In today's medical economic market place, the focus of patient care has shifted from the specialist's realm to primary care, and it is in this setting that practitioners are being asked to efficiently and competently manage the care of patients. Each day practitioners work in outpatient settings such as occupational health, primary care, secondary schools and colleges, and the emergency room, making clinical decisions that affect patient outcomes. These responsibilities speak to the necessity of the collaborative practice model.

Musculoskeletal Primary Care utilizes the community health preventive model to direct patient care. The prevention concept has three levels in which clinicians interact with patients: primary, secondary and tertiary (Leavell, H. R. et al., 1965). Primary prevention precedes dysfunction and has a twofold focus: (1) health promotion and (2) reduction of risks for illness. Primary intervention is aimed at educating a healthy population about adequate nutrition, exercise, and hygiene. Secondary prevention begins after dysfunction is recognized. It includes the screening of individuals thought to be at high risk for illness, follow-up after early detection, and treatment for existing illness and disability. Tertiary prevention (rehabilitation) begins when the dysfunction has stabilized and interventions focus on restoration of function and the prevention and limitation of further disability.

This manual is written to guide practitioners in the prevention and management of common regional musculoskeletal problems and to assist in the rehabilitation of patients with these problems. Where appropriate, it contains a review of basic anatomy and function, techniques of physical examination, and specific health management guidelines, presented in a problem-oriented format. Chapter One focuses on common age-related problems, beginning with the young child and continuing through the older adult. The following chapters are oriented around specific regional problems. This book provides quidelines to answer the most frequently asked patient care questions regarding prevention, evaluation, treatment, and predicted outcome.

S.J.G.
P.A.M.

Acknowledgments

W e wish to thank a number of our colleagues and associates without whom this publication would not have been possible.

We mention in particular Carol Hutelmyer, RN, CS, MSN, CRNP, Albert Einstein Medical Center, Nurse Practitioner HIV Program, Joint Appointee, LaSalle University School of Nursing, a visionary in collaborative practice; James E. Nixon, MD, for his recognition and promotion of the role of the nurse practitiner and the orthopedic surgeon; Tracey Hopkins, RN, BSN, Developmental Editor, for her detailed suggestions for Chapter 1; Robert Boutin, MD, Associate Professor, Department of Radiology, Veteran's Administration Hospital, San Diego, for his review of the lumbar MRI section; and lastly, Lippincott, Williams and Wilkins, especially Susan Glover, Senior Editor; Lisa Stead, Nursing Editor; Claudia Vaughn, Editorial Assistant; and Tom Gibbons, Associate Managing Editor.

Contents

MUSCULOSKELETAL
PRIMARY CARE

Chapter 1

Musculoskeletal Considerations Across the Life Span

Lynn McCullough, RNP, MNSc
Katherine S. Lyman, RNC, MSN, ANP, GNP

The musculoskeletal system consists of bones, muscles, ligaments, tendons, joints, and bursae. Injury and dysfunction of one part of the system often cause injury or dysfunction to adjacent structures. Although usually not life threatening, musculoskeletal problems have a significant impact on routine activities, self-concept, work capability, and, ultimately, independence. Musculoskeletal problems affect children, adolescents, adults, and mature adults; however, each group has specific challenges related to musculoskeletal health. This chapter reviews developmental tasks and physiologic characteristics associated with each group and covers conditions and diseases specific to age.

The Child

Psychosocial Factors That Influence Well-Being

Developmental Tasks

The developmental tasks of middle childhood, ages 6 to 12 years, involve finding a sense of industry and accomplishment versus a sense of inferiority (Erikson, 1963). School, where children learn to get along with peers, interact with authority figures, and identify gender-specific social roles, is key to the attainment of these tasks. Although thinking is still concrete, middle children are developing better reasoning abilities and learning to compromise. Gross and fine motor skills improve, and middle children begin to understand and enjoy competition. Expressing confidence in the middle child's ability to master new tasks and cope with new situations is important.

Adaptation to Illness and Injury

The middle child with an illness or injury is likely to feel guilty or think of it as a punishment for wrongdoing. Fear of loss of function, disfigurement, loss of control, and death (which is incompletely understood) is common. Explanations of the cause of the illness or injury, procedures, and treatments are very important and must be provided at a level the child can understand. Because children in this age group are beginning to develop their self-image and tend to be very self-conscious, it is important to respect their modesty.

The Child and Musculoskeletal Health

The epiphyseal plate is a unique feature of growing long bones (Fig. 1-1). Multiplying and enlarging cells in the epiphyseal plate push the articular cartilage away from the metaphysis and diaphysis. Concurrently, the cartilage cells located at the metaphyseal side of the epiphyseal plate become inactive and are replaced by bone. Trauma can separate the epiphyseal plate at the metaphyseal side because it is the weakest section of the growth plate. Disrupted blood supply to the plate can lead to termination of growth and a short extremity. Because the ligaments are stronger than the growth plate, epiphyseal injuries occur more often than ligamentous injuries in the immature skeleton.

Age-Related Issues and Challenges to Musculoskeletal Health

The musculoskeletal challenges experienced by children are due to trauma, congenital defects, and the sequelae of chronic illnesses such as cerebral palsy and spina bifida.

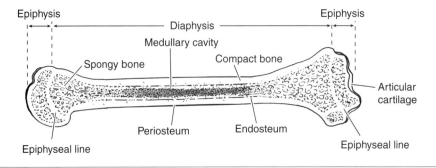

FIGURE 1-1. Basic long bone structure.

Fractures

Because the bones and ligaments of the immature skeleton have different biomechanical properties, they react differently to injuries and stresses. Fractures unique to the growing skeleton are plastic deformation, greenstick fractures, torus fractures, epiphyseal fractures, and apophyseal avulsions. Plastic deformation and greenstick fractures result from the ability of the immature bone to bend rather than break and are treated as complete fractures. Plastic deformation, if unrecognized and untreated, can result in permanent deformity. Torus fractures occur when the thin cortex of the metaphysis reacts to compression and tension forces by buckling outward. Epiphyseal injuries require long-term follow-up because sequelae (such as leg length discrepancies and angular deformities) will not be immediately evident. Apophyseal fractures occur where major tendon units attach to bone at large prominences or tuberosities. Sudden, contractile forces of the attached muscle may result in separation of the plate rather than the attaching tendon. For example, in the adult, a sudden extension of the knee with the hip flexed will create a pulled hamstring; in the immature skeleton, this maneuver results in an avulsion of the ischial tuberosity, which may require surgical intervention. Other areas where apophyseal fractures occur are the lesser trochanter where the iliopsoas muscle attaches, the anterior inferior iliac spine where the rectus muscle attaches, and the iliac crest where the lateral abdominal muscles attach.

Ligamentous injuries occurring in isolation are rare in the immature skeleton because the adjacent epiphyseal plate will fail before failure of the ligament (as discussed earlier). These differences in injury patterns make it important to assess the skeletal maturity of the athlete to determine injuries for which he or she is most at risk. Instruction in injury prevention increases the understanding of associated risks (Table 1-1).

Legg-Calvé-Perthes Disease

Legg-Calvé-Perthes disease (LCP), avascular necrosis of the femoral head of unknown etiology, is a hip disorder occurring in 1 out of 1200 children and is most often diagnosed between the ages of 4 and 8, although it can be diagnosed as

---

TABLE 1-1

Prevention of Overuse Injuries

1. Choose the right activity. Help the young athlete choose a sport that will be compatible with physical ability, skill level, and talent.
2. Evaluate equipment for proper working order. Teach the participant to change to new shoes as soon as wear is noticed (usually on the outside border first).
3. Obtain a preseason physical examination. Teach the participant that this will help to focus on both strengths and limitations allowing adequate time before the sport season begins to increase fitness with a proper exercise prescription.
4. Gradually build up body condition. Teach the importance of getting in shape 6 weeks before the season starts. Include strength, stretching, and cardiorespiratory conditioning in regimen. This will not only tone the body, but will also increase endurance. Fatigue is an important factor in injuries.
5. Warm-up before each practice or game.
6. Teach the importance of proper cool-down.
7. Help the young athlete understand not to play or practice when overtired.

young as age 2. Presenting symptoms are limp, pain (hip or knee), and sometimes shortening of the affected extremity. LCP is a self-limiting disease that takes several years to run its course. Two primary treatment modalities are used: (1) observation with radiographs every 3 to 4 months, restriction of activities that stress the hip, and treatment of synovitis, and (2) bracing in an abducted position while the disease goes through its stages. The former is the treatment of choice; the latter is used when there is significant loss of hip motion or recurrent synovitis not controlled by nonsteroidal anti-inflammatory drugs (NSAIDs) and activity restriction. Care should be taken to maintain the femoral head within the acetabulum and to observe for recurrent subluxation that suggests the need for surgery. Neither treatment affects the progress of the disease. After radiographs show the complete healing of the femoral head, the child is released to full activities.

Leg Length Discrepancies

Leg length discrepancies occur from hemihypertrophy or hemiatrophy, as sequelae from other conditions such as trauma that damages the growth plate, or from unknown causes. A variety of interventions are available for the treatment of discrepancies other than the traditional shoe lift (usually an unacceptable treatment modality to any but the young child), including procedures to shorten a long extremity or lengthen a short one. Determining which procedure is best in a given case is an individualized process. Regular, long-term follow-up beginning when the diagnosis is made is essential to the timing of the procedures so that equal leg length is achieved when growth ends. Significant leg length discrepancies (>2.0 cm) can lead to knee, hip, and low back pain.

The Adolescent

Psychosocial Factors That Influence Well-Being

Developmental Tasks

The primary developmental task of adolescence is identity establishment versus role confusion (Erikson, 1963). A favorable self-concept is part of identity establishment. Although the process of developing a self-concept continues throughout life, it is first examined, questioned, and revised during adolescence. Individuals with a favorable self-concept and high levels of self-esteem are successful, creative, independent, and well equipped to handle the problems that arise in their lives. Another key to identity establishment is acquiring and exercising independence.

Peer acceptance and maintenance of a positive body image are essential to the adolescent's developing self-esteem and self-concept. The many physical changes that occur at this age can be daunting. Encouraging the adolescent through this difficult period by reassuring him or her of the normalcy of these changes and the feelings he or she may have about them will help. Participating in sports also helps establish a healthy, positive body image. However, the adolescent believes that he or she is invincible. This, coupled with the desire for independence and peer acceptance, may lead the teenager to take risks that increase the likelihood of injury.

Adaptation to Illness and Injury

The effect of injury or illness on the adolescent is significant. Any illness, even if of short duration or acute, makes them different from their peers for that period. Children with a chronic illness or a permanent disability face different obstacles in establishing their identity and independence.

Loss of control during illness can affect the adolescent's attitudes and reactions to others. The issue of establishing independence and identity is so important that adolescents will find areas over which they can take control and make decisions. He or she may become uncooperative or belligerent and refuse to participate in treatment. Recognizing this and finding instances when they can safely make decisions are important to their development while sick or injured.

The Adolescent and Musculoskeletal Health

Age-Associated Physical Changes

The "adolescent growth spurt" is a phenomenon well known to both health care providers and parents of adolescents. This growth occurs in both height and weight and is accompanied by the changes in sexual and physical maturity. The increase in height may mean the appearance of weight loss for some and the appearance of weight gain for others. All adolescents should be assessed in both these parameters and assisted in dealing with the changes.

During growth spurts (between the ages of 12 to 14 years), epiphyseal injuries occur more frequently in obese or tall, thin boys. Participation in contact sports at this time increases the youngster's risk for injury. At-risk adolescents should avoid contact sports until maturity of muscle and coordination has been achieved. The Tanner stages of sexual development aid in assessment of skeletal maturity and development. Fewer injuries occur when teams are organized by height, weight, and general physical fitness (American College of Sports Medicine, 1995).

Age-Related Issues and Challenges to Musculoskeletal Health

Sports and the Preparticipation Physical Examination

It is estimated that twenty million or more children (25% of girls and 50% of boys ages 8 to 16) are engaged in competitive sports in any given year. It is often required that adolescents have a preparticipation physical examination.

The purpose of the preparticipation physical examination is to detect medical conditions that could predispose the athlete to serious injury or death during sports participation. The current recommendation of the American Academy of Pediatrics is to screen all adolescents beginning a new sports program and to obtain histories annually for athletes continuing in the program. The examination must be tailored to the sport, with particular emphasis on those areas of the body at risk.

The preparticipation physical examination (Fig. 1-2) should include a thorough history of previous illnesses and injuries, immunization records, general physical examination, maturational assessment, musculoskeletal examination, eye examination, and urinalysis. The general physical examination should pay particular atten-

Date of Exam _____

School Official _____

Exam Doctor _____

PREPARTICIPATION SPORTS EXAM

A B C
Contact: Coach ☐
School Nurse ☐
Family Doctor ☐
Family Dentist ☐

THIS IS NOT A SUBSTITUTE FOR A REGULAR PHYSICAL EXAM PERFORMED BY YOUR FAMILY DOCTOR

Name _____ Grade _____ Age _____ Birthdate _____

School _____ Sport _____ Sex _____

Parents _____ Address _____ Phone _____

Family Doctor _____ Address _____ Phone _____

HISTORY: Answer No or Yes with details and dates. Use reverse side if necessary.

I. Have you ever sustained an injury which prevented you from playing sports for more than one day and have you had any injuries such as (circle):   skull fracture—brain surgery; concussion—knocked out; neck pain/injury—arm/finger numbness; back pain/injury—leg/toe numbness; heatstroke/fainting—exhaustion; broken bone—fracture; joint dislocation—out of place; deep bruise—muscle pull; ligament sprains; tender kneecap/shin; trick knee—catching/locking;

_____

_____

II. Do you have a history of and/or take medicine (specify) for any medical problems such as (circle): asthma—allergy—wheezing—short of breath, heart murmur/palpitation—rheumatic fever—high blood pressure, diabetes—high/low sugar, fainting—seizure; yellow jaundice—hepatitis, severe influenza/ cold—mononucleosis—weakness, anemia—bruise easily—bleeding—sickle cell, loss of eyesight, hearing, testicle, kidney, etc., hernia—rupture—bulging, skin disease—boils—rash, or other?

_____

_____

III. Are you allergic to any medicine such as (circle) penicillin, iodine, novocaine or other?

_____

_____

IV. Any family history of medically unexplained or cardiac caused sudden death under age 50?

_____

V. L.M.P. _____

BP ___/___ P ____ Ht ____ Wt ____ Gross Vision: R ____ L ____ , Pupils R ____ L ____ Lab: UA ____

EXAM:

1. Upper Extr: AC jts _____
    Symm _____
    ROM _____
2. Spine: Neck _____
    Fwd Bend _____
    Curve _____
3. Lower Extr: Gait _____
    1-Hop _____
    Duck _____
    Symm _____
    ROM _____

4. Heart: _____
5. Lungs: _____
6. Skin: _____
7. Abdo: Spleen _____
    Liver _____
8. GU: Hernia _____
    Testicles _____
9. Dental _____
10. Other _____
    _____

IMPRESSION:
☐ Satisfactory Exam
☐ Recommend further evaluation/rehabilitation regarding: _____

Contact your: School Nurse—Coach—Family Doctor—Family Dentist

CLEARANCE:

A—Cleared for: Collision — Contact — Noncontact sports
B—Cleared for: Collision — Contact — Noncontact sports after completing evaluation
C—NOT cleared for: Collision — Contact — Noncontact sports due to: _____

FIGURE 1-2. Form for a preparticipation physical examination. (Permission to reprint granted by the Section of Sports Medicine, Department of Orthopaedic Surgery, Cleveland Clinic Foundation, Cleveland, Ohio.)

tion to the cardiovascular system to detect abnormalities such as congenital or acquired heart disease, hypertension, arrhythmias, mitral valve prolapse, idiopathic hypertrophic subaortic stenosis, a history of fainting, chest pain during exercise, family history of heart disease, and heart murmurs. Additional studies determine the fitness of such individuals for sports participation. Precautions are indicated for the athlete with any acute or chronic medical conditions (asthma, seizure disorders) that require special management, or the athlete recovering from an illness such as mononucleosis who may have an enlarged spleen and be in less than optimal physical condition. Strength, flexibility, muscular development, and joint mobility are tested. All joints should be put through a full range of motion. The preparticipation examination of the female athlete includes a gynecologic history and screening for eating disorders, iron deficiency, and risk factors for osteoporosis. The preparticipation examination should also include education to reduce the risk of injury.

PHYSICALLY CHALLENGED CHILDREN. More physically challenged children are participating in sports, and the health care provider must consider several factors when guiding them so they will have the least risk of injury and greatest chance of success. These factors include size, coordination, degree of physical fitness, physical health, stage of maturation, mental development, and emotional stability. Also to be considered are the physical and psychological benefits weighed against the potential frustration from repeated failure, the level of competition, and the need for special protective equipment. Careful physical assessment combined with consultation with family and the personnel who will be supervising the sports activity will allow most children to participate successfully.

Trauma and the Adolescent

MOTOR VEHICLE ACCIDENTS. Trauma is the primary cause of death in the adolescent age group, and motor vehicle accidents are the primary cause of this trauma. Injuries that result from motor vehicle accidents are frequently severe, often requiring a prolonged hospital stay and long-term care. The adolescent suffers a major unplanned interruption in his or her life with the loss of the control and independence for which he or she had been striving. These patients often exhibit the maladaptive behavior discussed earlier and to a much more dramatic degree. After discharge, he or she will need help reentering school and outside activities and coping with any sequelae of the accident, such as casts, external fixators, scars, and restrictions in activities and abilities.

Many accidents can be prevented or lessened in severity by using protective equipment, better driver education, and better judgment. Education is important in reducing the incidence of motor vehicle–related injuries, but equally important is helping the injured adolescent cope with his or her feelings about the accident. There is usually a feeling of guilt in the adolescent who was the cause of an accident in which a friend or family member was injured or killed. Friends and parents may feel guilt also. Unless such emotions are expressed in a therapeutic environment, they can become very destructive.

SOFT TISSUE INJURIES. Ninety-five percent of all injuries are soft tissue injuries. The most common are sprains, strains, and contusions. The likelihood of injury increases with the violence of the sport. *Sprains* affect ligaments, whereas *strains* affect tendons. Both sprains and strains are graded on a scale of I to III according to severity. The loss of joint stability determines the severity of sprains. Grade I sprains are mild with only overstretching of the ligaments and no loss of stability; Grade II sprains have some instability; and Grade III sprains have total loss of ligamentous continuity. The severity of strains relates to the extent of disruption. Grade I and II sprains and strains can often be treated symptomatically with rest and muscle rehabilitation. Grade III sprains and strains frequently require surgical repair. Stretching and strengthening exercises are important in maintaining muscle flexibility and strength. Contusions should be treated with ice and compression. Severe contusions may benefit from elevation and rest.

FRACTURES. Stress fractures result from repetitive stresses concentrated on a specific area of bone. These occur most often in the tibia, fibula, metatarsals, and calcaneus. The symptoms are local pain increased by activity and relieved by rest. Initial radiographs will show no bony disruption; 2 to 3 weeks later, however, periosteal new bone may be seen. If untreated, stress fractures can become complete fractures.

Complete fractures result from sudden, obvious trauma. Upper extremity fractures can most often be treated on an outpatient basis. Fractures of the tibia and ankle may require hospitalization and surgical treatment, but often they can be handled on an outpatient basis. Fractures of the femur will usually require hospitalization and surgical treatment. In all cases, follow-up care is imperative to ensure that the fracture heals properly and that no change in neurovascular status has occurred. The patient and family must be instructed in the care of the cast or fixator device, use of any assistive devices (see Appendices C and D), and signs and symptoms that should be reported to the primary care provider. Special arrangements for homebound schooling will frequently be necessary. Communication with the school throughout treatment is of great benefit in providing the student the opportunity to continue his or her education and to maintain contact with peers.

Conditions Affecting the Upper Extremity

Nontraumatic causes of problems in the upper extremity include infection, congenital defects, and sequelae of injuries sustained at a younger age. Most problems affecting the upper extremity are traumatic in origin.

THE SHOULDER. The most common injuries of the shoulder girdle are acromioclavicular (AC) joint separations, fractures of the clavicle and proximal humerus, and problems associated with the rotator cuff. Injuries to the proximal humeral epiphyseal plate ("Little League shoulder") are common in "throwing" sports such as baseball. Female athletes are also at increased risk for shoulder injuries because the upper extremities are weaker than the lower extremities and the arms are shorter in relation to the body. Shoulder dislocations are rare in skeletally immature individuals. It is more likely that injury to the shoulder will be seen as fractures to the proximal humeral epiphysis or metaphysis. Some individuals can voluntarily dislocate their shoulder; this should not be treated as an injury and can usually be ignored.

THE ELBOW. Fracture is a common injury of the elbow. This requires immediate medical attention because permanent damage can result when the swelling that accompanies these injuries compresses the nearby neurovascular structures. Dislocations of the elbow are not uncommon and may be accompanied by an avulsion of the medial epicondyle or a coronoid fracture. These should not be reduced except by trained medical personnel.

"Little League elbow" is a phenomenon occurring from the repetitive activity of the acceleration phase of pitching that applies abnormal stresses on the growth centers of the elbow. Chronic overstress can lead to tendonitis, or osteochondral fractures of the capitellum or radial head, and to permanent disability. New regulations governing how much children can pitch within a given time should reduce the number of individuals seen with this problem.

THE WRIST AND HAND. Wrist and finger fractures are also common. Baseball, or mallet, finger is a fracture that occurs when the ball hits the tip of the extended finger. This is a hyperflexion injury. Failure to recognize this injury can result in permanent flexion deformity of the distal phalanx. Gymnasts are especially prone to injuries of the distal radial growth plate because they use their upper extremities for weight bearing. These injuries have a significant potential for growth disturbances.

Conditions Affecting the Lower Extremity

THE HIP. Injuries of the hip result from a single macrotrauma or repetitive microtrauma. The most serious injuries involving the hip are acute fracture or dislocation. These injuries are true emergencies. The blood supply to the femoral epiphysis is easily compromised and can result in disruption of the flow to the femoral head and ultimately to avascular necrosis, a serious condition with permanent disability. Other injuries about the hip and pelvis include avulsion injuries, contusions, hip pointers (contusion of the iliac crest with subperiosteal hematoma formation), stress fractures, apophysitis, and snapping hip syndrome.

Another source of hip problems in adolescence is sequelae from earlier illnesses or injuries, some of which only become evident at adolescence. A septic joint or osteomyelitis at a young age can result in permanent damage if joint cartilage was destroyed or growth plates were involved. Growth arrest may also occur from traumatic injuries (fractures, dislocations, crush injuries) suffered before adolescence and could result in less than full range of motion of a joint, pain, or discrepancies in leg lengths. Obtain the patient's orthopedic history, the extent of follow-up care, and the duration of symptoms such as pain or limp.

Legg-Calvé-Perthes disease, as discussed earlier, is usually diagnosed before adolescence but continues to have an effect throughout life. In adolescence, surgical procedures may be necessary to correct trochanteric overgrowth or leg length discrepancy. The child treated for *congenital dysplasia* of the hip may also need additional procedures for similar sequelae.

Leg length discrepancies, as discussed earlier, will need continued follow-up through adolescence as the skeleton completes maturation. A procedure to shorten the long extremity will be done after growth is complete and measurements can be accurately obtained.

Slipped capital femoral epiphysis (SCFE) is the displacement of the femoral head in relation to the femoral neck. It occurs in 1 out of 50,000 children and adolescents. It can be chronic or acute or a combination of both (eg, a 2- to 3-month history of hip pain exacerbated after a fall or twisting injury to the hip). Early, accurate diagnosis is important to limit the amount of permanent disability. Any adolescent who presents with hip pain, limp, and external rotation of the leg should be assumed to have SCFE and referred for evaluation. Surgical intervention to prevent further slippage is necessary.

THE KNEE. Most knee complaints in adolescence are the result of trauma, especially overuse syndromes. *Patellofemoral arthralgia* (chondromalacia patellae) occurs frequently in adolescent girls and may or may not be related to overuse. The knee is often the site of injury in the form of fractures, ligamentous injuries, and various overuse syndromes.

Anterior knee pain is a common complaint in adolescence. Increased stress on the patella is a frequent cause. Pain is increased during activities that cause the knee to be flexed against pressure. This compresses the undersurface of the patella against the femoral condyles, resulting in pain. Tenderness is encountered on palpation of the undersurface of the patella. Having the athlete extend the knee and contract the quadriceps, while compressing the patella against the femoral condyles, will reproduce this pain. If there are no other associated conditions, this is usually a self-limiting condition, and symptoms disappear with stretching exercises and isometric exercises of the quadriceps and hamstrings. Isotonic exercises that bring the knee from a beginning flexed position into extension should be avoided.

Subluxation or recurrent dislocation of the patella is a common problem. Subluxation of the patella occurs in patellar malalignment syndromes where the patella moves down the intercondylar area unevenly. Quadriceps-strengthening exercises to improve patella femoral tracking are the mainstay of treatment. A patella stabilization sleeve is often beneficial. Surgery is indicated for persistent painful subluxation.

Dislocation of the patella occurs when the patella is completely displaced from the intercondylar joint. This is usually the result of a direct force that pushes the patella laterally and is accompanied by pain and swelling. The patella may spontaneously relocate or may require manipulation to relocate. Once the patella has dislocated, it is at risk to dislocate again. In the face of recurrent dislocations, the athlete must decide between surgery and modifying athletic pursuits.

Patellar tendonitis is usually due to overuse. It is known as "jumper's knee" because it is common in athletes participating in sports that involve jumping, such as basketball, modern dance, and high jumping. On examination, the inferior pole of the patellar tendon is tender. In chronic cases the patellar tendon may atrophy, and in severe cases it may rupture. Conservative treatment consisting of rest, heat, anti-inflammatory medication, and limitation of activity followed by progressive resistance exercises is usually all that is needed. A brace to restrain the patella should be worn when activity is resumed.

Apophysitis of the tibial tubercle is known as *Osgood-Schlatter's disease*. It develops during the period of most rapid growth (the prepubescent period in girls and early adolescence in boys). It is more common in boys and occurs bilaterally approximately 20% to 30% of the time. Symptoms include pain with activity, quadriceps atrophy, and a prominent, tender tibial tubercle. Treatment consists of limita-tion of activities, bracing, progressive resistive exercises, ice massage, and anti-inflammatory medication if necessary. Complete immobilization should be avoided because this increases muscle atrophy and lengthens rehabilitation time.

THE FOOT. Many complaints related to the foot can be treated with appropriate shoes. *Pes planus* (flat feet), which results in calf or foot pain, rarely requires more than a shoe with a good arch support or an insert with an arch. *Bunions,* although not extremely common at this age, are common enough to warrant mention. In their desire to be like everyone else, adolescents may wear shoes that are not comfortable and lead to hallux valgus (bunions). Bunions are treated by wearing shoes that fit well and allow room for the toes. Occasionally, a child presents with bunions resulting from metatarsus primus varus that are severe enough to require surgical correction to realign the metatarsal bone.

Sever's disease is a common cause of heel pain. It is frequently most noticeable after running and is seen usually in boys. The pain can be localized to the insertion of the Achilles tendon into the calcaneus or the plantar fascial insertions into the calcaneus. The use of heel cups inside the shoe and modification of activities (activity restricted until pain free) are usually all that is required as treatment.

Persistent complaints of foot pain that is worse with activity require a thorough evaluation to detect if a coalition between bones of the foot is present. Computerized tomography may be used to make this determination. If a coalition is found, surgical resection is necessary to prevent further pain or degenerative changes.

Conditions Affecting the Spine

The spine must receive special attention during the preadolescent and adolescent periods. Although uncommon, acute sprains and fractures of the spine are seen in children and adolescents and should be treated in the same manner as in the adult. Any injury to the spine must be treated as a fracture with immediate immobilization and transport to a medical facility. Improper handling of cervical spine fractures can increase or cause a neurologic deficit. Any athlete with a neck injury should be x-rayed. Persistent post-traumatic neck pain suggests spinal fracture or insta-bility.

SCOLIOSIS. The most common orthopedic problem of adolescence is scoliosis. Regular back screening examinations are necessary whether or not complaints related to the back exist. Scoliosis is a lateral curvature of the spine accompanied by vertebral rotation (Fig. 1-3). Scoliosis occurs from a variety of causes, including leg length discrepancies, spasticity, and structural anomalies, but typically the cause is idiopathic. Because scoliosis is usually not painful until a very large curve has developed, screening all children is important; often the adolescent and the parents are unaware of the curve. It is important that scoliosis be detected early, while the curve is small. Untreated, large curves will continue to progress throughout life and result in pulmonary and cardiac compromise, back pain, and severe cosmetic de-formity.

The first step in the evaluation for scoliosis is the history. Other important information includes complaints related to the back and any neurologic symptoms (numbness, tingling, loss of control of bowel or bladder, and so forth). Because

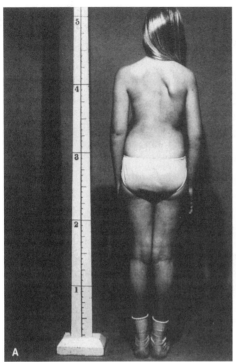 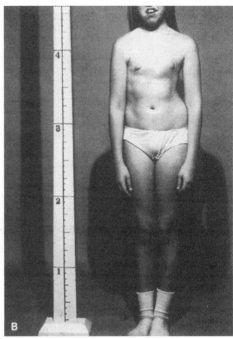

FIGURE 1-3. (**A**) A patient with a typical right thoracic curve as viewed from the back. The left shoulder is lower, and the right scapula is more prominent. The thorax is shifted to the right with a decreased distance between the right arm and the thorax. Because of the shift in the thorax to the right, the waistline is altered with the left iliac crest appearing higher. This crest asymmetry is apparent, not real. (**B**) A patient with a typical right thoracic curve as viewed from the front. The left shoulder appears lower. The thorax is shifted to the right with a decreased distance between the right arm and the thorax. The left hip appears more prominent secondary to the rightward shift of the thorax.

idiopathic scoliosis does not ordinarily cause pain or neurologic compromise, this information is important in differentiating the cause and determining if concurrent conditions exist. For females, knowing the date of menarche is important because 12 to 18 months of growth remain afterward.

Screening for scoliosis is simple and takes very little time. The patient should be undressed except for underwear. It is helpful, but not absolutely necessary, for girls to remove their bras to afford an unobstructed view of the back. The first part of the examination consists of having the patient stand straight but relaxed with feet together and hands by the sides. The signs to look for are:

1. Elevation of one shoulder
2. Elevation or prominence of one scapula
3. Elevation of the pelvis
4. Difference in the space between the arm and the body
5. Trunk shift with the head not aligned over the pelvis

Any one sign is probably not significant, but the presence of two or more raises suspicions for scoliosis and the patient should be referred to a spine specialist. The next step in the examination is to examine the patient from the side while he or she is still standing. Examine for the normal contours of thoracic kyphosis and lumbar lordosis. An exaggeration of these normal contours is a reason for referral, particularly if accompanied by complaints of pain. Next, have the patient place the hands together with the fingertips even and have him or her bend forward, dropping the head to the chest and allowing the arms to dangle (but keeping the hands together). Examine the back for an elevation of one side over the other. This unevenness is the result of a rib hump. As the vertebrae rotate and curve, the ribs are rotated as well, resulting in the rib hump. Have the patient bend slowly and examine the thoracic, thoracolumbar, and lumbar regions. This is a subjective examination, and a device called a scoliometer allows for a quantitated and specific examination. The scoliometer works on much the same principle as a carpenter's level and allows a numeric rating of rotation. It is simple to use and relatively inexpensive. Any child with a noticeable rib hump or with a scoliometer reading of 7 or more should be referred for further evaluation.

A very basic neurologic examination should also be completed. During the examination, look for any dimples or hairy patches on the back (indicative of spinal dysraphism) or other skin signs such as café au lait spots (indicative of neurofibromatosis). Scoliosis is more common in patients with spina bifida and neurofibromatosis. These patients may also have subtle neurologic findings.

Radiographs are vital for assessment of the curve. Serial films determine progression and are obtained at least twice a year, depending on the degree of curve and the remaining amount of skeletal growth expected. A curve lesser than 20 degrees requires semiannual or annual radiography depending on the skeletal maturity; a curve greater than 20 degrees requires more frequent radiologic observation, especially if significant growth remains. Obtain a standing anteroposterior view of the spine from the cervical area through the sacrum at the initial visit. A standing lateral view of the entire spine may be obtained as a screening film, but this view can often be omitted unless there is a specific indication (eg, back pain, kyphosis, or congenital deformity).

The treatment options for scoliosis include observation, bracing, and surgery. Treatment is based on many factors, including the degree of curvature, presence of structural abnormalities (hemivertebra), age of the child, skeletal maturity, location of the curvature, and psychosocial characteristics of the child and family. Generally, curves of 25 to 30 degrees are observed at 4- to 6-month intervals; curves between 30 and 40 degrees are braced; and curves greater than 40 to 50 degrees require surgery. These are very broad guidelines; it must be remembered that primary care providers' preferences vary, and curvature is not the only factor in determining treatment.

If bracing is prescribed, one of three types will be used. The Milwaukee brace consists of a pelvic girdle with a metal upper structure and attached pads. It is often poorly tolerated because of its restrictive nature and inability to be completely hidden by clothing. It is generally used on a full-time schedule, 22 to 23 hours daily. The Milwaukee brace can be used for any curve except those very high in the spine.

Low-profile braces (TLSO, Boston, Wilmington) are better tolerated. They can be better disguised under clothing because they do not have the metal upper structure and are less restrictive. They are worn on a full-time schedule. Low-profile braces are effective for curves with an apex of T8-9 or below.

The Charleston bending brace is the newest brace being used for scoliosis. Its advantage is that it is only worn at night. It can be used for most curves except those high in the spine and is most effective with single curves.

Bracing is instituted only in patients who have a year to a year and a half of growth remaining and is continued until skeletal maturity. The goal of bracing is to prevent progression of the curve; it does not provide correction. The curve present at the start of treatment will be the curve at the end of treatment. Therefore, bracing is only an option for curves less than 40 degrees.

A great deal of teaching is necessary for the patient and family (see Appendix C for brace care). The emotional and psychological aspects are as important as the physical aspects. Bracing makes the adolescent different from his or her peers, and the teenager must be helped in coping with the disorder and brace treatment. The family needs support also. If the brace is not tolerated for any reason, it is important that the adolescent and family do not feel as though they have failed.

Surgical correction is recommended for curves of 40 degrees or greater because they are biomechanically unstable and will progress significantly and result in complications. Surgery is the only treatment that will provide permanent correction. Surgery consists of spinal fusion in the corrected position using various types of instrumentation and bone grafting. The type of instrumentation and surgical approach used are determined by the surgeon's evaluation of the patient, the nature and flexibility of the curve, and which technique he or she believes yields the best results.

In most cases of idiopathic scoliosis, no postoperative immobilization is needed. If immobilization is needed, a polypropylene brace that can be removed on a daily basis for a shower is usually used. The average hospital stay is 5 days with a 1- to 2-week period of recuperation at home. The patient can resume all activities after 6 months.

BACK PAIN. Back pain in adolescents often results from overuse, lack of conditioning, or poor body mechanics. Most back pain is not serious, and treatment consists of a combination of rest, conditioning exercises, instruction in body mechanics, and anti-inflammatories. Some conditions that produce back pain are significant and include spondylolisthesis, spondylolysis, and spinal tumors (see Chapter 3).

The evaluation includes a pain history, sources of physical or emotional stress, and participation in activities that involve hyperextension of the back. Other components of the workup include a complete neurologic examination, complete x-rays, and often a bone scan. A magnetic resonance imaging (MRI) study can be helpful in some cases.

Chronic Conditions

Many chronic conditions result in permanent musculoskeletal disability. These include spina bifida, muscular dystrophy, and cerebral palsy. Surgical procedures, except spinal surgery, are usually done before adolescence. Neuromuscular scoliosis, different from idiopathic scoliosis, is a potential problem in all of the previously mentioned conditions. A latex allergy is more common in the spina bifida population, and health care providers should maintain latex precautions for all patients who have undergone multiple medical procedures.

The focus of the primary care provider is on helping these youngsters adjust to their limitations and accomplish the developmental tasks of adolescence. As much independence as possible is the primary goal. Help patients find areas in which they can excel and discover their personal strengths. Encourage competing in Para-Olympics or participating in other activities that give a sense of accomplishment.

Lesions of Bone

Because pediatric musculoskeletal malignant tumors are uncommon, they may be overlooked in the differential diagnosis of musculoskeletal complaints in adolescents. Considering neoplasms is important because a delay in diagnosis results in a poorer outcome. Lesions of bone usually present with a history of trauma or as a pathologic fracture. Pathologic fracture should be considered in the child who presents with pain and swelling after minor trauma, especially with a history of a lesion. These lesions may be benign (nonossifying fibroma, fibrous dysplasia, aneurysmal bone cyst, simple bone cyst, osteoid osteoma, exostoses) or malignant (Ewing's sarcoma, osteosarcoma). Any young person with pain, swelling, or tumor must be immediately referred to an orthopedic oncologist for complete evaluation. The use of limb salvage techniques, allografts, and prosthetic replacements has reduced the number of amputations done for malignant tumors. These surgical techniques, combined with radiotherapy and aggressive chemotherapy, have improved the prognosis for many malignant tumors, but the diagnosis must be made quickly for the optimum chance of success.

Exercise

Although children tend to be active, physical activity declines in adolescence (U.S. Department of Health and Human Services [DHHS], 1996). Instituting health-enhancing physical fitness behaviors should begin in childhood. Daily gym classes, regular family walks, and participation in team sports are examples of activities that can help establish a habit of exercise and provide multiple benefits (Box 1-1). Because the child or adolescent is at risk for overuse injuries and damage to epiphyseal plates, safety is a concern. The use of protective equipment, teams

---

Box 1-1 Potential Benefits of an Exercise Program for Children and Adolescents

Regular exercise can

- Improve self-confidence and self-image
- Provide an outlet for excess energy
- Improve cardiorespiratory efficiency
- Reduce risk factors associated with future coronary heart disease
- Develop motor coordination and flexibility
- Enhance social interaction through teamwork and participation
- Encourage prudent lifestyle habits

matched in height and weight, adequate conditioning, and an emphasis on skill development can reduce the risk of injury (American College of Sports Medicine, 1995).

The Adult

Psychosocial Factors That Influence Well-Being

Adulthood (18 to 60 years of age) has commonly been perceived as a time of stability and freedom. Adulthood, however, possesses its own difficult physiologic and psychosocial challenges. When evaluating the musculoskeletal risks and problems in the adult population, consideration must also be given to the developmental issues associated with this life stage.

Developmental Tasks

Young adulthood commences when there is closure on adolescent conflicts. It can be a turbulent transitional period as individuals continue to define their identities and establish themselves as productive members of society. Young adults face the challenges of completing their education, entering the labor force, determining career focus, and establishing intimate relationships. Deciding to marry, not to marry, or to defer marriage features prominently in the early adult years. Young adulthood is the time when many make the transition into parenthood, and the stress of balancing occupation, home, and family is a challenge.

In the middle years, the adult is cultivating and refining interpersonal relationships. Spouses may greatly modify their interaction with each other and focus their attentions from the children back to the marriage. Midlife crises may occur, and the potential for divorce is high. Intergenerational adjustments take much of the adult's time and energy. Becoming an in-law and a grandparent and remaining an adult child and a parent provide many roles. Considering the extended period of identity establishment for youth (Erikson, 1963) and the medically elongated life span of many aged individuals, middle-aged adults can expect more family responsibilities rather than less.

Emotional flexibility is needed in the middle years because it is a period in which children mature, parents die, and circles of friends may be broken by divorce, illness, and death. Jung (1971) described the last half of life as less oriented to pragmatic tasks and more toward aesthetic concerns, spiritual development, and ego transcendence. The adult's relationship with his or her aging parents may change as the adult child discovers the person behind the parent. The death of a parent has significant implications for the middle-aged person who must now assume the position of maintaining the family traditions and history.

The Adult and Musculoskeletal Health

Age-Associated Physical Changes

Biologic changes during the middle adult years occur gradually. This period represents a long plateau in the life span. The gradual but unrelenting physical signs of aging include graying of hair, wrinkling and sagging of flesh, and overall decrease in metabolic rate. Energy levels are no longer boundless; the adult now requires rest between strenuous activities. Skeletal muscle increases in bulk until age 50, with degeneration beginning by age 60. Because gross motor coordination depends on skeletal muscle, this decline increases the risk of injury for the middle-aged recreational athlete. There seems to be great uniformity among individuals regarding physiologic sense organ changes in adulthood. Presbyopia is the reduction in the elasticity of the lens of the eye, inhibiting accommodation for near points of vision. This means that middle-aged adults must now wear glasses to read. Adults experience a gradual deterioration and hardening of the auditory cells and nerves. Together, these sense organ changes place the adult population at risk for domestic, recreational, and work-related injuries.

Change of life often causes anxiety for middle-aged adults. Climacteric in males and menopause in females evoke both biologic and psychological states of change. Symptoms of menopause commence with hormonal shifts in females between the ages of 40 and 55 years. The shift is marked by reduction in ovarian and other gonadotropic organ activities. Physical symptoms include menstrual irregularities, changes in body contour (due to redistribution of fat), hot flashes, and hair loss. The cessation of menstruation for some women can be laden with intrapersonal and physical apprehensions. In contrast, many women adapt readily to the change.

There is no obvious physical change in males comparable to the change in females. It is hypothesized that the emotional lability experienced by some males in climacteric is attributable to the progressive aging process and diminishing sexual drive. Unlike their female counterparts, the male's reproductive function does not end until old age because androgen levels decline slowly.

In summary, the time of life defined as adulthood represents the greatest portion of our life. It is associated with considerable developmental and biologic challenges. From the standpoint of musculoskeletal health, the goal is to avoid injury and maintain fitness.

Age-Related Issues and Challenges to Musculoskeletal Health

Work-Related Injuries

ACUTE ACCIDENTAL INJURY. Accidents result from both direct and indirect causes. Direct causes are concrete, such as hazardous materials or poorly designed equipment. Indirect causes are unsafe acts or unsafe conditions in a system. They may be poor management or policy, inadequate controls, lack of knowledge, improper assessment of existing hazards, or other personnel factors. Specific examples of unsafe acts include improper use of equipment, improper lifting, and use of illicit drugs or alcohol. Unsafe conditions include defective equipment, poor housekeeping, bad lighting, or inadequate ventilation.

Many allied health disciplines have proposed and tested hypotheses suggesting that accident susceptibility is situational. An increased risk of injury occurs when coping mechanisms are taxed by life changes. Research suggests that accident risk during episodes of increased stress is even greater than the susceptibility to illness. Health care providers employed in settings where they may encounter accidental injuries should be aware of life changes and stressors when assessing causes of accidents.

Seemingly mild injuries can evolve into long-term residual disability resulting in lost work time and wages. Greater than one half of all workers' compensation cases involve musculoskeletal conditions. Workers' compensation law is designed to compensate injured workers for medical expenses and lost wages fairly. In exchange, the employer cannot be sued for additional monies beyond that provided by worker's compensation. A worker can qualify for benefits if three conditions exist simultaneously: there must be injury or illness; the injury or illness must arise from employment; and there must be medical/rehabilitative costs, lost wages, or disfigurement.

REPETITIVE STRESS AND CUMULATIVE LOAD INJURIES. Many musculoskeletal injuries that occur in the workplace are not the result of accidents but of repetitive motion and cumulative workload. Repetitive stress injuries (RSI) accounted for 63% of all illness reported to the Occupational Safety and Health Administration (OSHA) in 1993. Approximately two thirds of these claims were for back injuries and one third for upper extremity injuries, with the latter accounting for more lost work time and higher treatment costs (U.S. Department of Labor, 1996). At risk for RSI are workers whose jobs require heavy lifting, awkward postures, or postures that must be sustained for prolonged periods.

Causes of RSI in the upper extremities are not universally agreed on; however, musculoskeletal, psychosocial, and ergonomic factors all appear to contribute to its incidence (Tompkins, 1996). Besides the routine physical examination, the primary care provider should ask about the work space design; positioning of the hands, neck and shoulders during work; and time spent continuously engaged in a repetitive task or at the computer. Visiting the job site may be indicated. Psychosocial factors include heavy workload, lack of supervisory support, fear of job loss, job satisfaction, and deadline pressures. The examiner should question the patient about these issues and show empathy and support for the responses (Millender & Conlon, 1996).

The absence of objective findings to substantiate the symptoms can complicate the treatment of upper extremity RSI. Patients may present with complaints of aching or burning pain, numbness, upper extremity weakness and fatigue, stiffness, hypersensitivity, and/or loss of grip strength (Millender & Conlon, 1996; Thompson & Phelps, 1990). Adding to the controversy about treatment and prevention of RSI is the lack of strong scientific data regarding risk factors for many disorders. Early intervention (within 8 to 16 weeks of onset) with appropriate medical and job management will usually result in a positive outcome (Millender & Conlon, 1996). Treatment includes anti-inflammatory medications, restricted activity of the affected part, aerobic exercise, upper body strengthening exercises, stress reduction, patient education regarding proper body mechanics, and ergonomic assessment of the worker and workplace (Millender & Conlon, 1996).

The cost of injuries and illness in the workplace is estimated to be more than $100 billion per year. Given the overall social and economic implications of work-related injuries, the prudent health care provider will carefully assess all of the variables when eliciting histories and strategizing treatment programs for the patient injured in the workplace. The goal of treatment is to reduce disability, restore function, and return the patient to work.

HISTORY AND PHYSICAL EXAMINATION OF THE INJURED WORKER. Reconstructing a detailed and accurate scenario of events precipitating the injury and systematically describing the mechanism of insult is crucial to the evaluation of work-related injuries. Envisioning the patient in the work environment is compulsory. The provider may be asked to comment on psychosocial influences. A history that includes a thorough evaluation of work activities will guide the clinician in treatment planning (Table 1-2).

The physical examination of the patient presenting with work-related musculoskeletal injury requires only minor modification from standard technique. Patients experiencing work-related injury may present for evaluation and treatment earlier than the general population. Subtle indications of trauma can be overlooked if the examiner is not sensitive to the time sequence and mechanism of injury. For example, the patient with an eversion type first- or second-degree ankle sprain may present to the on-site industrial accident clinic minutes after injury and before the onset of pain, swelling, ecchymosis, or deformity. Hours, or even days later, the physical

TABLE 1-2
Outline of Industrial Orthopaedic History

I. Presenting complaint
  A. Complete and accurate description. Patient's words in quotes.
  B. If extremity, double check whether right or left and make sure all entries in the record are consistent.
  C. Mode of onset
    1. Sudden or gradual?
    2. Associated with single injury? Unaccustomed activity? Repetitive motion? Sudden pressure or temperature change?
    3. If associated with injury
      a. Detailed description (time, date, circumstances)
      b. Immediate effects? (deformity, swelling, discoloration, loss of function)
      c. If symptoms delayed, time and circumstances of onset
  D. Progress of condition since onset
  E. Effect of treatment, if any
    1. Local heat or cold application? Medication? Manipulation?
    2. Mobilization versus immobilization?
    3. Best position for comfort? Worst?
II. Past history
  A. Similar symptoms in past? When? Circumstances?
  B. Other musculo-skeletal symptoms? (contralateral area, arthritic, bursitic, rheumatic symptoms)
III. Family history (parents and siblings)
  A. Condition similar to patient's?
  B. Arthritis, bursitis, rheumatism, gout?
  C. Congenital musculoskeletal defects?
IV. Socioeconomic history
  A. Kind of work? Work record? Time on same job? Relationships in department? Job satisfaction?
  B. Evidence of adaptive resilience (medical record)
    1. Frequency of visits? Lost time? Frequency and duration appropriate to medical condition?
    2. Level of complaints versus objective findings in past?
    3. Home and family situation?
  C. Possible significance of present complaints in above areas?

From Rowe, M. L. (1985). *Orthopaedic problems at work.* New York: Perinton Press.

manifestations of trauma would be easily identifiable to even the novice examiner. Timely follow-up can avoid this dilemma and is crucial to all aspects of work injury treatment.

Because more than one provider interacts with the patient through the course of rehabilitation, accurate descriptive physical examination is essential. Accepted physical assessment terminology and global abbreviations should be used when documenting. Objective tools such as tape measures, goniometers, pin wheels, and reflex hammers assist precision in documentation. Six key assessment techniques are necessary for the thorough documentation of physical findings from the patient with a work-related injury (adapted from Rowe, 1985).

Recording *negative findings* is as important as recording positive ones. The potential for full joint range of motion at initial encounter (before the onset of swelling and spasm) precludes a diagnosis of tendon rupture. Documenting the untraumatized state of associated structures may avert unwarranted claims in the future. If the first examiner omits documenting negative findings, subsequent concerns regarding the actual diagnosis may arise.

Recording areas of *point tenderness* should be as routine to the objective assessment as the recording of gross changes such as swelling, discoloration, deformity, and functional loss. Because tender points become diffusely distributed with the passage of time and may be evident only to the first examiner, the value of point tenderness assessment is lost days or weeks after the initial insult.

Comparison of the injured or symptomatic extremity part with the opposite or unaffected part is called *comparison to the contralateral.* This contralateral comparison can inform the examiner that what he or she perceives as "deformed" may be a normal variant.

Another important assessment tool is *range-of-motion* measurement. Degree measurements of maximum angles of extension and flexion of the unaffected joint should precede the analysis of the injured part. Contralateral comparison of range of motion will take into account the normal standard for each patient.

Circumference measurements of the affected extremity can objectify the amount of soft tissue swelling sustained and help with chronicling progress. Passing the tape measure around the extremity perpendicular to its long axis and performing a similar measurement contralaterally will help with quantifying degree of disability.

Radiographic examination is almost uniformly indicated in acute trauma situations. The health care provider should be familiar with the optimal views for visualizing the affected and associated parts (see specific anatomic regions for guidelines). Comparison of old films may be helpful when there is a question of an old fracture or joint space narrowing.

PREVENTION OF WORK-RELATED INJURY. Industrial management, health care providers, and workers share the responsibility for the occurrence and prevention of accidents in the workplace. Federal regulations and guidelines (NIOSH), state laws, OSHA standards, and regional ordinances serve as guides for management. A commitment to the worker and the work environment will enhance overall safety. Comprehensive job training, periodic on-site inspections, and expedient emergency care demonstrate this commitment.

The provider employed in industry is confronted with the task of individualizing preventive programs for "at-risk" employees in the work milieu. Employee screening programs, physical education, and the ergonomic design of manual jobs illustrate primary prevention efforts. Gross strength testing systems are predictive screening tools in the occupational setting. Several studies have suggested that a worker's likelihood of sustaining a back injury or other musculoskeletal disorder is three times greater when job lifting requirements approach or exceed strength capability (Nordin et al, 1997). Quantitative analysis of the physical energy demands of a particular activity (eg, lifting patients, mopping floors, or operating a drill) can help in reducing strain disorders. The provider can ease the newly employed individuals' adaptation to their work duties by carefully correlating the screening data obtained with knowledge of the physical demands of the job.

Another way to prevent injury in the workplace is by educating workers. This includes instruction on the proper methods for lifting and the need for maintaining good physical health, muscle strength, and endurance. Proper lifting techniques include keeping the object close to the body, using the large muscles of the legs, and lifting slowly and smoothly without twisting.

Ergonomic redesigning of manual handling jobs to reduce bending, twisting, and excessive weight is another primary prevention measure (Box 1-2). With many compensable low back and upper extremity injuries resulting from manual handling job design problems, modification of the physical space to fit the worker's anatomic, biomechanical, and behavioral characteristics should be considered. Interventions such as raising counter spaces or adding foot rests are inexpensive but very effective.

The occupational health care provider achieves short- and long-term objectives for prevention of musculoskeletal injuries in the workplace by assessing for workplace hazards, providing education and training that will help prevent worker fatigue and awkward posturing, and promoting safe behavior.

Box 1-2 Ergonomically Sound Work Design

Some simple and relatively inexpensive interventions to reduce work-related repetitive stress injury include:

- Chairs with adjustable armrests, seat height, and back height
- Work station design that prevents reaching more than 16 inches or abducting shoulder greater than 30 degrees
- Padded work surface edges
- Adjustable keyboard holders with wrist rest to keep wrists in a neutral position
- Ergonomically designed tool handles that prevent extremes of wrist or finger motion
- Headsets to prevent cradling the telephone receiver
- Computer monitor positioned so first line of type is at eye level
- Pivoting footrests
- Training in proper lifting techniques

Recreational Athletes and Novice Exercisers

Recreational athletes and novice exercisers present diverse challenges to the primary care provider. Exercise-induced asthma, heat-related illness, sprains, tendon ruptures, stress fractures, exacerbation of arthritis, hematuria and myoglobinuria, and frostbite are a few of the potential outcomes faced by these adults. Treating the recreational athlete and supporting the novice exerciser in maintaining his or her program will require intervention from the primary, secondary, and tertiary preventive perspectives.

Advertisements depicting finely toned torsos and intriguing exercise regimens within the confines of luxurious health spas contribute to the number of people engaging in strenuous physical activity. A conflict arises when the novice exerciser is exposed to the disparity between the image of physical fitness and the reality of exercising to attain fitness. The clinician can be helpful in both assessing the potential athlete's readiness for strenuous exercise and educating the patient in a sensible exercise regimen.

The first step toward fitness in the apparently healthy individual is the careful assessment by the primary care provider of exercise limitations and risk factors. Providing an exercise program tailored to the individual's initial fitness level will promote safety and enthusiasm for exercise and decrease attrition. Factors that must be considered when recommending exercise programs and advising patients on athletic activity include age, usual physical activity, activity preferences, coronary heart disease risk factors, and underlying disease states.

The positive effects of a regular exercise program will not be realized if injuries, excessive fatigue, and soreness discourage the exercise beginner or the recreational athlete. The provider can suggest an appropriate program that will promote overall fitness and reduce the risk of injury by directly educating the patient in exercise methodology, rate of progress, adequate warm-up and cool-down periods, and use of proper footwear and equipment.

Pregnancy

Pregnancy induces many physiologic alterations. Changes in hemodynamics, resting oxygen requirements, basal metabolic rate, heat production, posture, and joint stability all exert an influence on the pregnant woman's musculoskeletal system and exercise tolerance (American College of Obstetricians and Gynecologists [ACOG], 1994; Rungee, 1993). Musculosketal pain is common in pregnancy and is thought to be a result of mechanical, vascular, and hormonal changes.

LOW BACK PAIN. As many as 50% to 90% of women develop low back pain during pregnancy (Rungee, 1993). Physiologic changes thought to combine and contribute to low back pain are increased secretion of relaxin, which softens the pelvic and cervical ligaments; increased lumbar lordosis and compensatory thoracic kyphosis, to accommodate the changed center of gravity; and increased circulatory volume coupled with venous stagnation (MacEvilly & Buggy, 1996; Östgaard, 1996; Rungee, 1993). Back pain may originate from the lumbar spine, the posterior pelvis, or the pubic symphysis. Treatment differs according to the source (Östgaard, 1996).

Assessment of the pregnant woman presenting with low back pain begins with a good standard history. Other causes, such as urologic problems or premature labor, must also be considered as causes of flank, low back, or pelvic pain. After the history, the examiner does a complete physical examination, including a posterior pelvic pain provocation test. This test (Fig. 1-4) differentiates between pain arising from the posterior pelvis and lumbar pain. With the patient supine and the hip and knee flexed at 90 degrees, the examiner places his or her hand on the patient's iliac crest and exerts gentle force on the long axis of the femur. This

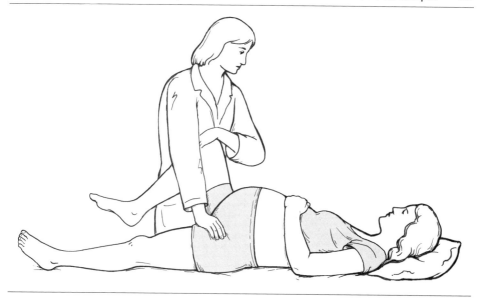

FIGURE 1-4.   Posterior pelvic pain provocation test.

maneuver will reproduce posterior pelvic pain on the examined side and is both sensitive (81%) and specific (80%). Pain from the symphysis pubis occurs in combination with posterior pelvic pain and is not treated separately. Östgaard (1996) outlines assessment findings for patients with lumbar versus posterior pelvic pain:

Posterior Pelvic Pain
- Positive provocation test
- No history of lumbar pain before pregnancy
- Pain in the gluteal area (which may or may not radiate to the posterior thigh and knee, but not to the foot)
- Full range of motion in the spine

Lumbar Pain
- Negative provocation test
- History of low back pain before pregnancy
- Pain above the sacrum in the lumbar spine
- Decreased range of motion in the lumbar spine
- Pain on palpation of the erector spine muscle

Treatment for pregnant women with lumbar back pain is the same as for nonpregnant women. Mixed pain types should be treated for the posterior pelvic pain first and for lumbar pain after the posterior pelvic pain resolves. Treatment of posterior pelvic pain consists of patient education in proper body mechanics; relaxation exercises; use of a pelvic belt that supports the back and abdomen, an abdominal pillow when lying down, and support hose; avoidance of stairs and extremes of movement in the hips or spine; and avoidance of physical monotony (MacEvilly & Buggy, 1996; Östgaard, 1996; Rungee, 1993). The pregnant woman may also be referred to a physical therapist for fitness classes and/or joint rotation maneuvers (Östgaard, 1996; MacEvilly & Buggy, 1996; McIntyre & Broadhurst, 1996).

EXERCISE AND PREGNANCY. Recreational sports and active physical fitness programs are important aspects of many women's lives and may often be continued throughout pregnancy. However, pregnancy and its physiologic changes can limit involvement in certain activities or preclude them completely.

Thermoregulatory, metabolic, respiratory, cardiovascular, and mechanical changes must be considered when planning an exercise program for the pregnant woman. The pregnant woman's lower fasting blood glucose levels and increased use of carbohydrates during exercise make her more prone to hypoglycemia, whereas increased resting oxygen requirements and increased work of breathing decrease the oxygen available for aerobic activity. Activities in which balance is important may be hazardous, and some studies suggest that intensive exercise is correlated to decreased birth weight. The increased levels of norepinephrine associated with exercise can potentially precipitate preterm labor in at-risk individuals (ACOG, 1994). Women with chronic hypertension, thyroid, cardiac, vascular, or pulmonary disease require very careful evaluation before recommending exercise. Additionally, certain obstetric conditions are contraindications to exercise, including pregnancy-induced hypertension, premature rupture of membranes, preterm labor during the prior or current pregnancy, incompetent cervix/cerclage, persistent second- or third-trimester bleeding, and intrauterine growth retardation (ACOG, 1994).

Despite these important considerations, most pregnant women can exercise safely throughout their pregnancy. Target heart rate, the accepted measure for cardiovascular conditioning, should be approximately 70% of the target heart rate for the nonpregnant woman (ACOG, 1994). ACOG has issued guidelines for exercise during the pre- and postpartum periods (Box 1-3), and the reader is referred to their general recommendations for guidance.

Exercise

An accumulating body of research suggests that regular exercise can reduce the risks of cardiovascular disease, colon cancer, falling, overall mortality, and obesity (DHHS, 1996). Regular exercise can improve mental health and physical functioning (Box 1-4). Despite this knowledge, more than 60% of American adults are not regularly active, and 25% of the adult population is not active at all (DHHS, 1996, p 5). Inquiring about level of activity and prescribing exercise if indicated should be a routine feature of provider/patient interactions. Formal training is not necessary for deriving health benefits, and programs that are realistic and achievable can be developed on an individualized basis. Emphasizing regular, moderate activity such as gardening or walking and encouraging varying activities may help patients incorporate exercise into their lives.

Some people will require a supervised program of activity. Many health care providers have not been formally educated about how to prescribe exercise to their patients. The exercise prescription should include written instruction for the type, intensity, duration, and frequency and progression of exercise, and the goals or expected outcomes of exercise.

TYPE. Activity types can be classified according to their conditioning effects and include cardiorespiratory, flexibility, and strength training. The exercise prescription recommends a combination of all three types of exercise training. Aerobic activity,

Box 1-3 American College of Obstetricians and Gynecologists Guidelines for Exercise During Pregnancy and Postpartum

There are no data in humans to indicate that pregnant women should limit exercise intensity and lower target heart rates because of potential adverse effects. For women who do not have any additional risk factors for adverse maternal or perinatal outcome, the following recommendations may be made:

1. During pregnancy, women can continue to exercise and derive health benefits even from mild-to-moderate exercise routines. Regular exercise (at least three times per week) is preferable to intermittent activity.
2. Women should avoid exercise in the supine position after the first trimester. Such a position is associated with decreased cardiac output in most pregnant women; because the remaining cardiac output will be preferentially distributed away from splanchnic beds (including the uterus) during vigorous exercise, such regimens are best avoided during pregnancy. Prolonged periods of motionless standing should also be avoided.
3. Women should be aware of the decreased oxygen available for aerobic exercise during pregnancy. They should be encouraged to modify the intensity of their exercise according to maternal symptoms. Pregnant women should stop exercising when fatigued and not exercise to exhaustion. Weight-bearing exercises may under some circumstances be continued at intensities similar to those prior to pregnancy throughout pregnancy. Non-weight-bearing exercises such as cycling or swimming will minimize the risk of injury and facilitate the continuation of exercise during pregnancy.
4. Morphologic changes in pregnancy should serve as a relative contraindication to types of exercise in which loss of balance could be detrimental to maternal or fetal well-being, especially in the third trimester. Further, any type of exercise involving the potential for even mild abdominal trauma should be avoided.
5. Pregnancy requires an additional 300 kcal/d in order to maintain metabolic homeostasis. Thus, women who exercise during pregnancy should be particularly careful to ensure an adequate diet.
6. Pregnant women who exercise in the first trimester should augment heat dissipation by ensuring adequate hydration, appropriate clothing, and optimal environmental surroundings during exercise.
7. Many of the physiologic and morphologic changes of pregnancy persist 4 to 6 weeks postpartum. Thus, prepregnancy exercise routines should be resumed gradually based on a woman's physical capability.

American College of Obstetricians and Gynecologists (1994). *ACOG technical bulletin* (number 189).

Box 1-4 Potential Benefits of Exercise for the Adult

Regular exercise can

- Reduce risk factors associated with heart disease
- Maintain weight control
- Improve cardiorespiratory endurance
- Improve muscular strength and endurance
- Improve energy level
- Improve sleeping habits
- Improve tolerance to stress
- Improve self-confidence and self-image

such as walking, swimming, cycling, or rowing, will foster cardiorespiratory fitness. Flexibility activities help with maintaining and extending joint range of motion and should be done before and after strengthening and cardiovascular activities to reduce the risk of soft tissue or muscle injury. Strengthening activities refer to effort against heavy resistance, as in weight lifting, or isometric exercises that tense one set of muscles against a static object. These activities will deliver overall muscle hypertrophy, but do little for cardiovascular toning.

INTENSITY. There is an intensity in aerobic exercise that is sufficient to condition the musculature and cardiovascular system without exceeding safe limits. Metabolic calculation of exercise duration is represented by a target zone. Oxygen consumption will determine intensity of exercise. Exercise physiologists have selected exercise target heart rate as the most practical measure for cardiovascular fitness and conditioning. Target heart rate is determined by the following formula:

$$(220 - \text{age}) \times 60\% \text{ to } 80\% = \text{target heart rate range}$$

Pregnant women should exercise at a heart rate that is 70% of the range determined by the above formula. A 6-second radial pulse rate should be taken periodically throughout the session.

DURATION. Duration of exercise refers to the time allocated per exercise session to the three basic components of each workout session. Exercise sessions should include a 5- to 10-minute warm-up period. The warm-up period serves to prevent musculoskeletal strain and readies the cardiovascular system for the cumulative work. It consists of stretching, flexibility, and slow-paced activity. Heart rate should be below the target rate. A stimulus period follows the warm-up phase. It is the time of moderate to intense exercise when the target heart rate is maintained. New exercise subscribers should aim for 15 to 20 minutes of stimulus activity with an eventual increase to 40 to 50 minutes. The cool-down period lasts 5 to 7 minutes. Stretching for 5 to 10 minutes follows the cool-down. As we age, both warm-up and cool-down periods need to be extended. If not performed, symptoms of vertigo, nausea, or even syncope may occur. Again, pulse should be monitored. The type of exercise performed in the cool-down period is similar to those in the warm-up period.

FREQUENCY. Frequency of exercise refers to the number of exercise sessions per week included in the program. The usual recommendation is minimally to exercise at least three times weekly with no more than 2 days between workouts. Maintenance of this exercise prescription requires a lifetime of commitment, because fitness rapidly deteriorates with program fluctuations.

PROGRESSION. The rate of progression depends on many factors. Functional ability, health status, individual preferences and response to exercise, and preestablished goals all influence progression. The initial conditioning phase takes 4 to 6 weeks and includes low-level aerobic exercise (40% to 60% of maximum heart rate) and light muscle strengthening. The improvement stage takes 4 to 5 months and includes more intense aerobic activity (50% to 85% of maximum heart rate). The maintenance stage is usually reached after 6 months of progressive conditioning.

Reviewing goals and selecting enjoyable activities that will maintain fitness are features of the maintenance phase (American College of Sports Medicine, 1995).

The importance of regular exercise cannot be overstated. Its benefits go far beyond cosmetic improvements and can effectively combat both the physical and psychological stressors of aging.

The Mature Adult

Psychosocial Factors That Influence Well-Being

The mature adult population is a diverse and heterogeneous group that, contemporary stereotypes and misconceptions aside, defies easy characterization. The physical health characteristics, self-care abilities, and social and psychological assets of the working 62-year-old woman will differ markedly from those of her 87-year-old mother for whom she is the primary caregiver.

Demographics of Aging

The mature adult population is commonly divided into subgroups based on age. Thus the "older population" denotes those people ages 55 to 60 years, the "elderly" those age 65 years and older, the "aged" those ages 75 to 84 years, and the "extreme aged" or "old old" those age 85 years and older. These differentiations are often useful in comparing certain characteristics between groups, such as morbidity and mortality or functional characteristics. More commonly, though, population statistics are reported for the "elderly" in general.

In 1990, the U.S. population numbered approximately 250 million people, and about 13% (31 million) were age 65 years or older (U.S. Bureau of the Census, 1996). The absolute and proportional numbers of the elderly have been growing steadily since the turn of the century, with the groups 75 to 84 and age 85 and older experiencing the greatest growth. From 1980 to 1990, the growth of the elderly population was three times that of the U.S. population in general. This trend will continue until about 2030 when the effect of the post–World War II "baby boom" will taper off. One in every five Americans will be age 65 or older. Using the "middle population series" estimates, the U.S. Census Bureau has predicted that by 2050 (1) the number of elderly will increase to more than 78 million, and (2) about 30% of the population will be over age 64 years.

There is no typical mature adult, but certain demographic characteristics are well documented and are useful in identifying potential problems and related areas of prevention. These characteristics include (1) gender differences, (2) racial differences, (3) socioeconomic status, and (4) physical health and functional abilities.

There are more older women than older men, and the ratio of men to women decreases with age. In 1995, there were 69 men for every 100 women age 65 and older (U.S. Bureau of the Census, 1996). The older man is much more likely to be married and living with a spouse than is the older woman. In 1995, 75% of men, but only 41% of women, age 65 and older were living with a spouse, whereas 47% of women were widowed and 42% lived alone.

Almost 14% of the U.S. white population is 65 years or older compared with 8.2% of the black population (U.S. Bureau of the Census, 1996). This is due in part to the greater mortality rate for blacks than whites at most ages. Certainly other factors are involved, such as different patterns of health care utilization and socio-economic status.

The economics of aging in the United States is an issue that has generated much debate for decades. Although most of us look forward to our retirement and the subsequent years of freedom and independence, for many older Americans the retirement years portend a gradual or precipitous attrition in financial resources. For some, retirement means simply an exacerbation or acceleration of an ongoing cycle of poverty.

Most of American elderly are not poor, but only a small minority can be considered affluent. In 1994, less than 7% of households headed by an elderly American had an annual income exceeding $50,000 (U.S. Bureau of the Census, 1996), and 12% of elderly lived below the poverty level. Moreover, for certain racial groups poverty is pervasive. In 1994, 28% of elderly blacks and 23% of elderly Hispanics were impoverished. Certainly, the economic status of most elderly Americans falls somewhere between affluence and poverty. Their incomes meet, or to varying degrees exceed, their cost of living. Nevertheless, such factors as the rising cost of health care, heavy reliance on government sources of income (eg, Social Security), and increasing out-of-pocket medical expenses threaten their economic viability.

Perhaps no characteristics of the mature adult population are more stereotyped and misconstrued than general physical health and functional abilities. The visual media tend to portray older adults dichotomously as either loving, retired, bespecta-cled grandparents or as dependent, disfigured, incapacitated octogenarians. Although the former may be closer to reality than the latter, such generalizations belie the diversity of this population and perpetuate the myths of aging.

Studies have shown increasing functional dependency with age. Activities of daily living (ADLs) are descriptors of everyday functional self-care abilities and are commonly divided into two categories: basic ADLs and instrumental ADLs. Basic ADLs include mobility (walking and transferring), bathing, dressing, eating and toileting. Instrumental ADLs include a variety of tasks such as shopping, meal preparation, managing finances, housekeeping chores such as cleaning and laundry, and the use of transportation. In a study based on longitudinal data from a national probability sample of American elders, a hierarchical progression of disability across basic ADLs emerged. In descending order of progression were walking, bathing, transferring, dressing, toileting, and feeding (Dunlop et al, 1997). Housekeeping is the instrumental ADL most likely to be limited, followed by shopping and meal preparation (U.S. Bureau of the Census, 1996).

Most mature adults are in good health and have few limitations in their activities or functional abilities. The vast majority live independently and require little or no outside help. Nevertheless, advanced age is associated with declining function and increased dependence on others. For a small but growing minority of elders, institutionalized care becomes necessary. In 1990, 1% of those age 65 to 74, 6% of those age 75 to 84, and 24% of those age 85 and older lived in skilled nursing facilities (Ham, 1997). A variety of alternatives other than nursing homes exist, and they represent a growing sector of long-term care. However, all long-term care options are expensive, and personal assets can be drained rapidly.

The home care industry has been expanding rapidly, in large part due to the shorter length of hospital stays. For every person over 65 years old in a skilled care nursing facility, approximately four similarly frail elders are being cared for in the community. Families, most commonly females of the immediate or extended family, provide approximately 80% of care to elders in the home (Keenan & Hepburn, 1997). The physical, psychological, emotional, and economic burdens of caregiving are great, and the social consequences are complicated (Cochran, 1994).

Developmental Tasks

Mature adults are survivors. Sixty or more years ago, when they were born and growing up, death by the fifth or sixth decade was usual. Over several decades, unprecedented global political, economic, and social changes have influenced their lives. Through maturation and adaptation, they gained the psychosocial skills needed to endure and thrive in the face of those changes. "Normal" human growth and maturation explain only part of this developmental process; changing social norms and attitudes have further influenced their lives. Knowledge of the developmental tasks of aging and its associated hazards is prerequisite for successful interaction and collaboration with the mature adult.

The mature adult must make many adjustments throughout the advancing years. Many types of losses characterize old age. The death of a spouse often forces the survivor to learn new skills, adjust to the loss of significant support systems, and sometimes to find a new home. Once considered a highly productive member of a fast-moving society, the mature adult must now face retirement. Coupled with retirement is a decrease in income and often a decrease in perceived self-worth. Days that were never long enough may now be too long and inadequately filled with meaningful activities.

Erikson reminds us that psychosocial development is a lifelong process. The psychosocial development task for mature adults is to confront the ends of their lives. Erikson termed this final stage of development Integrity versus Despair (Erikson, 1963). If the previous stages of life have been satisfactory, then old age is colored with a sense of integrity, a sense of a life well lived, a sense of tranquillity, wholeness, and quiet confidence. The elderly attain ego integrity when they can adapt positively to the constant changes throughout their lives. However, if reflection brings disappointment and regret and they view life as a series of lost opportunities and failures, then the final years will be years of despair.

Mature adults must adjust to physiologic and psychological changes. Poor health, chronic illnesses, loss of bodily functions, and lack of autonomy contribute to feelings of grief, loss, helplessness, and increased isolation. Loneliness may be associated more with loss than with isolation; the recently widowed have been found to be the most lonely. This feeling of loneliness is more significant if the widowed people are childless or rarely interact with their children.

An intact social support network, both formal and informal, is necessary to help mature adults maintain well-being. Assessment of the role family and friends play in an elder's life is basic to establishing plans of care. Without such supports, formal systems may be needed to replace the losses of significant others. Such support systems must be available, affordable, reliable, and effective. Because services for the elderly are often complex and overlapping, case management (the process of matching assessed needs with resources) is often warranted if the older adult is not able to advocate for himself or herself.

Not all mature adults successfully adapt to, or cope with, the physical and emotional challenges of aging. Inadequate coping can be manifested behaviorally in many ways, such as preoccupation with physical changes and discomforts, social withdrawal and isolation, and overt depression. Although depression is a highly treatable disease once diagnosed, one half of all depressed patients seen by internists are not identified as having depression (Butler & Lewis, 1995). The most effective way to screen for depression and suicide risk is a direct one. Within the context of any patient encounter, a brief but thorough psychosocial assessment can be completed. Questions to consider include: Is the patient expressing feelings of loneliness, helplessness, or hopelessness? Have there been any recent significant losses? Are effective support systems in place? Has the patient lost interest in or demonstrated poor compliance with the treatment regimen? The responses to those questions will identify patients for whom direct questions are indicated: Are you depressed? What does it mean to you? Have you ever considered suicide? Have you thought about how you might take your life? Acknowledgment of depression or related symptoms mandates further evaluation and treatment. Patients with a history of attempted suicide or who admit suicidal ideation are at particular risk of suicide and demand immediate intervention. Referral to a mental health worker or crisis intervention team should be made. Informing the patient and family or significant other as to why measures are needed and how these people should participate in the plan of care is an integral part of crisis intervention.

The Mature Adult Body and Musculoskeletal Health

Cardiovascular Changes

Cardiovascular disease remains the most frequent cause of death among persons over age 65. Cardiac output at rest and with exercise decreases with age, so that by age 70 preload (ventricular filling) is half the value compared with age 30. Thus, a 70-year-old adult has approximately one half the cardiac reserve of a young adult (Wei, 1992). With increasing age, there is a decreased ability to raise heart rate in response to exercise, systolic blood pressure has a greater increase, and both heart rate and blood pressure have a prolonged recovery time after exercise (Kane et al, 1994). In addition, aging baroreceptors in the carotid sinus are less sensitive to decreased arterial blood pressure that results from postural changes, consumption of a meal, or defecation; thus, orthostatic hypotension (defined as a drop in systolic blood pressure of at least 20 mm Hg from supine to standing) becomes increasingly prevalent in the elderly. The cardiovascular system is a good example of how aging, given a pattern of gradual functional limitations, is best considered within the framework of thresholds. The diminution of organ function is not important until a given boundary has been crossed, and then it is how the organ system can adapt to external stressors that becomes the critical measure of functional performance.

Musculoskeletal Changes

There is a gradual, progressive decrease in muscle mass by 30% with aging, but the decrease of muscle strength and endurance should be considered because of the specific muscle groups being tested. Many studies have suggested that disuse of muscles is likely as important a factor as aging itself (Sloane, 1997). Aging joints show changes of articular cartilage and intervertebral discs related to decreased water content that ultimately account for many arthritic problems in older adults. Thus, although these degenerative joint changes cannot be reversed, the human body can compensate by strengthening muscles through exercise training, thereby helping affected joints to move and ultimately maintaining or improving functional mobility.

Changes in bone structure and composition affect all aging adults. Most notable of these changes is the decrease in bone density that, although affecting more women than men, is also influenced by race and coexisting factors. Osteoporotic bone is brittle, less dense than normal bone, and contributes significantly to fractures primarily of the hip, shoulder, wrist, and vertebral bodies. Loss of vertebral bone mass results in varying degrees of spinal kyphosis (the "dowager's hump" common in many older women) and ultimately affects stature, posture, gait, and balance.

Neurologic and Sensory Changes

Loss of neurons begins in young adulthood at the rate of approximately 50,000 to 100,000 neurons/day; lost neurons are not regenerated. There is a gradual decrease in brain size and a concurrent increase in the size of the ventricles. Nevertheless, cortical function remains normal and, except for mild short-term memory loss, any cognitive impairment indicates pathology and warrants investigation. "Senility" is not part of normal aging.

Peripheral nerve conduction gradually slows and deep tendon reflexes frequently diminish, especially in the lower extremities. Certain superficial reflexes may disappear (eg, cremasteric and abdominal). Vibratory and tactile sensations decline, especially in the lower extremities, and may be accompanied by peripheral neuropathy resulting from chronic disease such as diabetes and peripheral vascular disease. Sensitivity and responsiveness to extremes of temperature decline significantly and place the mature adult at increased risk for hypo- and hyperthermia. Mobility is affected by a gradual but variable impairment of balance, diminished body-orienting reflexes and posture control, and decreased ability in the height the adult can step. Intermittent, rapid, low-amplitude muscle tremors and fasciculations in the lower extremities may occur normally, but muscle fibrillation is an abnormal finding.

The abilities to see, hear, taste, and smell decline with age as the result of specific anatomic changes. Presbyopia, or loss of accommodation and near vision, typically occurs by age 50 and results from loss of elasticity of lens and ciliary muscle. There is a decrease in the number of retinal receptors, gradual corneal degeneration, and decreased tear production. Aging pupils are smaller and less reactive to light. Visual acuity, the ability to adapt to the dark properly, and the range of visual field decline. Color vision is impaired; this affects discrimination between greens and blues more than between yellows and reds. Typical eye disorders include cataracts, macular degeneration, glaucoma, and retinopathy. Visual changes that are abnormal and require investigation include blurred vision, diplopia, and perception of halos or rainbows around lights, and may result in frequent eyeglass prescription changes.

Presbycusis, the degenerative bilateral sensorineural hearing loss that accompanies normal aging, affects more than 50% of people 65 years and older. Loss of high-frequency (high-pitched) sounds occurs first. A sudden or acute change in hearing is abnormal and merits investigation. Frequently, a buildup of cerumen in the external auditory canal will produce a "sudden" conduction hearing loss that resolves after removal of the blockage.

The physiologic, anatomic, and functional changes that accompany normal aging predispose the mature adult to certain hazards and pathologic conditions. Many of these common hazards and conditions affect, directly or indirectly, basic activities of daily living in general and mobility specifically. Epidemiologically, a limited number of age-related problems predominate and account for most acute and chronic orthopedic conditions. These problems include (1) falls, (2) fractures, and (3) degenerative problems (eg, osteoporosis and arthritis).

Age-Related Issues and Challenges to Musculoskeletal Health

Alcohol Abuse

Despite an overall decrease in alcohol consumption in later life, hospitalized elders have the highest proportion (roughly 60%) of alcohol-related diagnoses in conjunction with a separate primary diagnosis (Banys, 1996). Such factors as the normal physiologic changes of aging, the probability of these changes coexisting with chronic health problems, and the use of medications mean the consequences of alcohol use may be more detrimental in the mature adult. Reductions of lean body mass and total body water, with diminished hepatic mass and blood flow, decrease the rate of elimination of alcohol, increase its toxic effects at lower doses, and prolong its action compared with younger adults (Banys, 1996). Alcohol-induced changes in liver enzyme systems may decrease the elimination of some drugs while increasing the toxicity of others. Combined with the expected gait changes and slowing of reflexes encountered in the mature adult, alcohol use can be particularly hazardous and is often a factor in falls.

In interactions with patients, the provider must be attuned not only to signs of alcohol abuse but also to evidence of apparently normative social manner (Adams, 1996). Patient education is indicated whether alcohol is used problematically or responsibly. Referral to a substance abuse counselor or mental health agency should be made when appropriate.

Falls

Falls are a leading cause of morbidity and mortality in the mature adult population. One fourth of elders ages 65 to 74 and one third of those 75 and older fall annually. Subsequent falls within 6 months of a previous fall occur in approximately two thirds of elders (Tideiksaar, 1996). Not surprisingly, the death rate from falls increases with age. Most falls are not fatal but result in significant physical, psychological, and economic trauma. Falls affect independence, self-esteem, and mobility, and a fall often precipitates institutionalization. Effective primary and secondary prevention of falls requires an understanding of the characteristics of people at risk to fall, the multiple causes of falls, and the identification and implementation of appropriate preventive and corrective measures.

Mature adults at risk to fall are likely to be incontinent, use several medications, have impaired gait and balance, have arthritis or history of stroke, or experience significant orthostatic or postprandial hypotension. Causation is often separated into two main categories: host ("intrinsic") and environmental ("extrinsic") factors (Tibbetts, 1996). Host factors include normal physiologic changes of aging, pathologic conditions, and drug effects. Environmental factors include both home and community hazards (Table 1-3). Rarely can a fall be attributed to only one factor or cause; falls usually result from the interaction of several factors. Adults who "simply tripped" on a throw rug when getting up at night to go to the bathroom may, on closer questioning, recall that (1) they did get up suddenly, experiencing some lightheadedness (orthostatic hypotension); (2) were not wearing their eyeglasses (visual impairment); (3) the night light was off (environmental hazard); and (4) they had taken a sleeping pill 3 hours earlier (drug effect). Because most falls occur in the home, a home hazard assessment is mandatory (Table 1-4). The assessment and interventions must be accomplished with considerable tact, concerned objectivity, and respect for the autonomy of the person.

TABLE 1-3
Causes of Falls in Mature Adults

I. *Host factors*
  A. *Physiologic changes of aging*
     1. Impaired gait, balance, and righting mechanisms
     2. Decreased height of stepping
     3. Decreased flexibility of trunk and extremities
     4. Decreased muscle mass, strength, and tone, especially in lower extremities
     5. Sensory changes—impaired vision, hearing, proprioception, tactile sense
     6. Orthostatic hypotension
     7. Impaired mechanoreceptors in cervical facet joints
     8. Sedentary lifestyle
     9. Inability to rise from chair without using arms
     10. Poor self-assessed health
  B. *Pathologic conditions*
     1. Chronic conditions (eg, DJD, RA, Parkinson's disease, dementia, peripheral neuropathies, depression, vertebral basilar insufficiency)
     2. Acute and episodic conditions (eg, cardiac dysrhythmia, syncope, drop attack, transient ischemic attack)
  C. *Drug effects*
     1. "Normal" side effects (eg, orthostatic hypotension)
     2. Adverse reactions—electrolyte imbalance, secondary diuretics, digitalis toxicity
     3. Drug interactions (eg, OTC anticholinergic drugs plus anxiolytic or antidepressant)
     4. Alcohol
II. *Environmental factors*
  A. *Outside home*
     1. Community obstacles, high curbs without wheelchair type ramp; timing of traffic light "walk—don't walk" cycle; use of escalators over elevators in malls; mass transit vehicles with high steps; lack of wheelchair lifts; poor street lighting
  B. *Home hazards*
     1. Entrance ways—stairs in good repair and negotiable height? hand rail sturdy? adequate lighting? path to/from driveway or garage unobstructed?
     2. Floors/hallways—slick? scatter or throw rugs secured? electric cords in pathway? adequate lights?
     3. Kitchen—linoleum or waxed floor? are top or high shelves used?

TABLE 1-4
Home Hazard Assessment and Intervention

Hazard	Intervention
I. *Outside*	
Uneven, cracked, or cluttered walk	Repair; remove obstacles
Loose, slippery steps on porch	Repair; paint porch with nonskid paint
Inadequate lighting	Walkway, porch, steps should be well lit
Loose or absent railing	Provide railing, well secured to house or steps; one on both sides best
Tight, "sticky," or cumbersome storm or main door	Repair; lever-type handle superior to round knob or push button
II. *Inside*	
Hallways	
Extension cords, furniture, or other obstacles	Remove
Loose scatter or throw rugs	Remove or secure to floor
Inadequate lighting	Ceiling or floor lighting with light switch at each end of hallway greater than or equal to 100 watt
No railing	Installation of railing secured to underlying wall studs
Living Area	
Furniture on casters	Remove casters or place furniture against wall
Low chairs without arms	Suggest chairs with arms and high seat; electric lift chair when appropriate (may be covered by Medicare)
Kitchen	
Linoleum or slick floors	Table, chairs with rubber nonskid tips; avoid waxing
High shelves	Move items to shelves preferably shoulder height or lower
Bathroom	
Low toilet seat	Raised toilet seat with arms
Slick tub, absence of mat or grab bars	Rubber nonskid mats; grab bars; bath seat or shower stool
Excessively high hot water temperatures	Adjust hot water heater to temperature of 120° to 130°
Stairways	
No railing	Railing on both sides secured to underlying wall studs
Carpeting on floor same color as walls/ceiling	Red or yellow paint or reflection strip on first and last riser

Certain host factors are readily modified, and these modifications result in a significant risk reduction. Simple remedies are often the most important (eg, the use of appropriate shoes and keeping canes and walkers accessible and in good repair). Exercise influences many potentially deleterious normal physiologic changes by improving strength, flexibility, gait, and balance. Correction of sensory impairment through the appropriate use and maintenance of adaptive devices (eg, eyeglasses) is a simple but crucial measure.

Orthostatic hypotension and/or postprandial hypotension are common in the elderly and are frequently precipitating factors of falls (Bludau & Lipsitz, 1997). Patients with persistent orthostatic hypotension must be educated in methods to reduce the frequency and severity of disabling symptoms. Adaptive behaviors include rising slowly from a lying to sitting position, then sitting for a minute before standing, especially in the morning; remaining seated while dressing; and using a recliner chair when possible. Activities that result in vasodilation and venous pooling should be avoided (eg, hot baths and prolonged exposure to hot or humid conditions, prolonged lying or standing, and very large meals). For some adults, the use of elastic support garments and drug treatment may be necessary.

Pathologic conditions often play a role in falls, including the impact of chronic disease on mobility and impaired function due to acute episodic conditions. Neurologic and cardiovascular conditions are often implicated in falls. Thorough medical evaluation is indicated to identify and correct the underlying disorder. The risk of drug effects as a factor for falls must be suspected, with particular emphasis on certain classes of drugs (antihypertensives, diuretics, antidepressants, hypnotics, all central nervous system medications) and the use of over-the-counter drugs.

With increasing age there is the probability of multiple etiologies of any given fall and, as such, it should be considered a symptom rather than a diagnosis (Bludau & Lipsitz, 1997). Taking this idea a step further, it has been suggested that geriatric syndromes such as delirium, dementia, urinary incontinence, and falls may share a set of predisposing factors that may require a more unified therapeutic approach if functional dependence is to be modified (Tinetti et al, 1995).

Fractures

Fractures are a common orthopedic problem for mature adults, and the incidence of fractures increases with age. Normal physiologic changes of aging, osteoporosis, and falls are the most important etiologic factors related to fractures. Loss of bone density, a stiffened and weakened musculoskeletal system, and impaired gait accompany normal aging and increase the risk of fractures. Certain lifestyle behaviors, medications, and other pathologic conditions further accelerate bone demineralization (Table 1-5). Secondary to aging and osteoporosis, alcoholism exacerbates the decrease in bone density. Corticosteroids, often used in chronic lung disease and arthritis, and furosemide, often used in hypertension and heart disease, increase bone loss and urinary excretion of calcium, respectively. Metastatic disease from

TABLE 1-5
Chronic Conditions Affecting Skeletal Integrity

Osteoporosis
Hyperparathyroidism
Hyperthyroidism
Adrenal insufficiency
Alcoholism
Nutritional deficiencies (calcium, vitamin D)
Metastatic carcinoma
Hypogonadism
Diabetes mellitus
Immobility
Corticosteroids

primary breast, prostate, thyroid, and kidney cancers, and multiple myeloma often result in lytic bone lesions.

Each encounter provides an opportunity to assess the patient's relative risk of fractures. All patients should be assessed for dietary deficiencies (eg, calcium and vitamin D). Alcohol abuse remains underdiagnosed but, when recognized, mandates appropriate referral. A review of medications may identify the need for adjustment (eg, reducing steroids or substituting hydrochlorothiazide for furosemide). The activity and functional level of all patients should be assessed, with the goal of establishing baseline data and developing an exercise program directed toward optimal function. Special attention should be directed to those with certain chronic conditions (eg, cancer, thyroid, and parathyroid disorders).

The most common fracture sites for mature adults are the hip, wrist, and vertebrae. Hip fractures predominate, with an annual incidence in the United States greater than 250,000. More than 90% of hip fracture patients are over age 70 (Greenspan et al, 1994). Hip fracture is associated with a 12% to 20% increase in mortality for elders, a 25% increased probability of long-term institutionalization, and a less than 50% chance that the individual will independently ambulate again (Pollak et al, 1997). Wrist fractures are generally of the Colles' type (ie, fractures of the distal radius within 1 inch of the articular surface that result in the characteristic "silver fork" deformity with the wrist displaced dorsally and radially). Typically, such a fracture occurs when the victim falls on outstretched arms. Vertebral fractures may also result from trauma, although the responsible event may be minor and unrecognized for some time.

The cardinal signs and symptoms of fractures include deformity, swelling, bruising, muscle spasm, tenderness, pain, impaired sensation, impaired function, crepitus, and abnormal mobility. Their presence and magnitude depend on the site, type, and severity of the fracture; other structural injury; general physical condition; and psychological factors (eg, mental status). Compared with younger patients, mature adults are much more likely to present atypically, particularly with fractures of the hip and vertebrae. The injury may be disproportionately greater than the pain or initial functional limitation might suggest. The patient may not seek medical attention for days until the pain resulting from weight bearing or the inability to perform basic activities of daily living forces him or her to seek help.

The absence of obvious trauma does not exclude the possibility of fracture, particularly in the presence of advanced osteoporosis. Frequently, older adults, especially the "old old," may present with a gradual decline in specific functional abilities and a reluctance to perform what had been routine activities (eg, dressing, grooming, or ambulation). There may be an associated complaint of arthritis "flaring up" or a similar attribution to some chronic condition that may or may not explain the change. Physical examination should focus on the (apparently) involved extremity, assessing for any pain to palpation or with motion, range of motion, muscle strength and tone, and circulation and neurologic function. Any abnormal findings merit more thorough diagnostic evaluation, but especially erythema, swelling, pain with motion, or limitation in range of motion. A minor infection, monoarticular arthritis, or superficial soft tissue injury will often be a fracture in disguise.

The provider should expect the presentation of fractures to vary greatly from person to person and according to site (Table 1-6). Fractures are often the first and most prominent clinical sign of osteoporosis. Yet, although 90% of hip fractures

TABLE 1-6
Clinical Presentation of Fractures by Site

Site	Signs and Symptoms
Hip	Pain on weight bearing and/or ambulation Increased pain with percussion of sole of foot on involved side Decreased ROM—but may be normal except for extremes of rotation, especially internal rotation Point tenderness Leg abducted, externally rotated, may be shortened compared to noninvolved side
Vertebrae	Sudden acute back pain or slow, insidious increase in chronic back pain Usually thoracic or lumbar spine Pain increased by sitting, relieved when lying supine Alteration in respirations Decreased bowel sounds, ileus Silent progression of kyphosis and decrease in stature
Wrist (Colles' fracture)	Pain with all ROM, especially flexion and extension, supination and pronation Decline in ADLs, such as personal hygiene New onset of preferred use of nondominant hand

result from falls, fewer than 5% of falls result in hip fracture, suggesting that fall characteristics and body habitus are important factors for hip fracture beyond bone mineral density (Greenspan et al, 1994). Hip pain after a fall (or any other traumatic event), no matter how benign the event may seem, should lead to the presumption that a fracture has occurred until an evaluation proves otherwise.

When there is no apparent history of trauma and a patient complains of a gradual increase in pain over a period of days or weeks, the possibility of a metastatic or pathologic fracture must be considered. Multiple myeloma frequently presents with back pain secondary to a pathologic vertebral fracture. Over one half of malignant bone lesions originate from primary carcinoma elsewhere, yet the bone lesion may be the presenting complaint. Such lesions are commonly in the vertebrae and pelvis and are rarely below the knee.

After a fracture, the primary goal should be the earliest possible resumption of normal activities and ambulation. This is essential for the patient to achieve the highest possible level of functioning and independence and to maintain muscle action and joint function. The approach to rehabilitation after a fracture will vary according to fracture site and severity, prefracture functional abilities, and coexisting medical problems. Involving the patient and family (or support system) is crucial in planning the postfracture treatment and rehabilitation program and in setting realistic and attainable goals.

The type of fracture and the method of repair will have the greatest impact in determining rehabilitative goals. Hip fractures usually require some surgical intervention and, particularly in the "old old," often require a hip prosthesis. There will usually be a limited period of relative immobility postoperatively, which significantly increases the risk of such complications as pneumonia, pressure ulcers, generalized muscle weakness and atrophy, impaired bowel function, and changes in mental status such as acute confusional states. The primary care provider, rehabilitation therapists, and patient must collaborate in actively preventing such complications by the implementation of a care plan that emphasizes early activity and adequate analgesia. From the onset, patients must be encouraged to participate in self-care to the greatest extent possible.

The clinician must assume responsibility for anticipating potential obstacles to recovery and for adjusting the treatment plan accordingly. This responsibility presumes a thorough knowledge and understanding of the patient, especially the pre-fracture physical, functional, and psychosocial characteristics.

Although rehabilitation and care plans must be different for each patient, certain guidelines can be applied to all patients. Such topics as cast care, potential complications and their signs and symptoms that must be reported (eg, thrombophlebitis, compromised circulation), appropriate use of analgesics, comfort measures, correct use of mobility aids (crutches, canes, walkers), and a thorough description of allowed and contraindicated activities should be reviewed. Caregivers should be present when possible, and written instructions should be provided. Allow sufficient time for the patient and caregiver to express fears and concerns, ask questions, and acknowledge understanding of instructions. Arrangements for supportive services such as in-home skilled nursing care, physical therapy, or occupational therapy should be reviewed so no misconceptions or misunderstandings occur.

Early resumption of normal activities and ambulation is extremely important. Although fractures often result in some residual functional impairment, appropriate rehabilitation can reduce the degree of that impairment, so the patient may continue to live independently.

Arthritic Disorders

No chronic condition affects more people than arthritis. Rare indeed is the mature adult who does not have symptoms of one of the arthritides: osteoarthritis (OA, or degenerative joint disease), rheumatoid arthritis (RA), gout, pseudogout, polymyalgia rheumatica, or soft-tissue rheumatism. Certainly osteoarthritis and rheumatoid arthritis predominate, but all arthritic conditions can result in chronic pain and functional impairment, and complications resulting from treatment can be serious. Arthritis generally cannot be prevented. The clinicians' efforts will be most effective if aimed at limiting pain and disability and helping patients in the accomplishment and maintenance of appropriate rehabilitative measures. These efforts require insight into the prevalence, clinical presentation, natural history, and clinical management of osteoarthritis and rheumatoid arthritis.

Osteoarthritis is the second most common cause of disability in this country. It is widely assumed to be a normal consequence of aging, given its prevalence (40 million Americans) and increasing incidence with aging. Some research has suggested, however, that osteoarthritis is truly a disease process of articular cartilage, not simply an inevitable age-related change (Fife, 1994). The clinical presentation of osteoarthritis is one of slowly progressive, intermittent, aching joint pain, stiffness, and deformity involving primarily the cervical and lumbar spine, shoulders, hips, knees, and interphalangeal joints; rarely are elbows, wrists, or ankles involved (Fife, 1994). The process is diffuse and generalized in women (who typically have multijoint involvement) but usually localized in men to the hips and knees. Pain is directly related to deterioration of articular cartilage, joint stress, and bone proliferation. Joint stiffness is common in the morning and after prolonged periods of sitting or standing. Treatment is symptomatic; most patients respond well to physical measures, mild analgesics such as acetaminophen, or NSAIDs. Severely damaged joints may require surgical intervention.

Rheumatoid arthritis differs from osteoarthritis. Rheumatoid arthritis is a systemic, autoimmune problem that may have a sudden or subacute onset. Inflammation to varying degrees is always present, but in the elderly fewer joints tend to be affected compared with younger patients. Older people with rheumatoid arthritis tend to have larger proximal joint involvement, especially knees, rather than the small joints of hands and feet as is typically seen in younger patients (Sewell, 1997). Treatment is aimed primarily at reducing acute inflammation, usually with NSAIDs, corticosteroids, gold, antimalarial drugs, immunosuppressive medications, and penicillamine. Physical therapy and the use of adaptive devices often result in marked improvement of functional abilities.

Patients with arthritis can assume primary responsibility for the management of their rehabilitation program. They are the experts in understanding how their condition affects them, what activities are most limited, the type and severity of pain and discomfort, and the relative success of different treatment modalities. Health care providers can best help the patient by providing ongoing assessment, education, and consultation.

Assessment and education should occur simultaneously. The patient who presents with an arthritic complaint for the first time must have a thorough nursing and medical assessment to identify the nature of the problem. What appears to be "arthritic" back pain may be a vertebral compression fracture, peptic ulcer disease, pneumonia, or cardiac ischemia. Once the diagnosis is made, education should focus on the natural history, treatment options, and expected outcomes. The rehabilitative measures and goals should be addressed, both generally and specifically about how they relate to the patient's particular manifestations of disease (Table 1-7).

Based on the findings of the medical and nursing assessments and the specific problems identified, the patient and primary care provider can develop a plan of care that is individualized, goal directed, and flexible. Specific instructions must often be given, and written guidelines may be necessary. Anyone involved in the provision of care for an older adult should be involved from the initial history taking and physical assessment to the identification of short- and long-term goals. More than one perspective on a problem often helps its resolution.

Ongoing assessment and evaluation of the patient's condition and plan of care are necessary due to the chronicity of arthritic conditions and the potential for functional decline. With older patients, it is often necessary for the provider to ask directly and explicitly about their status if "false-negative" histories are to be avoided. Poor pain control, gradually declining self-care abilities, and social isolation may go unreported if patients fear that acknowledgment would signal the need for institutional care. Similarly, problems in paying for, taking, or tolerating medications may be an embarrassment or presumed sign of inadequacy that is difficult to verbalize. The time spent reviewing the medication regimen is never wasted and, in the typical geriatric scenario of multiple medications and potentially adverse reactions, this time will often identify previously unrecognized, serious complications.

TABLE 1-7
Rehabilitative Measures for Arthritis

Intervention	Purpose/Goal
Rest	
Bedrest indicated only for acute phase of inflammatory arthritis; must be accompanied by ROM exercises and short periods of rest for DJD	Eliminate effects of gravity and weight bearing Minimize hazards of immobility Reduce stress on joints
Splinting	
Immobilization of inflamed or deformed joints Optimal effect for acute inflammation requires continuous use for at least 24 hours	Mechanical support and stabilization Maintain anatomic alignment Stretch joint, stimulate muscle activity
Exercise/Activity	
Slowly progressive isometric exercise Maintain physical activity and ADLs through work simplification and energy conservation	Muscle strengthening Maintain muscle strength and mass; joint flexibility; prevent/delay functional decline
Physical Therapy	
Active and or passive ROM	Maintain joint flexibility Gradual release of contractures
Application of cold/heat	Cold to relieve acute pain; inflammation Heat to relieve chronic pain, inflammation

From Portnow, J. & Helfgett, S. (1987). Rehabilitation of the elderly arthritic patient. *Geriatric Medicine Today,* 6(9), 63.

Medications and Associated Problems

For many reasons, advancing age is associated with an increase in the use of both prescription and over-the-counter medications. Older adults usually have one or more chronic conditions managed in part by drug therapy. Normal changes of aging, such as impaired bowel function, result in the use of many nonprescription drugs. Receiving health care from more than one provider or using several pharmacies to fill prescriptions may result in drug duplication, or polypharmacy. Drugs are not innocuous and are associated with frequent noxious or deleterious side effects and/ or adverse reactions (Table 1-8). Primary care providers must be aware of the normal changes of aging that impact on drug therapy. These include both changes in body composition and in organ systems that alter drug absorption, metabolism, excretion, and distribution (Table 1-9). In general, older adults are more sensitive to drugs, require lower doses, are more likely to experience adverse reactions, and may react in a paradoxical or unexpected fashion. Therefore, the cliche "start low and go slow" is an important caveat when prescribing drugs for older patients. Equally important is careful attention to individual patient characteristics (such as presence of chronic disease) that may interact with normal changes of aging and result in a greater impact on pharmacokinetics and pharmacodynamics. The malnourished patient with a greater than "normal" decrease in serum albumin is likely to have higher serum concentrations of highly protein-bound drugs.

TABLE 1-8
Commonly Used Drugs and Related Problems

Drug	Problem
Digitalis	Cardiac dysrhythmias Nausea and vomiting
Diuretics	Dehydration Electrolyte imbalance Hyperuricemia Hyperglycemia Ototoxlcity (furosemide)
Beta blockers	Orthostatic hypotension Depression Masked hypoglycemia
CNS drugs Benzodiazepines	Oversedation Paradoxic response (agitation) Impaired gait/balance Altered sleep cycle
Antipsychotics/ antidepressants	Oversedation Paradoxic response Tardive dyskinesia Disturbed temperature control Orthostatic hypotension Constipation Urinary retention Dry mouth
NSAIDs	Nausea Diarrhea Constipation Stomatitis Gastritis Active peptic ulceration Sodium retention

Adverse drug reactions are a significant hazard for older patients. Drugs with the highest incidence of adverse effects include psychotropics, antibiotics, antihypertensives, digitalis, and NSAIDs. The rate of adverse reactions is two to three times that of younger adults and accounts for approximately 10% of geriatric hospital admissions (Lonergan, 1996). People over age 65 consume one third of all prescriptions and 40% of all over-the-counter medications. One of the most important factors for the incidence of adverse drug reactions is the number of medications taken by the patient. New studies suggest that co-morbidity is an equally important factor, rather than chronologic age alone, in determining risk and probability for adverse drug reactions (French, 1996).

Despite the many potential hazards associated with their use, drugs are often essential in the management of chronic and acute conditions that accompany aging. Clinicians must ensure that patients use prescription and nonprescription medication safely and appropriately. Elderly patients may have difficulty managing complicated drug regimens, although often they may not acknowledge this or even be aware a problem exists unless specifically asked. Such mismanagement may present as poor control of chronic conditions, presence of side or adverse effects that are dose

TABLE 1-9

Normal Changes of Aging Affecting Drug Therapy

Change	Consequences
Body Composition	
Decreased total body water	Increased sensitivity to water-soluble drugs
Decreased lean body mass/increased total body fat	Delayed onset and prolonged action of fat-soluble drugs (eg, psychotropics)
Decreased serum albumin	Elevated serum levels of highly protein-bound drugs (eg, warfarin, phenytoin)
Decreased homeostatic abilities	Increased risk of adverse reactions and side effects
Impaired baroreceptors	Orthostatic hypotension
Kidney Function	
Decreased ability to concentrate urine and conserve sodium	Tendency to dehydration with diuretics
Decreased glomerular filtration	Delayed drug clearance, longer half-life of
Decreased creatinine clearance	*most* drugs
GI Function	
Decreased bowel perfusion	Decreased drug metabolism by liver—
Decreased motility	increased serum levels (eg, propranolol,
Decreased hepatic perfusion and metabolism	acetaminophen, tricyclics)
Decreased amount/acidity of gastric secretions	Decreased absorption of weak acids (eg, ASA, theophylline)

related, or inappropriate requests for refills indicating over- or underutilization. In some cases, drug regimens can be simplified (eg, by using a NSAID with daily or twice-a-day doses and accepting the associated hazards of a longer half-life). For many patients, the correction of minor problems may be all that is needed to improve compliance. In prescribing medications, it may be useful to specify nonchildproof containers, large-print labeling, and explicit instructions for drug use (eg, not "take as directed," but "take one tablet every 4 hours as needed for pain, not to exceed 6 tablets in 24 hours"). A variety of "pill reminders" are available commercially and often result in improved "compliance." Finally, perhaps the most important intervention is to involve the patient's spouse, family, and support systems. Some patients will require no prompting and supervision;, some will need the implementation of elaborate systems or direct administration of drugs by others, especially if cognitive impairment is a problem.

Exercise

The mature adult population can benefit from exercise in terms of maintaining function and independence (Box 1-5). Appropriate and effective education should focus on the specific benefits of exercise, the development of an exercise prescription or program, and individualized exercise recommendations based on specific chronic problems.

Box 1-5 Potential Benefits of Exercise
for the Mature Adult

Regular exercise can

- Improve quality of life
- Reduce anxiety and depression
- Improve sleeping habits
- Improve self-confidence and maintain independence
- Maintain weight control
- Improve flexibility and coordination
- Improve muscular strength and endurance
- Retard osteoporosis
- Sustain libido

Convincing patients that they will benefit in measurable ways is important for health professionals. Ironically, this may be easier with mature adults, who often have some degree of physical or functional limitation, than with younger patients, who generally are in good health. Life expectancy, a measurable criterion that older patients tend to pay more attention to, has been shown to correlate with exercise. In a prospective study of more than 16,000 Harvard alumni ages 35 to 74, physical activity was examined in relation to mortality and longevity (Paffenbarger et al, 1986). Exercise was found to have an inverse relationship to mortality, particularly to cardiovascular and respiratory disease. In general, the greater the level of exercise, as measured by the number of calories expended per week, the greater the decrease in death rates. Mortality rates were lower for those people who were physically active, despite the presence or absence of hypertension, cigarette smoking, or extremes of body weight. By the age of 80 years, adequate physical activity and exercise were found to result in an increase in life expectancy of 1 to more than 2 years.

Exercise will often improve the quality of the patient's life by ameliorating physical and functional changes that accompany normal aging (Table 1-10). How much improvement clearly will be a result of the level, frequency, and type of exercise and the patient's general condition and physical capabilities. However, all patients can benefit from exercise if the program is geared to their capabilities and aimed at realistic goals.

Before embarking on an exercise program, all patients should have a complete health history and physical examination. This is important to (1) obtain baseline data regarding fitness, (2) highlight health conditions such as cardiac disease that will affect and be affected by a physical exercise program, (3) outline medication profiles that may require titration once exercise is initiated, and (4) identify elders for whom vigorous aerobic training would pose an unacceptable risk (Fiatarone, 1996). An exercise tolerance test (ETT) for the "younger old" (65 to 75 years old) may be considered if thought is being given to moderately vigorous exercise. For the older, more frail elder, the ETT is not necessary when exercise is a means of maintaining or improving functional mobility and increasing independence (Barry & Eathorne, 1994). Exercise, although beneficial, does have some risks and complica-

TABLE 1-10

Normal Changes of Aging and Related Physiologic Benefits

Aging Change	Exercise Benefit
Cardiovascular	
Decreased maximum cardiac output and maximum work capacity	Increased maximum aerobic capacity
Increased total peripheral, resistance	Decreased vascular resistance
Increased systolic BP	Decreased BP
Respiratory	
Decreased maximum ventilation	Increased maximum voluntary ventilation
Endocrine	
Impaired glucose tolerance	Improve glucose tolerance
Increased incidence of hypercholesterol-emia and hyperlipidemia	Decreased serum lipid levels; increased HDL fraction
Increased total body fat	Decreased body fat
Musculoskeletal	
Decreased muscle mass/strength	Increased muscle strength
Decreased flexibility	Increased flexibility
Decreased bone density	Decreased involutional bone loss
	Increased bone mineral content

tions. Older patients are more prone to develop problems of dehydration, heat intolerance, cardiac ischemia, and overuse musculoskeletal injuries than younger patients. They should be instructed about the signs and symptoms of exercise intolerance and complications that indicate the need to stop the activity. Given the normal aging changes associated with total body water and thermoregulatory functions, dehydration and hyperthermia are of particular concern for elders. Moreover, clinically significant dehydration often occurs long before the onset of thirst. Specific guidelines for exercising in hot and/or humid conditions should be provided. The type of activity should be based on patient preference and abilities, cost, and the goals of the program. If exercise is to become a routine part of the care plan, it should be enjoyable and should fit into the patient's pattern of daily living.

Instructions should be given on the purpose and methods of warming up before exercise and cooling down after exercise. A gradual stretching of muscles and supporting structures, particularly those muscle groups most involved in the specific activity, can prevent injuries such as sprains and strains. Rhythmic, repetitive exercises, beginning at a slow pace that is gradually increased, will allow the cardiovascular system to adjust to the increased functional demands put on it and will optimize vasodilation. If walking is the main exercise activity, the pace should be slow at first and gradually increased during the first 10 to 15 minutes to the desired maximum pace, then gradually decreased over 10 to 15 minutes at the end of the session. Stretching exercises should precede the warm-up and follow the cool-down periods.

For older patients, the intensity level of exercise should be based on attaining between 50% and 80% of the maximum heart rate (Ulfarsson & Robinson, 1997). Some patients may require lower levels of intensity. Conditioning benefits are achieved by increasing the duration of the activity. The patient should begin with shorter periods and slowly increase the duration over several weeks. Exercising three to five times per week achieves optimal conditioning. However, a flexible schedule should be encouraged. This might consist of daily exercise sessions of alternating vigorous and less intense activities. On a daily basis, vigorous exercise is potentially harmful and should be avoided.

Clearly, many older patients cannot engage in vigorous or strenuous exercise. Still, nearly all patients can benefit from exercise if realistic and attainable goals are developed. Remind these patients that exercise can make everyday life easier and more enjoyable.

References and Recommended Readings

Child and Adolescent

Cook, P. (1995). Issues in the pediatric athlete. *Orthopedic Clinics of North America, 26*(3), 453.

Erikson, E. (1963). *Childhood and society* (2nd ed.). New York: W. W. Norton.

Gerbino, P., & Micheli, L. Back injuries in the young athlete. *Clinics in Sports Medicine, 14*(3), 571.

Ginsburg, G., & Bassett, G. (1997). Back pain in children and adolescents: evaluation and differential diagnosis. *Journal of the American Academy of Orthopaedic Surgeons, 5*(2), 67.

Koop, S., & Quanbeck, D. (1996). Three common causes of childhood hip pain. *Pediatric Clinics of North America, 43*(5), 1053.

Letson, G., & Greenfield, G. (1996). Evaluation of the child with a bone or soft-tissue neoplasm. *Orthopedic Clinics of North America, 27*(3), 431.

Morrissy, R. & Weinstein, S. (Eds.). (1996). *Lovell and Winter's pediatric orthopaedics* (4th ed.). Philadelphia: Lippincott-Raven.

Outerbridge, A., & Micheli, L. (1995). Overuse injuries in the young athlete. *Clinics in Sports Medicine, 14*(3), 503.

Paletta, G., & Andrish, J. (1995). Injuries about the hip and pelvis in the young athlete. *Clinics in Sports Medicine, 14*(3), 591.

Roemmich, J., & Rogol, A. (1995). Physiology of growth and development. *Clinics in Sports Medicine, 14*(3), 483.

Rome, E. (1995). Sports-related injuries among adolescents: when do they occur and how can we prevent them? *Pediatrics in Review, 16*(5), 184.

Saperstein, A., & Nicholas, S. (1996). Pediatric and adolescent sports medicine. *Pediatric Clinics of North America, 43*(5), 1013.

Teitz, C., Hu, S., & Arendt, E. (1997). The female athlete: evaluation and treatment of sports-related problems. *Journal of the American Academy of Orthopaedic Surgeons, 5*(2), 87.

Van de Loo, D., & Johnson, M. (1995). The young female athlete. *Clinics in Sports Medicine, 14*(3), 687.

Weinstein, S. (Ed.). (1994). *The pediatric spine: principles and practice.* New York: Raven Press.

Adult

American College of Obstetricians and Gynecologists. (1994). *Exercise during pregnancy and the postpartum period.* ACOG Technical Bulletin 189. Washington, DC: ACOG.

American College of Sports Medicine. (1995). *Guidelines for exercise testing and prescription* (5th ed.). Baltimore: Williiams & Wilkins.

Gassett, R. S., Hearne, B., & Keelan, B. (1996). Ergonomics and body mechanics in the workplace. *Orthopedic Clinics of North America, 27*(4), 861.

Goroll, A., & Mulley, A. (1995). *Primary care medicine: office evaluation and management* (3rd ed.). Philadelphia: Lippincott.

Jung, C. (1971). The stages of life. In Campbell, J. (Ed.). *The portable Jung.* New York: Viking Press.

MacEvilly, M., & Buggy, D. (1996). Back pain and pregnancy: a review. *Pain, 64,* 405.

McIntyre, I. N., & Broadhurst, N. A. (1996). Effective treatment of low back pain in pregnancy. *Australian Family Physician, 25*(9; Suppl. 2), 565.

Millender, L., & Conlon, M. (1996). An approach to work related disorders of the upper extremity. *Journal of the American Academy of Orthopaedic Surgeons, (4)*3, 134.

Nordin, M., Pope, M. H., & Anderson G. (1997). *Musculoskeletal disorders: principles and practice.* St. Louis, MO: Mosby.

Östgaard, H. (1996). Assessment and treatment of low back pain in working pregnant women. *Seminars in Perinatology, 20*(1), 66.

Rowe, M. L. (1985). *Orthopedic problems at work.* New York: McGraw-Hill.

Rungee, J. (1993). Low back pain during prenancy. *Orthopaedics, 16*(12), 1339.

Thompson, J., & Phelps, T. (1990). Repetitive strain injuries. *Postgraduate Medicine, 88*(8), 143.

Tompkins, N. C. (1996, May). Office ergonomics: focusing on the problem. *Occupational Health and Safety,* 93.

U.S. Department of Health and Human Services. (1996). *Physical activity and health: a report of the Surgeon General.* Atlanta, GA: DHHS, Centers for Disease Control and Prevention, National Center for Chronic Disease and Health Promotion.

U.S. Department of Labor, Bureau of Labor Statistics. (1996). *Occupational injuries and illnesses: counts, rates, and characteristics, 1993* (Bulletin 2478). Washington, DC: Author.

Mature Adult

Adams, W. (1996). Alcohol use in retirement communities. *Journal of the American Geriatric Society, 44*(9), 1082.

Banys, P. (1996). Substance abuse. In Lonergan, E. (Ed.). *Geriatrics.* Stamford, CT: Appleton & Lange.

Barry, H., & Eathorne, S. (1994). Exercise and aging. *Medical Clinics of North America, 78*(2), 357.

Bludau, J., & Lipsitz, L. (1997). Falls in the elderly. In Wei, J., & Sheehan, M. (Eds.). *Geriatric medicine.* Oxford University Press.

Butler, R., & Lewis, M. (1995). Late-life depression: when and how to intervene. *Geriatrics, 50*(8), 44.

Cochran, J. (1994). Family caregivers of the frail elderly: burdens and health. *Nurse Practitioner, 19*(5), 5–6.

Dunlop, D., Hughes, S., & Manheim, L. (1997). Disability in activities of daily living: patterns of change and a hierarchy of disability. *American Journal of Public Health, 87*(3), 378.

Erikson, R. (1963). *Childhood and society* (2nd ed.). New York: W. W. Norton.

Fiatarone, M., O'Brien, K., & Rich, B. (1996). Exercise: Rx for a healthier old age. *Patient Care,* 145.

Fife, R. (1994). Osteoarthritis. In Hazzard, W., Bierman, E., Blass, J., Ettinger, W., & Halter, J. (Eds.). *Principles of geriatric medicine and gerontology.* New York: McGraw-Hill.

Fink, A., Hays, R., Moore, A., & Beck, J. (1996). Alcohol-related problems in older persons. *Archives of Internal Medicine, 156*(11), 1150.

French, D. (1996). Avoiding adverse drug reactions in the elderly patient: issues and strategies. *Nurse Practitioner, 21*(9), 90.

Greenspan, S., Myers, E., Maitland, L., Resnick, N., & Hayes, W. (1994). Fall severity and bone mineral density as risk factors for hip fracture in ambulatory elders. *Journal of the American Medical Association, 271*(2), 128.

Ham, R. (1997). Demographics. In Ham, R., & Sloane, P. (Eds.). *Primary care geriatrics.* St. Louis, MO: Mosby.

Kane, R., Ouslander, J., & Abrass, I. (1994). *Essentials of clinical geriatrics* (3rd ed.). New York: McGraw-Hill.

Keenan, J., & Hepburn, K. (1997) Home care. In Ham, R., & Sloane, P. (Eds.). *Primary care geriatrics.* St. Louis, MO: Mosby.

Lonergan, E. (1996). Medications. In Lonergan, E. (Ed.). *Geriatrics.* Stamford, CT: Appleton & Lange.

Paffenbarger, R., Hyde, R., Wing, A., & Hsieh, C. (1986). Physical activity, all-cause mortality, and longevity of college alumni. *New England Journal of Medicine, 314*(10), 605.

Pollak, R., Sheehan, M., & Gerhart, T. (1997). Osteoporosis and hip fractures in the elderly. In Wei, J., & Sheehan, M. (Eds.). *Geriatric medicine.* Oxford: Oxford University Press.

Sewell, K. (1997). Arthritis in the elderly. In Wei, J., & Sheehan, M. (Eds.). *Geriatric medicine.* Oxford: Oxford University Press.

Sloane, P. (1997). Normal aging. In Ham, R., & Sloane, P. (Eds.). *Primary care geriatrics.* St. Louis, MO: Mosby.

Tibbetts, G. (1996). Patients who fall: how to predict and prevent injuries. *Geriatrics, 51*(9), 24–31.

Tideiksaar, R. (1996). Preventing falls: how to identify risk factors, reduce complications. *Geriatrics, 51*(2), 43.

Tinetti, M., Inouye, S., Gill, T., & Doucette, J. (1995). Shared risk factors for falls, incontinence, and functional dependence. *Journal of the American Medical Association, 273*(17), 1348.

Ulfarsson, J., & Robinson, B. (1997). Falls and falling. In Ham, R., & Sloane, P. (Eds.). *Primary care geriatrics.* St. Louis, MO: Mosby.

U.S. Bureau of the Census. (1996). *Statistical abstract of the United States: 1996* (116th ed.). Washington, DC: Author.

Wei, J. (1992). Age and the cardiovascular system. *New England Journal of Medicine, 327*(24), 1735.

Chapter 2

The Cervical Spine

Paul A. Glazer, MD
Kathy Taft, MSN, RNC

The cervical spine is a unique anatomic structure. It enables us to move our head in order to see, hear, and speak directly to our environment. Furthermore, it performs this important function while protecting the delicate spinal cord. An examination of a patient's cervical spine requires a detailed neurologic examination and knowledge of the bony and soft tissue structures in this area.

Anatomy

The cervical spinal column consists of seven cervical vertebral segments. They serve with their articulation with the occiput to support and protect the spinal cord. When the cervical spine is viewed in the sagittal plane, there are two curves. A small kyphotic (concave anteriorly) segment occurs between the occiput and the axis or C2. The larger lordotic segment occurs between C2 and T2—the second thoracic vertebra (Fig. 2-1).

The occiput is the bony covering for the cerebellum and borders the opening to the cranium (foramen magnum) where the spinal cord and brain stem join the brain. An elevated ridge of bone present in the midline of the squamous portion of the occiput is known as the external occipital protuberance or inion. This is the thickest region of occipital bone and is a useful palpable landmark. Transverse landmarks, extending caudally from the inion, include the nuchal lines. The posterior border of the foramen magnum is referred to as the opisthion; the anterior border is known as the basion or clivus and is formed by the basilar portion of the sphenoid and occipital bones. Lateral to the foramen magnum bilaterally are the convex occipital condyles, which articulate with the superior articular facets of the atlas, together forming the atlanto-occipital joints.

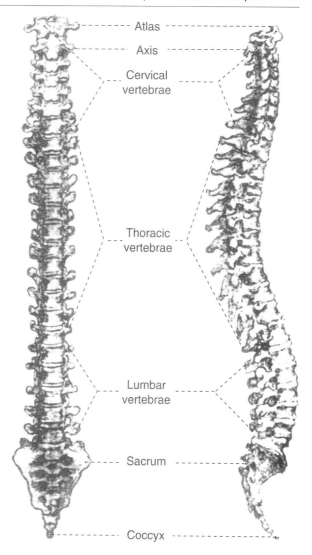

Atlas

Axis

Cervical
vertebrae

Thoracic
vertebrae

Lumbar
vertebrae

Sacrum

FIGURE 2-1. The vertebral column, drawn by Leonardo da
Vinci, as seen from the *front*
and the *side*.

Coccyx

The first two cervical vertebrae are atypical in structure in comparison to the others. The first cervical vertebra or atlas (C1) lacks a body and a spinous process. It consists of a ring through which the spinal cord passes. The anteroposterior diameter of the spinal canal is divided into three regions (Steel's rule of thirds) with the anterior third occupied by the odontoid process of the axis (C2), the middle third occupied by the spinal cord, and the posterior third filled with epidural fat and blood vessels. The arch of C1 articulates superiorly with the occipital condyles, which allows for the movements of flexion, extension, and some lateral bending. The atlanto-axial articulation allows for significant rotational movement (Fig. 2-2).

Each transverse process has a foramen (foramen of the transverse process) for passage of the vertebral arteries, which are the largest of the cervical region (Fig. 2-3). The arterial supply of the cervical region derives primarily from the paired vertebral arteries, which ascend the vertebral column bilaterally within the

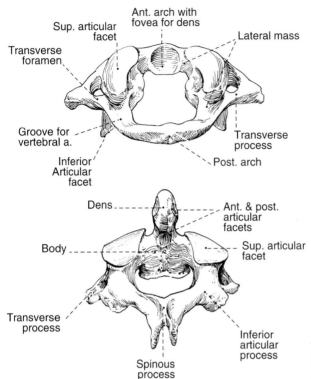

FIGURE 2-2. The atlas and axis seen from behind.

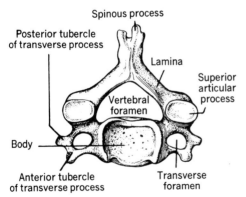

FIGURE 2-3. View of the fourth cervical vertebra, superior aspect.

transverse foramina of the cervical vertebral bodies, usually bypassing the C7 level. The vessels then enter the foramen magnum, where they unite to form the basilar artery. This forms the blood supply for the upper portion of the cervical spinal cord.

The stability of the craniovertebral region depends on the integrity of the upper cervical spinal ligaments. The spinal ligaments, common to all areas, include the anterior and posterior longitudinal ligaments; the ligamentum flavum; and the supra-spinous, interspinous, and intertransverse ligaments. The stability of these ligaments is determined by flexion/extension radiographs.

Patient Evaluation

The evaluation consists of taking a detailed history, a thorough, focused physical examination, and interpretation of any other objective data such as x-rays. This should proceed in an organized fashion, the one following the other. You will do your patients a disservice if you review a radiology report or film and base your diagnosis and treatment solely on this finding. The history and physical examination are the major determinants of your diagnosis, and the laboratory data are your supporting evidence.

The History

It is essential to observe the patient carefully during the history taking. Posture, facial expression, eye contact, and clothing give clues to the differential diagnosis. As with any medical history, it is essential to know the duration and type of symptoms. Establishing the location of the pain is also critical (see Eight Critical Questions for Data Gathering). What is the quality of the pain? Is the pain aching and dull in nature, or sharp and radiating? Is there any numbness or tingling? Was there any preceding trauma? Neck pain after trauma may develop within several hours, or it may be delayed 24 to 48 hours. Has the patient received any prior treatment for this problem? What medications is he taking? What makes the pain better or worse? Is the pain worse when awaking or at night? Does the patient have any arm or neck pain? Does the patient have headaches? Are there any changes in muscle strength? Any difficulty opening doors or jars? Has he had recent changes in handwriting? Does the patient have a gait disturbance or problems controlling his bowel or bladder? The answers to these questions can focus your evaluation and physical examination.

Arthritic, nontraumatic neck pain is mechanical in nature. It is typically worse in the morning. Patients complain of neck stiffness and aching that improves throughout the day. Does the patient have any associated arm pain? If arm pain is associated with neck pain, determine the nature of this pain, the location, and intensity. Patients with degenerative neck conditions may also complain of shoulder pain that may or may not radiate down the arm. It is important to establish the motion of the shoulder and strength of the shoulder muscles to rule out a possible rotator cuff problem. A patient experiencing paresthesias (tingling sensations) indicates a possible nerve compression. Does the patient experience any "electric shock" sensations in his upper extremities? Does he experience any muscle twitching or

Eight Critical Questions for Data Gathering

1. Was there a precipitating event?
   A. Trauma
   B. Lifting
   C. Bending
2. What was the onset?
   A. Gradual
   B. Sudden
3. How long has the pain persisted? (duration)
4. Where exactly is it? (location)
   A. Neck, back, buttocks
   B. Extremities
5. What is the nature of the pain?
   A. Aching
   B. Burning
   C. Radiating
6. What are the aggravating and relieving factors?
   A. Worse with coughing, sneezing, straining, and sitting
   B. Relieved by lying down
7. Are there associated complaints?
   A. Paresthesias of extremities
   B. Weakness or numbness of extremities
   C. Bowel or bladder dysfunction
8. Occurrence: when is the pain worse?
   A. Morning
   B. Afternoon/evening
   C. Night

"jumping," particularly at night? This should heighten your suspicion of cord compression.

Physical Examination

Observation

Examine the position and posture of the head. Normally the head is held erect, perpendicular to the floor (Hoppenfeld, 1976). A forward flexed posture may be observed in normal individuals, but it can also represent a soft tissue injury to the neck or fixed spinal deformity.

Have the patient disrobe to the waist to allow observation of the neck and upper extremities. The arc of motion during the process of undressing should be unrestricted. The patient with significant muscle spasm splints the neck and leans toward the spasm to avoid pain. With the patient seated comfortably on the examining room table, inspect the neck for scars, blisters, and discoloration.

Examine the spine for symmetry of the cervical musculature and for the normal cervical lordosis. A loss of lordosis can indicate paravertebral spasm, degenerative changes related to normal aging, or prior injury.

Palpation

It is essential to try to have the patient's muscles relaxed. With the patient supine, palpate the anterior and posterior soft tissues, including the paracervical musculature, the cervical nodes, and the thyroid gland. Identify the area of maximal tenderness. Carefully palpate the carotid pulse and listen for bruits. (Carotid massage has been known to precipitate cardiac events.)

Gross neck tenderness can be related to emotional or functional factors. Tenderness of the triceps occurs with C6–7 problems. Tenderness of the biceps and pectoralis major is associated with C5–6 lesions. This is often associated with tenderness of the costochondral junction of the first six ribs at the origin of the pectorals, imitating Tietze's syndrome (costochondritis). Tenderness of the sternocleidomastoid muscle can occur with hyperextension injuries of the neck.

Paravertebral muscle spasm occurs with soft tissue injury and cervical disc herniation. Enlarged lymph nodes resulting from upper respiratory infection can cause wryneck (torticollis).

Range of Motion

Caution: Do not attempt range of motion with a suspected unstable neck (ie, fracture). If there is no history of acute trauma, one can evaluate active and passive range of motion. Have the patient sit and face the examiner. Active motion should be recorded in flexion, extension, lateral flexion, rotation, and rotation with extension. To test active flexion, have the patient touch the chin to the chest. Extension is tested by asking the patient to look directly at the ceiling. Soft tissue trauma can result in a decrease in both flexion and extension.

Test rotation by having the patient turn his head to the right and then to the left. Normally the chin should line up with the shoulder; note any restriction in the arc of motion.

To test lateral flexion, have the patient attempt to touch each ear to the near shoulder. (Be aware that the patient often attempts to compensate for lack of lateral bending by bringing the shoulder up to the ear.) Normal lateral bending is 45 degrees. Test for rotation and extension by asking the patient to rotate to either direction, and while rotated, extend the chin. The patient may report shooting pain down his thorax or a reproduction of his symptoms. Some examiners prefer to examine for passive range of motion with the patient supine. With the muscles supported and relaxed, the range of motion may increase.

Neurologic Examination

MOTOR STRENGTH. To test neck flexion, stabilize the sternum with one hand, and with the opposite hand placed against the patient's forehead, offer resistance as the patient flexes the neck forward. Record the result, using the 0 to 5 motor grading scale (Table 2-1). To test neck extension, stabilize the posterior thorax and scapula with one hand, place the opposite hand over the occiput, and gently offer resistance as the patient extends the neck. For lateral bending, place one hand on the patient's right shoulder and offer resistance with the palm of the opposite hand placed on the patient's temple as the patient brings the ear to the shoulder. Note maximum resistance. To test lateral rotation, place the left hand on the patient's left shoulder, and with the right hand placed on the right side of the mandible, offer resistance as the patient rotates the head in a "no" motion (Hoppenfeld, 1976).

TABLE 2-1
Muscle Grading Chart

Muscle Gradations	Description
5—Normal	Complete range of motion against gravity with full resistance
4—Good	Complete range of motion against gravity with some resistance
3—Fair	Complete range of motion against gravity
2—Poor	Complete range of motion with gravity eliminated
1—Trace	Evidence of slight contractility, no joint motion
0—Zero	No evidence of contractility

NEUROLOGIC LEVEL. In a systematic manner with the patient seated on the edge of the examination table, legs dangling over the side, evaluate the neurologic levels from C3–T1 (Fig. 2-4).

C5 LEVEL. The deltoid and biceps muscles have both C5 and C6 innervation. Test deltoid strength by offering resistance against the shoulder motions of forward flexion and abduction. Test biceps strength by offering resistance against elbow flexion. An abnormal biceps reflex and altered sensation over the proximal lateral deltoid muscle are indicative of C5 innervation disturbance.

C6 LEVEL. The wrist extensors and the biceps are innervated by C6. Evaluate the wrist extensors by offering resistance and comparing the strength of both extremities. The brachioradialis reflex is examined, and the lateral forearm, thumb, index finger, and one half of the middle finger are examined for sensation.

C7 LEVEL. The triceps, wrist flexors, and the finger extensors are innervated by C7. Test triceps strength by offering resistance against elbow extension. Test the wrist flexors by resisting against the palmar aspect of a closed fist. Test the strength of the finger extensors by asking the patient to resist downward pressure on the dorsum of the extended fingers. With C7 dysfunction, the triceps reflex may be decreased or absent, and the middle finger may have altered sensation.

C8 LEVEL. The finger flexors are innervated by C8. Test the patient's grip strength bilaterally. There is no reflex innervated by C8. The ulnar side of the distal half of the forearm, the ulnar side of the little finger, and the ring finger are tested for sensation.

T1 LEVEL. The finger abductors are innervated by T1. Test finger abduction strength by having the patient extend and spread them against resistance. No reflex is able to be tested. T1 dermatomal innervation corresponds to sensation along the medial side of the upper half of the forearm. Table 2-2 describes the symptoms associated with compromise of the nerve roots of C3, C4, C5, C6, C7, and T1.

It is essential to attempt to distinguish cervical myelopathy from cervical radiculopathy. The patient with upper motor neuron disease or cord compression often presents with hyperreflexia. Long tract signs (indicating cord compression) include clonus, the Hoffman and Babinski signs, and the cremasteric and abdominal reflexes. In addition, lower extremity spasticity and bowel and bladder control should be documented.

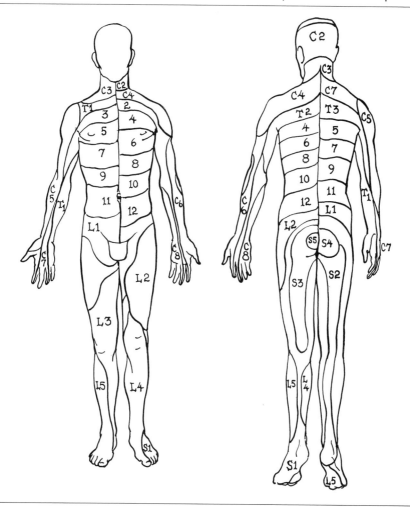

FIGURE 2-4. Distribution of spinal dermatomes. Considerable overlap occurs; consequently, involvement of a single spinal segment may not be evident.

The pain of radiculopathy is described as aching, and the pain follows a sensory dermatome. It may be accompanied by weakness, loss of tone and bulk of the upper extremity muscles, and absent or diminished reflexes. The signs and symptoms of myelopathy may be preceded by radicular symptoms with great variability. Paresthesias of the hands are common. There may be evidence of progressive lower extremity weakness. Ataxia may also be present.

Special Tests

COMPRESSION. With one hand, press down upon the top of the patient's head. Note if neck pain increases and if it recreates the patient's pain. This compression reduces the space of the neuroforamen, which can aggravate radicular pain.

TABLE 2-2
Cervical Radiculopathy

Nerve Root	Disk Level	Sensory and Pain Symptoms	Motor and Reflex
C3	C2-C3	Pain and numbness in back of neck, especially around ear	No changes; electromyelographic findings only
C4	C3-C4	Pain and numbness in back of neck; radiation to intracapsular area and down anterior chest	No changes; electromyelographic findings only
C5	C4-C5	Pain radiating from side of neck to supraspinous shoulder; numbness chevron or middeltoid (axillary nerve) area	Deltoid weakness; shoulder abduction; biceps reflex
C6	C5-C6	Pain lateral arm and forearm, into thumb and index; numbness tip of thumb and first dorsal interosseous muscle	Weak biceps, elbow flexion and supination; wrist extension; brachioradialis reflexes
C7	C6-C7	Pain middle of forearm to long finger; index and ring may be involved	Triceps elbow extension; finger extension; wrist flexion; triceps reflex
C8	C7-T1	Pain medial forearm to ring and little fingers; numbness ulnar side of ring finger and little finger	Triceps elbow extension, finger flexion at metacarpophalangeal joints and distal joints; reflex—none
T1	T1-T2	Medial arm	Finger intrinsics, dorsal interrossei, abduction, and palmar interrossei adduction; reflex—none

VALSALVA MANEUVER. Have the patient take a deep breath and strain as if to have a bowel movement. This maneuver increases intrathecal pressure. An increase in intrathecal pressure increases pain in the presence of a space-occupying lesion such as a tumor or a herniated nucleus pulposus. If the test is positive, the patient will complain of neck pain or radiating pain that follows a definable dermatome.

Difficult or painful swallowing may arise from esophageal trauma, bony osteophytes of the anterior vertebral bodies, hematomas, infection, or tumor. A hoarse voice may be due to involvement of the laryngeal nerve, which may be injured during anterior cervical spine surgery.

ADSON MANEUVER. Take the patient's radial pulse at the wrist. While you extend, abduct, and externally rotate the arm, have the patient take a deep breath and hold it while turning the head toward the arm being tested to determine if the pulse is still present. A diminished or absent pulse is a positive Adson's test. This evaluates the presence of compression of the subclavian artery (Hoppenfeld, 1976).

Evaluate associated areas that can mimic cervical spine problems: the shoulder, the upper extremities, the lower jaw, and the temporomandibular joint.

General Referral Guidelines: When to Refer

1. Intractable pain
2. Signs of extremity weakness
3. Indication of cord compression
4. Meningeal signs
5. Suspected cardiac or thyroid disease
6. Lymph node
7. Vertebral artery insufficiency
8. Suspicion of brachial plexus lesion, stinger, burner
9. Trauma
10. Suspected fracture, infection, or tumor
11. Failure to respond to therapy

Differential Diagnosis of Neck Pain

Several tests will assist in differentiating the causes of neck pain (see Differential Diagnosis of Neck Pain).

Diagnostic Tests

RADIOGRAPHS. Routine radiographic evaluation of the cervical spine usually begins with plain x-rays. Cervical spine x-rays should be ordered when a patient without preceding trauma has a history of pain greater than 6 weeks' duration that

Differential Diagnosis of Neck Pain

Ligamentous/muscular disorders
  Spasm
  Strain/sprain
  Contusion
  Wryneck (torticollis)
Skeletal disorders
  Cervical disk degeneration
  Cervical disk herniation
  Shoulder joint (rotator cuff tendinitis)
  Fracture
  Atlantoaxial instability secondary to RA
  Discitis
  Cervical stenosis
Psychogenic
  Secondary gains
  Litigation pending
Neurologic disorders
  Nerve root lesions
  Brachial plexus lesions ("stingers")
  Thoracic outlet syndrome
  Neurogenic pain syndromes
Spinal cord/brain
  Meningitis
  Spinal cord compression
  Cervical myelopathy
Cardiac disorders
  Angina

is not responding to conservative therapy. X-rays should be ordered only after performing a detailed physical examination. This will decrease the amount of radiation exposure to the patient and tailor the radiographic examination to the area in question. Routine views will include anterior-posterior and lateral views of the cervical spine. If there is any history of trauma, an open-mouth or odontoid view should also be ordered. If there is significant pain on range of motion, one should obtain flexion and extension views as well. One needs to evaluate these radiographs for the presence of a fracture, subluxation, ligamentous instability, spinal stenosis, and soft tissue abnormalities. Common radiographic findings seen include the following:

1. Narrowing of the interspace with associated symptoms suggestive of disc degeneration. Remember that a great percentage of the population will show degenerative changes after the age of 30, and radiographic evidence of degenerative changes is not diagnostic in and of itself.
2. Loss of normal cervical lordosis resulting from paravertebral muscle spasm, which may suggest an acute injury or disc disruption.
3. Cervical instability (ie, translation of more than 3.5 mm or 11 degrees angulation of one vertebral body relative to the next; White & Punjabi, 1990).

Obtain an electrocardiogram if the patient complains of chest pain that radiates to the neck or jaw, or in any patient who is in a high-risk group for coronary disease.

OTHER TESTS. Aids to diagnosis of persistent or worsening symptoms after 6 weeks include the following:

1. Electromyography—for cervical radiculopathy, electromyography will evaluate for nerve root involvement. This distinguishes peripheral nerve involvement from nerve root involvement and is diagnostic of either radiculopathy, a brachial plexus lesion, or peripheral neuropathy. Electromyography aids in the differentiation of organic from inorganic (functional) problems.
2. Magnetic resonance imaging (MRI)—for suspected nerve root or cord involvement, tumor, infection, or fracture.
3. Computerized axial tomogram (CAT)—for suspected herniated disc, for suspected stenosis, and patient reassurance.
4. Laboratory studies—for hemoglobin, hematocrit, complete blood count with differential, urinalysis, erythrocyte sedimentation rate, blood chemistry studies, immunologic studies, serum protein electrophoresis, and TB skin tests to rule out underlying systemic disease.

The Adolescent With Neck Pain

Neck symptoms in the adolescent are unusual. Complaints of neck pain need careful evaluation.

Predisposing Factors

1. Immaturity of the cervical spine
2. Mobility of the young cervical spine (under age 20)

3. Congenital instability of C1–2, C4–5, C5–6 (which may occur with Down's syndrome)
4. Long, thin necks (increased susceptibility to sports-related injuries)
5. Participation in certain competitive and contact sports (wrestling, swimming, diving, football, rugby, and gymnastics)
6. Motor vehicle accidents (all terrain, motorcycle, and automobile)

Etiology

1. Acute or chronic muscle, tendon, or ligamentous strain that results from head-on tackling during football when trauma to the head is transferred to the neck. Athletes playing as defensive backs or wide receivers risk violent flexion (most dangerous), extension, and lateral stretch injuries (most common; Micheli, 1995).
2. Localized acute muscle strain resulting from motor vehicle accidents
3. A direct blow to the cervical spine causing a contusion, which can mimic cervical strain.
4. Cervical disc herniation can occur on impact with sports or motor vehicle accidents but is rare in this age group. Evaluate the athlete to distinguish cervical radiculopathy (nerve root compression) from a brachial plexus (stinger type) injury.

Prevention

The injured athlete must be assessed immediately. The team primary care provider or trainer must be drilled in the proper techniques for evaluation, on-field treatment, and transportation. Education in this age group is the key to preventing many of the cervical spine injuries.

Prevention can be aided by the following:

1. Preseason screenings of the cervical spine to identify high-risk individuals. These screenings should include determination of general fitness, strength testing, evaluation of range of motion, evaluation of cervical tenderness, axial compression test, and information about previous injury. Obtain cervical spine x-rays on all individuals with a history of pain or prior neck injury. An athlete with prior injury and a positive physical examination is at increased risk for injury. Athletes with a normal examination and a history of prior injury have a slightly increased risk.
2. Utilize a strict criterion for returning to competition.
3. Establish a 12-month conditioning/training program to include neck exercises. Recommend isometric resistance and isotonic resistance (Nautilus) to build the strength of the supporting neck musculature.
4. Bar trampolines from regular gymnastic classes.
5. Educate the coaching staff and athletes about the associated risks for injury and the prevention techniques.
6. Insist that athletes wear seat belts at all times, adjust car headrests to protect the head and neck, and do not drive under the influence of alcohol, sedatives, or tranquilizers.

Common Management Problems

Pinched Nerve Syndrome (Brachial Plexus Lesion, Stinger, and Burner)

ETIOLOGY

This is a common football or wrestling injury. The head is flexed as in a spearing injury in football or forced to one side while the opposite shoulder is depressed.

SYMPTOMS
1. Sudden onset
2. Burning sensation in the shoulder
3. Paresthesias of entire arm, hand, and fingers
4. Possible pain and weakness in the arm and hand
5. Possible complete transient paralysis of affected arm

SIGNS
1. Sensation loss over multiple (two to four) dermatomes
2. Tenderness over the brachial plexus
3. Increased symptoms with passive movement of head and neck to the opposite side
4. No posterior neck tenderness
5. No increased symptoms with compression test

TREATMENT (ACUTE)
1. Ice
2. Anti-inflammatory medications
3. Muscle relaxants
4. Splinting (rolled towel, hard collar, sandbags)

REFERRAL
1. Immediate

Outcome

RETURN-TO-PLAY CRITERIA
1. No pain with full active neck range of motion
2. No pain during resistance testing of neck movements
3. Full strength of shoulder shrugs, abduction, elbow flexion and extension, and grip
4. Normal sensation along all dermatomes

The Adult With Neck Pain

Degenerative change in the cervical spine is a part of the aging process. This phenomenon can begin in adolescence and can affect the discs and/or the facet joints. By age 40, some individuals have narrowing of the interspace between C5–6 and C6–7, osteophyte formation, and sclerosis of the facet joints. These changes, which can be seen on the x-ray, can compress and irritate the nerve roots, the spinal cord, and the vertebral arteries.

Adult problems may originate in the workplace. The worker with a neck injury loses more work time than one with a back injury, although neck injury occurs only

20% as frequently. Often the most common cause of upper-extremity pain in middle age is osteoarthritis of the cervical spine (Wiesel & Boden, 1995).

Predisposing Factors

1. Static arm postures, such as those used by dentists, hairdressers, and bike riders
2. Repetitive arm movements, such as those used by coal miners, assembly line packers, meat cutters, and swimmers
3. Static sitting postures, such as those assumed by computer terminal operators, secretaries, and students
4. Motor vehicle accidents

Etiology

1. Acute or chronic muscle, tendon, or ligamentous strain that results from work-related postures or recreational activities
2. Localized acute muscle strain resulting from motor vehicle accidents
3. Cervical disc herniation occurring as a result of the impact on the aging spine after a fall or motor vehicle accident. Most herniations will resolve with conservative management within 6 weeks, although the patient may be left with residual aching and limitation of movement.
4. Changes associated with aging—a sedentary lifestyle, work-related postures, and recreational activity. The "weekend athlete" syndrome presents as either overuse (acute), degenerative, or chronic pain.

Prevention

1. Identify at-risk groups in the work environment. Conduct educational programs targeting at-risk occupational groups to emphasize the importance of alleviating static postures. Workers should be able to change their postures at least every hour. On-site institutional aerobic programs are effective in promoting fitness to reduce injury.
2. Foster the wearing of seat belts at all times and adjustment of car headrests to protect the head and neck.
3. Educate post-trauma victims about the long-term nature of their illness and the need for protracted treatment. Provide continuous support through active listening, and encourage patients to return as soon as possible to normal activities to promote a successful outcome.
4. Educate patients about the decreased risk of injury with proper training techniques, including a regular exercise regimen for 30 to 40 minutes five times a week. Each exercise session should begin with 15 minutes of warm-up and end with 15 minutes of cool-down.

Common Management Problems

Cervical Spondylosis (Degenerative Arthritis and Osteoarthritis)

Commonly found at C4–5, C5–6, and C6–7, cervical spondylosis affects more males than females, usually between the ages of 40 and 70. The problem can follow a precipitating event and cause sudden, severe pain with splinting of the neck, or it can begin gradually without a precipitating event and become chronic over a period of months or years. Patients complain of pain and neck stiffness that is localized in the middle or upper neck and radiates to the occiput area and shoulder (the levator scapulae muscles), causing headache and pain. Motion, especially extension, increases the pain, and the pain is worse at the end of the day.

ETIOLOGY

1. Excessive axial loading of the head and neck
2. Static postures
3. Repetitive movements
4. Extreme movements
5. Minor injuries
6. Chronic strain of ligaments or joints

SYMPTOMS

1. Recurring neck stiffness
2. Mild aching of the neck musculature and associated structures, especially in the cervical scapular region
3. Limitation of neck motion that the patient has noticed for months or years
4. Headache (migratory, with a typical pattern from the temple to the forehead), sensory dermatome of the first trigeminal nerve, accompanied by discomfort behind the eye, dizziness, visual blurring, alteration in hearing, disassociation from the environment
5. Vertigo
6. Radicular pain, pain radiating to the arms, back, and head, and associated with tingling, numbness, and weakness; the pain pattern typically proceeds along the ulnar side of the upper extremity, posterior aspect of the forearm, or radial side of the hand
7. Spastic weakness of the legs, which could indicate silent cord involvement
8. Complaints of neck constriction, difficulty swallowing, and voice changes as a result of swelling of the esophagus and associated structures

SIGNS

1. Limitation of cervical flexion, rotation, and extension
2. Tenderness/pain with anterior palpation
3. Crepitus
4. Reproduction of pain in the upper to mid cervical spine with movement
5. Long tract signs indicating cord compression (eg, hyperreflexia)

TREATMENT (ACUTE)

1. Initial weekly appointments to help develop trusting provider–patient relationships, lessen anxiety, and foster early return to normal activities. Maintain communication with the employee's supervisor because an early return to work is encouraged.
2. Education using a three-dimensional model to increase knowledge of spinal structure, the disease process and its causes, and the potential long-term treatment and chronic nature of the problem. Increased knowledge decreases apprehension. Distinguish between hurting and harm; teach that all pain does not necessarily mean permanent damage. Underscore the

need to increase physical fitness and avoid postures or movements that increase risks.

3. Decreased inflammation resulting from immobilization with a soft cervical collar continuously (including sleep) from several days to weeks, if it relieves the symptoms.

The neck must be maintained in a neutral position with the head held in slight to moderate flexion. The usual collar height is 3½ inches. If the collar is too high, the neck will be forced into hyperextension; if too low, there will be no support. During the acute phase, collars are to be worn 24 hours a day for 2 to 3 weeks or until the pain subsides. Rigid supports are contraindicated; they can increase muscle stiffness and result in muscle atrophy. Nonsteroidal anti-inflammatories, ice or heat, phonophoresis (ultrasound with cortisone cream), and cervical traction for 2 to 3 months at home for 20 minutes three times a week are helpful for many patients.

REHABILITATION
1. Physical therapy provides instruction about isometric exercises to strengthen paravertebral musculature, and modification of home/work environment to reduce the chances of exacerbation.
2. Review activities of daily living with specific advice on how to avoid extension-producing strain. Do not restrict activities unnecessarily, but base restrictions on personal tolerance. General guidelines to avoid increasing neck pain follow.
   a. Avoid reaching overhead or looking up at the ceiling.
   b. When driving an automobile, adjust the seat and headrest to keep the spine in proper alignment; the seat should be close to the steering wheel to avoid craning the neck. Driving should be avoided with acute pain.
   c. Avoid lifting or carrying packages over 10 lb (eg, women with capacious handbags); avoid moving heavy loads and wearing heavy overcoats.
   d. When sitting, avoid resting the chin on the hand.
   e. Sleep with either several pillows to keep the head and shoulders supported or with a cervical neck roll.
   f. Sports should be avoided with severe symptoms; golf, bowling, and swimming (except on the back) may aggravate neck pain.

Be sure the patient understands what has been taught, and provide written instructions to eliminate confusion. Keep a copy of the instructions with the patient's record.

REFERRAL
1. Intractable pain
2. Signs of extremity weakness
3. Indications of cord compression (long tract signs)
4. Meningeal signs (fever, stiff neck, severe occipital headache, positive Brudzinski, positive Kernig)
5. Suspected cardiac or thyroid disease
6. Lymph node involvement

7. Vertebral artery compression syndrome (intermittent dizziness, diplopia, syncope, headaches, tinnitus and momentary loss of consciousness that is induced by head and neck movements of rotation, extension, and lateral flexion; Jones & Mayer, 1994)

OUTCOME
1. 60% improve with resolution in 3 to 4 months.
2. 20% have symptomatic relief.
3. 20% have no improvement.

Cervical Disc Disease (Cervical Radiculopathy)

This is part of the syndrome of cervical osteoarthritis. Faulty forward head posture can be contributory. It can be acute or chronic.

ACUTE SYMPTOMS
1. Sudden, severe pain along the involved sensory dermatome
2. Radiation of pain to the neck and shoulders or down the arm, forearm, and to the fingers
3. Possible anterior or posterior chest pain
4. Possible paresthesias along the involved sensory dermatome

ACUTE SIGNS
1. Pain that increases with all movement, especially rotation, lateral flexion, and extension
2. Possible loss of motor strength
3. Possible diminished or absent reflexes
4. Possible presence of muscle atrophy with fasciculations

CHRONIC SYMPTOMS
1. Insidious pain, usually after repetitive work or exercise that is performed in an awkward position
2. Symptoms similar to those of acute disc disease

CHRONIC SIGNS
1. Possible loss of cervical lordosis
2. Mild muscle atrophy
3. Loss of motor strength rarely
4. Limitation of motion to the affected side in rotation and lateral flexion
5. Increased pain with extension, lateral flexion, and rotation toward the affected side
6. Increased pain with palpation of the cervical muscles
7. Increased pain with bony palpation of the spinous process over the affected disc
8. Possible pain that radiates in the distribution of the affected nerve root
9. Possible leg weakness

TREATMENT
1. Patient education regarding probable, usually good, outcome
2. Ice or heat to affected area
3. Physical therapy for instruction in gentle stretching, strengthening, and range-of-motion exercises

4. Immobilization with a soft collar
5. Nonnarcotic analgesics (aspirin)
6. Anti-inflammatory drugs
7. Cervical spine pillow
8. Therapeutic massage by either a physical therapist, massage therapist, or primary care provider

REFERRAL
See Cervical Spondylosis.

OUTCOME
Prognosis is usually good, with improvement in 3 to 4 months.

Stiff Neck, Acute Torticollis (Wryneck)

This usually occurs in children but may occur in individuals above age 15. It involves muscles, ligaments, tendons, and discs. The differential diagnosis includes spinal cord or cerebellar tumors, lymphadenitis, herniated disc, rheumatoid arthritis, typhoid fever, tuberculosis, multiple sclerosis, osteomyelitis and fractures, subluxations, and dislocations of the cervical spine, especially C1–C2.

ETIOLOGY
1. Trauma
2. Awkward positions held for many hours (especially sleeping positions in which the neck is unsupported and tilted toward one side)
3. Occupational postures of secretaries and computer terminal operators who glance to the side
4. Recreational stressors (following a ball during a tennis match), overuse syndrome (particularly in swimming), and playing tennis (when out of shape or without warming up)
5. Occurrence before the onset of an upper respiratory infection

SYMPTOMS
1. Awakening with a ''crick'' in the neck (stiff neck)
2. Pain, usually unilateral and constant, that increases with rotation toward painful side
3. Neck, fixed to the side, either toward or away from the affected side and held rigid
4. Patient looking sideways by turning body or eyes, not the neck

SIGNS
1. Exquisite tenderness of the sternocleidomastoid, levator scapulae, and trapezius muscles
2. Restricted rotation and flexion with pain at the end point of movement
3. Possible flattening of the normal cervical lordotic curve
4. Possible limitation of shoulder motion

TREATMENT
Patients who have experienced trauma or those with a prior malignancy should undergo definitive testing, particularly cervical spine films, with open mouth view (if pain worsens or does not improve after 2 weeks), a bone scan (if there is a high

suspicion of infection, fracture, or tumor) and a CBC with differential, SMA 12, ESR, SPEP, and Tine test (if infection or tumor is suspected).

1. Initial rest (in a supine position with the head on a small pillow or in a semireclining position with the head and neck supported by several large pillows) alleviates the muscles from supporting the head.
2. Ice is applied with massage (see The Ice Massage), or an ice pack is applied to the painful area 15 to 20 minutes several times a day for the first 48 hours.

The Ice Massage

1. Freeze water in a paper cup
2. Position patient lying on the unaffected side, with a small pillow supporting the head.
3. Peel down the top of the cup.
4. Using a circular motion, apply to the painful neck area.

---

3. After 72 hours, moist heat may be applied for 20 minutes per hour; caution the patient not to lie on the heating pad.
4. Gentle stretching exercises several times daily promote the return to normal function by decreasing stiffness (see Appendix E). Physical therapy may be indicated for passive exercises or if the patient is reluctant to exercise.
5. Medications including nonnarcotic analgesics (aspirin, two to three tablets four times a day with meals) or nonsteroidal anti-inflammatories. Muscle relaxants are centrally acting and tend to produce unpleasant side effects, such as drowsiness. It is unclear whether the various drugs effectively relax the muscles; however, they do help the patient remain on bedrest.
6. A three-dimensional model and an illustration of the supporting musculature increase the patient's understanding of the injury and treatments.

Educate the patient in methods to decrease side effects of medications (ie, take anti-inflammatories with meals); review the importance of proper posture, especially during sleep; and adjust the height of chairs, work surfaces, and keyboards to reduce strain (see Chapter 1). Instruct the patient to continue exercises indefinitely and to take a rest period after work if aching persists. Instruct the patient to apply warm, moist heat or ice to the affected area as needed at the end of the work day.

REFERRAL
1. Failure to respond to therapy
2. Trauma
3. Suspected fracture
4. Suspected infection
5. Suspicion of a tumor

OUTCOME
1. Complete resolution in 7 to 15 days
2. Return to work as soon as the pain subsides or as able

Muscle Strains

Tension Neck (Middle and Lower Trapezius Muscle)

ETIOLOGY
Continuous contraction of the muscle, combined with poor posture, results in a rounded upper back. This commonly occurs as a result of leaning forward while sitting at or standing over a desk or using a microscope. Heavy breasts that are poorly supported are also a contributing factor. Tension neck is usually seen after the age of 30 years.

SYMPTOMS
1. Soreness and fatigue along the muscle
2. May be accompanied by a burning pain
3. Intermittent pain
4. Relief with position change or lying down

SIGNS
1. Point tenderness where the trapezius muscle attaches to the thoracolumbar spine, pectoral muscles, and tendons
2. Adaptive shortening of the pectoral muscles
3. Rounding of the upper back (may have thoracic kyphosis)
4. Pain in posterior neck
5. Forward head posture
6. Hyperextension of the cervical spine

TREATMENT
1. Ice or heat to painful area
2. Emphasis on correct posture that maintains the normal spinal curves
3. Correction of round shoulder posture with the following exercise: Stand erect with the back to the wall. To improve posture, abduct both shoulders, pressing elbows against the wall. To strengthen the trapezius, pull arms back against the wall in a diagonal overhead position. Hold for a count of 10, release; repeat five times twice a day.
4. Instructing female patients to wear properly fitted bras
5. Reviewing patient's job-related activities and, if necessary, referring the patient to an occupational rehabilitation specialist for job retraining

OUTCOME
Relief of symptoms with readjustment of occupational movements or correction of other underlying problems.

Strain of the Upper Trapezius Muscle

ETIOLOGY
This is caused by overstretching of the trapezius muscle while reaching for an object with the head tilted in the opposite direction. The condition may be acute or chronic.

SYMPTOMS
1. Pain in the posterolateral portion of the neck (from the occiput to the acromial process of the scapula)
2. Tenderness of the muscle
3. Excessive spasm and contraction of the muscle

SIGNS
The muscle may be tight, tense, or very tender along its insertion, from the occiput to the acromion.

TREATMENT
1. Massage with an upward stroke (downward stroking increases tension)
2. Use of a soft collar

OUTCOME
Resolution in 2 to 7 days.

Acute Cervical Strain/Sprain (Whiplash)

Whiplash is a soft tissue injury of the neck involving a sudden acceleration of the head and neck into hyperextension, followed by hyperflexion beyond the normal range of motion. This results in a tear of one of the musculotendinous units in the neck: the trapezius, sternocleidomastoid, erector spinae, scalenes, levator scapula, or rhomboids (Spitzer et al, 1995).

ETIOLOGY
1. Motor vehicle accident, especially a rear-end collision
2. Competitive sports, especially wrestling, football, and gymnastics
3. Work-related accidents

SYMPTOMS
Onset may be delayed from 2 to more hours after the precipitating event.

1. Headache
2. Aching neck pain, soreness, stiffness
3. Pain that radiates to the upper shoulder, scapula, occiput, or eyes
4. Possible difficulty with swallowing
5. May be associated with visceral symptoms, dizziness, ringing or buzzing in the ears, blurring of vision

SIGNS
1. Spasm and pain of the paravertebral muscles
2. Restricted range of motion
3. Flexion of the neck to the contralateral side producing pain
4. Local tenderness and swelling
5. Numbness and radiating pain (if present, does not follow a dermatome)
6. Possible tilting of head toward the affected side

TREATMENT (ACUTE)
To promote an active patient role, involve the patient in the recovery process and avoid passive treatment such as massage. This can cause further irritation of the muscles and promote the sick role. The management regimen should be based

on a careful evaluation of the nature and severity of the injury, the magnitude of the symptoms, the physical findings, the emotional makeup of the patient, and the psychosocial environment. Additional diagnostic tests should be performed on victims of trauma, occupational, or sports-related injuries, or if there is potential for litigation. Patients with suspected fracture, nerve root pain, and/or a neurologic deficit also should have definitive testing.

1. Reassurance, support, active listening with a relaxed manner
2. Explanation of the problem, its course, and expected outcome in detail
3. Application of ice to the painful area for 15 minutes several times a day, until symptoms subside. After 72 hours, ask the patient to stand under a warm shower to increase muscle relaxation. Avoid deep radiating heat because it can increase muscle and ligament irritation.
4. Immobilization that allows soft tissues to heal by decreasing the work of the head's supporting musculature. This is initially accomplished with 2 to 4 days of bedrest, soft collars, or intermittent traction.

   If cervical traction is indicated for severe injury, use 6 to 10 lb applied in a sitting position for 20 to 30 minutes two to four times a day. Initial instructions should be given by a physical therapist; the traction is then applied at home. Additional physical therapy should be avoided unless nerve impingement is suspected or the therapy reduces the symptoms because it promotes the sick role.
5. Medication as indicated under Stiff Neck (above), decreasing medication as symptoms subside

REFERRAL
1. No improvement within 10 days
2. Neurologic symptoms
3. Intractable pain
4. Significant weakness
5. Pressure on spinal cord as indicated by long tract signs on physical examination
6. Meningeal signs
7. No improvement in 6 weeks and x-rays are normal; a bone scan, medical evaluation, and psychosocial evaluation should be done

REHABILITATION
The patient can increase activity as tolerated and can be encouraged in early return to normal activity and work. When the patient is asymptomatic for 2 weeks, it is time to begin isometric exercises (see Appendix E) and gradually to wean the patient from the collar by omitting daytime wear. The patient may perform range-of-motion exercises and isometric exercises twice a day, beginning with 5 repetitions of each exercise and increasing to 10 with tolerance. A warm shower or warm, moist towel should be used to warm the neck before exercising. It is important to bear in mind that exercises are to increase the strength of the cervical musculature, not to increase the range of motion.

OUTCOME
1. Most patients respond to treatment within 10 days. Allow 6 weeks for healing; at 6 weeks, most symptoms are relieved. Most patients return to

normal activity within 2 months. Occasionally, patients exhibit a reluctance to return to normal activities with no evidence of objective findings.
2. Symptoms may return with fatigue. Daily rest periods lessen chances of exacerbation.
3. Return to light-duty work if pain is tolerable in 0 to 7 days.
4. Return to noncompetitive sports when pain is tolerable and activity does not increase pain (usually 10 to 14 days).
5. Return to competitive sports when full painless range of motion in all planes and strength have returned (usually by 6 weeks).

Thoracic Outlet Syndrome (TOS)

TOS describes a group of symptoms caused by compression of the brachial plexus and the subclavian artery and vein (usually between the clavicle and first rib). It can be associated with a cervical strain.

ETIOLOGY
1. Bony abnormality of the first rib (cervical rib)
2. C7 elongated transverse process
3. Overuse related to athletics (basketball and swimming)
4. "Whiplash" injury
5. Occupational postures, especially those requiring overhead work
6. Postural fatigue
7. Emotional stress (sagging shoulders)
8. Carrying heavy shoulder loads

SYMPTOMS
1. Pain in the arm in certain positions
2. Color changes in the hand
3. Aching pain across the shoulder
4. Pain that may be felt in the side of the neck and down the arm
5. Pain that may be associated with heaviness, sensation of weakness, and fatigue when using the arm, especially above shoulder height (ie, when combing or washing the hair)
6. A sensation of cold, pallor, and swelling of the hand (less common)

SIGNS
1. Sensory loss of the fourth and fifth fingers of the affected hand (ulnar nerve)
2. Weakness of the fourth and fifth fingers (ulnar nerve)
3. Positive Adson's test
4. May have reflex changes (usually reflexes present)
5. May have bruits heard over the subclavian artery

TREATMENT
Care must be taken to differentiate TOS from Raynaud's phenomenon, ulnar nerve entrapment at the elbow, pulmonary tumor (compression of the brachial plexus can result from neoplasm or fibrosis due to radiation), or Horner's syndrome. Definitive diagnostic tests for TOS are plain cervical spine films, EMG, and ultrasound of the subclavian artery.

At the initial office visit, carefully explain the source of the symptoms. Use line drawings of the anatomy to increase patient understanding. Listen carefully to allay anxiety, fear, and frustration. Teach progressive relaxation training. Provide shoulder exercises (see Appendix E).

OUTCOME
Early recognition and treatment of TOS result in a better outcome; after 2 years, little improvement can be expected.

The Mature Adult With Neck Pain

Chronic degenerative changes account for most of the neck problems encountered by the older adult.

Predisposing Factors

1. Aging spine
2. Increased susceptibility to injury and strain from lack of muscle strength and flexibility
3. Decreased mobility that increases the risks for accident-related trauma
4. Lack of energy to participate in a regular exercise program
5. Lack of understanding of the importance of physical fitness
6. Lack of financial resources and fear of the environment that may keep the mature adult homebound and unable to join in group activities that may aid prevention

Etiology

1. Chronic degenerative disease such as osteoarthritis of the facet joints, discogenic syndrome, and cervical stenosis
2. Episodes of torticollis that occurred when patient was a young adult

Prevention

Instruction focuses on recognition by the mature adult that aches and pains are not normal expectations of aging and that simple remedies such as regular exercise and aspirin (taken on a regular basis) will help to foster a sense of wellness and improve or maintain function.

Common Management Problem

Cervical Osteoarthritis (Discogenic Syndrome)

ETIOLOGY
Etiology is the degeneration of the cervical discs.

SYMPTOMS
1. Constant aching in the scapular area
2. Most intense pain in the morning
3. Painless restriction of motion (stiffness)

4. May have paresthesias in the hands
5. May have pain in both upper limbs

SIGNS
1. Limitation of cervical spine movement, especially extension; severe pain with hyperextension
2. Preservation of forward flexion
3. Tenderness on compression of the facet joints

TREATMENT
See patient at 6-week intervals and monitor for myelopathy (may present as ataxia or difficulty in walking).

1. Soft collar as needed with neck in 15 degrees of flexion; avoid hyperextension, try narrow part of collar anteriorly to increase comfort
2. Nonnarcotic analgesics (mild) or nonsteroidal anti-inflammatories
3. Neck exercises
4. Patient reassurance
5. Development of short-term, easily attainable goals that will encourage compliance with suggested regimen

REFERRAL
1. Primary care provider referral for local anesthetic and steroid injection into trigger points
2. When there is progressive neurologic deficit, a referral is required

OUTCOME
This is a chronic problem, and the patient needs constant supervision and interaction with the health management team primary care provider.

General Treatment Guidelines for Cervical Spine Disease

Treatment for cervical spine disease may be either surgical or conservative. As newer treatment modalities are introduced, the likelihood of surgical intervention is diminished. Most (>95%) cervical spine problems can and should be treated conservatively. Do not be misled by reports of abnormalities on radiographs if the patient does not have supporting signs and symptoms. Surgery should be reserved for those patients at clear risk for functional impairment due to an identifiable target and who are not responding to conservative therapy. The primary care provider's role as patient advocate can be crucial in assisting patients in the decision-making process.

Conservative Treatment

The available therapies for treating cervical spine problems are extensive if one considers traditional and nontraditional approaches. The provider needs to be broad-minded in approach. Keep in mind the "hurt" versus "harm" dictum. No single therapy is indicated for any specific problem, and it is useful to have "a big bag of tricks."

Treatment Pearls

1. Involve patient in the plan
2. Patient education regarding problem, treatment, and probable outcome
3. Use of ice and heat
4. Judicious use of cervical collars
5. *Temporary* rest from aggravating factors, if possible
6. Physical therapy, which may include ice, heat, phonopheresis, electrical stimulation, massage, stretching range of motion, conditioning, traction
7. Ergonomic adjustments in work or home environment
8. Cervical spine pillow
9. Trigger point injections
10. Nonsteroidal anti-inflammatory drugs (may need to try several to effect pain relief)
11. Muscle relaxant drugs
12. Serotonergic drugs (antidepressants, anticonvulsants)
13. Steroid therapy, typically epidural injections
14. Acupuncture
15. Relaxation techniques
16. Biofeedback
17. Hypnosis
18. Magnet therapy
19. Exercise (Although some exercise may cause an increase in pain, it is not likely to harm, even in the presence of known disc herniations.) The rule of thumb is, if it hurts, stop, at least temporarily.

References and Recommended Readings

An, H. S., & Simpson, J. M. (eds.). (1994). *Surgery of the cervical spine.* London: Martin Dunitz.

Blakney, M., & Hertling, D. (1996). In Hertling, D., & Kessler, R. M. *Management of common musculo-skeletal disorders (physical therapy and principles)* (3rd ed.), pp. 528–558. Philadelphia: Lippincott-Raven.

Bland, J. H. (1994). *Disorders of the cervical spine.* Philadelphia: W. B. Saunders.

Cramer, G. D., & Darby, S. A. (eds). (1995). *Basic and clinical anatomy of the spine, spinal cord, and ANS.* St. Louis: Mosby–Year Book.

Crandall, P. H., & Batzdorf, U. (1996). Cervical spondylotic myelopathy. *Journal of Neurosurgery, 25,* 57–66.

Crock, H. V. (1993). Applied anatomy of the spine. *Acta Orthopaedica Scandinavica, 25*(1 suppl), 56–58.

Hales, T. R., & Bernard, B. P. (1996). Epidemiology of work-related musculoskeletal disorders. *Orthopedic Clinics of North America, 27*(4), 679–709.

Hohl, M. (1975). Soft tissue injuries of the neck. *Clinical Orthopedics and Related Research, 109*(4), 42–49.

Hoppenfeld, S. (1976). *Physical examination of the spine and extremities.* East Norwalk, CT: Appleton-Century-Croft.

Jones, E. T., & Mayer, P. (1994). Regional disorders of the musculoskeletal system. In Weinstein, J. N., & Buckwalter, J. A. (eds.). *Turek's orthopaedics* (5th ed.). Philadelphia: J. B. Lippincott.

Lees, F., & Aldren Turner, J. W. (1963). Natural history and prognosis of cervical spondylosis. *British Medical Journal, 2,* 1607–1610.

Lindgren, K. A. (1997, April). Conservative treatment of thoracic outlet syndrome: a 2-year follow-up. *Archives of Physical Medicine and Rehabilitation, 78*(4), 373–378.

MacNab, I. (1975). Cervical spondylosis. *Clinical Orthopaedics and Related Research, l09*(1), 69–77.

MacNab, I., & McCulloch, I. (1990). *Backache* (2nd ed.). Baltimore, MD: Williams & Wilkins.

Micheli, L. J. (1995). Sports injuries in children and adolescents. *Clinics in Sports Medicine, 14*(3), 727–745.

Nurick, S. (1972). The natural history and the results of surgical treatment of the spinal cord disorder associated with cervical spondylosis. *Brain, 95,* 101–108.

Panjabi, M. M., Duranceau, J., Goel, V., et al. (1991). Cervical human vertebrae: quantitative three-dimensional anatomy of the middle and lower regions. *Spine, 16,* 861–869.

Parke, W. W. (1992). Development of the spine. In Rothman, R. H., & Simeone, F. A. (eds.). *The spine* (3rd ed.), pp. 1–17. Philadelphia, PA: W. B. Saunders.

Smith, G. W., & Robinson, R. A. (1958). The treatment of certain cervical spine disorders by anterior removal of the intervertebral disc and interbody fusion. *Journal of Bone and Joint Surgery, 40A,* 607–624.

Spitzer, W. O., Skovron, M. L., Salmi, L. R., et al. (1995). Scientific monograph of the Quebec Task Force on Whiplash—Associated Disorders: redefining "whiplash" and its management [see comments; published erratum appears in *Spine, 20*(21), 2372, 1995]. *Spine, 20*(8 suppl), 1S–73S.

Torg, J. S., Truex, R. C., Jr., & Quedenfeld, T. C. (1979). The national football head and neck registry report and conclusions. *Journal of the American Medical Association, 241,* 1477–1479.

Travell, J. G., & Simons, D. G. (1995). *Myofascial pain dysfunction: the trigger point manual* (vols. I and II). Baltimore, MD: Williams & Wilkins.

Vasseljen, O. Jr., Westgaard, R. H., & Larsen, S. (1995). A case-control study of psychological and psychosocial risk factors for shoulder and neck pain at the workplace. *International Archives of Occupational and Environmental Health, 66*(6), 375–382.

Watkins, R. J., Dillin, W. H., & Maxwell, J. (1990). Cervical spine injuries in football players. In Hochschuler, S. H. (ed.). *The spine in sports.* St. Louis: C. V. Mosby.

White, A. A., & Panjabi, M. M. (1990). *Clinical biomechanics of the spine* (2nd ed.). Philadelphia, PA: J. B. Lippincott.

Wiesel, S. W., & Boden, S. D. (1995). Diagnosis and management of cervical and lumbar disc disease. In Weinstein, J. N., Rydevik, B. L., & Sonntag, V. K. (eds.). *Essentials of the spine.* Philadelphia, PA: Lippincott-Raven.

Wiesel, S. W., Feffer, H. L., & Rothman, R. H. (1985). The development of a cervical spine algorithm and its prospective application to industrial patients. *Journal of Occupational Medicine, 27*(4), 272–276.

Chapter 3

The Spine: Thoracic and Lumbar

Sharon J. Gates, RN, CS, MSN

Back pain in the lumbar region occurs commonly in the general population. Although seen less frequently, musculoskeletal pain in the thoracic region can be persistent and hard to manage. Often, patients with musculoskeletal spine pain present with confusing symptoms, making the diagnosis difficult. A systematic approach to problem solving, moving from the history and physical examination to the appropriate tests and studies, ensures the best possible clinical outcome. Spine problems are often enigmatic; therefore, they require a trusting provider/patient partnership for a successful clinical conclusion.

In early life, the spine is a straight column. As the developing child sits and walks, this straight column develops three separate curves: the lordotic curves of the cervical and lumbar spine and the kyphotic curve of the thoracic or dorsal spine. This curved column comprises 24 individual vertebrae that rest on a bony base called the sacrum (see Fig. 2-1). The motion provided by the cervical and lumbar spine is flexion, extension, lateral bending, and rotation. The primary motion of the thoracic spine is rotation. The facet joint functions to limit motion, restricting movement beyond the normal range. Between each vertebra lies the intervertebral disc. The disc comprises two parts. The outer portion, the annulus, consists of concentric rings of fibrocartilage. The central portion, called the nucleus, consists of a hydrophilic gelatinous substance that distributes applied stresses to the annulus, allowing the disc to function as a shock absorber. The disc also aids the gliding movement between each of the vertebrae. As part of the normal aging process, the nucleus becomes less hydrophilic and is less able to resist compressive and torsional forces. The smooth gliding motion of the vertebrae over the disc is disrupted. The disc space narrows, altering the mechanics of the posterior facet joints. Osteophytes (bone spurs) form on the facet joints and vertebral bodies in response to the altered mechanics. The combination of a narrowed disc space and osteophytes in the intervertebral foramen can cause nerve root impingement (Fig. 3-1).

Disc degeneration can begin as early as adolescence in the cervical spine, is seen in the middle years in the thoracic spine, and usually occurs in the lumbar spine

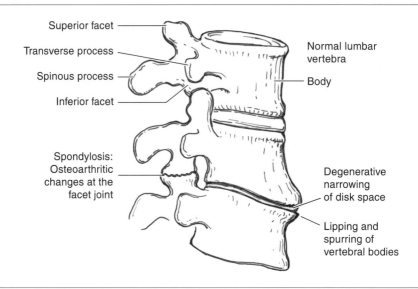

Superior facet

Transverse process

Spinous process

Inferior facet

Normal lumbar vertebra

Body

Spondylosis: Osteoarthritic changes at the facet joint

Degenerative narrowing of disk space

Lipping and spurring of vertebral bodies

FIGURE 3-1. Degenerative spondylosis. (Reilly, B. M. [1991]. *Practical strategies in outpatient medicine.* Philadelphia: W. B. Saunders.)

after age 25. By 50 years of age, most individuals will have radiographic changes demonstrating this phenomenon. These aging changes in the disc can result in pain and limited mobility.

The Thoracic Spine

The thoracic spine, due to its bony attachment to the ribs and sternum, is the part of the spine least vulnerable to trauma or to the problems of aging (Fig. 3-2). Muscle strains from overuse are the frequent problem in this region. Athletic participation in contact sports and gymnastics increases the risk for injuries. Vertebral fractures can occur from direct or indirect blows or as a result of osteopenia (osteoporotic fractures) or metastatic disease (pathologic fractures). Herniated discs are rare but do occur. Differential diagnosis is critical to the evaluation of the thoracic spine. The clinician must distinguish between musculoskeletal problems, cardiac problems, and pulmonary problems.

History

The history for both the child and adult begins with observation. Posture, facial expression, eye contact, and clothing are clues to the differential diagnosis. The younger child will be accompanied by a parent or guardian who may provide many of the answers to the questions. Often parents will report abnormal gait patterns or postural deformities. Identifying a failure to achieve milestones and/or regression from established milestones is crucial. Children who fail to achieve milestones or suffer from regression may have an underlying systemic inflammatory, infectious, or neoplastic disease. Although adults usually present with complaints of pain,

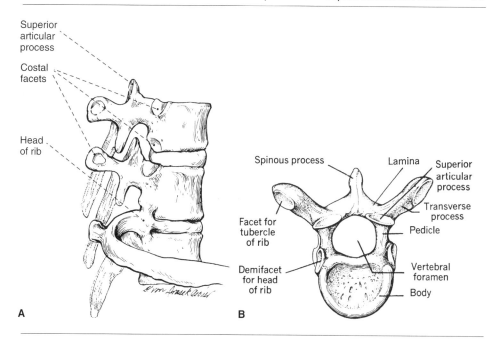

Superior
articular
process

Costal
facets

Head
of rib

Spinous process

Lamina

Superior
articular
process

Transverse
process

Facet for
tubercle
of rib

Pedicle

Demifacet
for head
of rib

Vertebral
foramen

Body

A   B

FIGURE 3-2. (**A**) Thoracic vertebrae and one associated rib. (**B**) Sixth thoracic vertebrae.

children may not complain of pain. Establishing the location of pain is critical. Be careful not to lead the patient or parent, but if necessary offer hints of description. Does the pain feel aching and dull, hot and bursting, or lancinating or knifelike? Is the pain worse with activity? Is the pain relieved by rest? Was there a precipitating event? Musculoskeletal problems in the thoracic region are described as sharp, aching, or dull. The pain can last from seconds to days to months. Musculoskeletal pain may be localized or diffuse, may increase with deep inspiration and coughing, and can be precipitated by direct palpation, movement, and exercise. Costochondritis (Tietze's syndrome) can present with unilateral anterior chest pain that can be confused with cardiac pain. The patient with costochondritis presents with localized tenderness and swelling over the costal cartilages.

Cardiac pain can occur suddenly or gradually. The pain of a myocardial infarction (MI) is described as heaviness or tightness in the chest. The pain is usually substernal and may extend to the arms, neck, jaw, or back. Often, it is associated with weakness, diaphoresis, nausea, or vomiting.

The sudden, severe pain of aortic dissection is described as knifelike. Patients report a sense of impending doom. The pain can occur in the anterior chest, lower chest, interscapular region, back, flank, or abdomen. Symptoms suggestive of dissecting aortic aneurysm are neurologic (ie, syncope), vascular (ie, absent pulses), cardiac (ie, diastolic murmur and blood pressure greater in left arm than right arm). The patient with these symptoms requires *immediate* medical referral.

Pulmonary pain can be distinguished from musculoskeletal pain because pulmonary pain is localized anteriorly and increases with inspiration, and the patient is able to relieve the pain by leaning forward while sitting. Costovertebral joint dysfunction can mimic pleuritic chest pain.

Is there radiating pain or associated sensations of tingling and numbness? Is there any weakness? Is the gait pattern changed? The pain of thoracic disc herniation may present as pain and/or paresthesia radiating across the chest or abdomen. Is there night pain that is relieved by aspirin? Back pain at night relieved by aspirin in a child may be suggestive of an osteoid osteoma or osteoblastoma. Night pain in the adult may be indicative of tumor or infection. Is there a history of trauma or sudden, sharp, unrelenting pain without a precipating event? The mature adult may or may not recall a specific event. Suspect a compression fracture in a patient at risk for osteoporosis.

Physical Examination

The physical examination begins with observation. Observe the patient's stance, gait, and coordination. Have the patient stand with the disrobed back facing the clinician. The female child may be more comfortable in a two-piece bathing suit. Inspect the skin for any abnormal markings (café au lait) or tags that could indicate an underlying bony abnormality. Note the posture. What is the position of the head in relation to the floor? Normally, it should be aligned directly above the shoulders. Look for the normal outward kyphotic, dorsal curve. An increased curve or round shoulders can be symptomatic of Scheuermann's disease, scoliosis, degenerative disc disease, a compression fracture, the kyphosis of old age suggesting osteoporosis, or longstanding poor posture. A lateral curve is suggestive of scoliosis; note the convexity of the curve and the level of the shoulders and iliac crests. Normally, both should be level.

Unequal shoulders are observed in scoliosis; note which shoulder is higher and whether there is a compensatory or second curve. An unequal pelvis can reflect a true leg length discrepancy. With the patient supine and knees straight, place a measuring tape from the anterior iliac crest to the medial malleolus to measure leg lengths. Compare the right leg with the left leg. A significant discrepancy is greater than $\frac{1}{2}$ to $\frac{3}{4}$ inch.

Look for symmetry of the spinal musculature. Palpate bony structures of the spinous processes and the costovertebral joints for areas of tenderness. Palpate the soft tissues in the midline from the level above the iliac crests. Examine the rhomboids, the trapezius, and the latissimus dorsi muscles, and note areas of spasm and tenderness. Observe the motion of flexion as the patient bends forward and then returns to erect posture. Bend the patient forward and look from head to tail to evaluate for a rotational spinal curve; note the convexity of the curve, if present. Examine chest expansion with the patient facing the examiner. Place a tape measure around the largest diameter of the chest. Have the patient inhale and measure the chest. Ask the patient to exhale, and measure the chest. Note the difference between inspiration and expiration (chest excursion). Normally, it is between 6 and 10 cm. Patients with ankylosing spondylitis have a decreased ability to expand their chests.

Perform the neurologic examination with the patient seated on the examining room table. Figure 2-4 depicts the spinal dermatomes.

Ask the patient to twist at the waist; note any restriction of movement. Evaluate for sensation, motor strength and reflex in the medial forearm (T1), medial side of upper arm (T2), medial side of upper arm and axilla to the nipple line (T3), umbilicus (T10), triceps (C7), upper abdominal (T8, T9, T10), and lower abdominal (T11,

T12). Examine for long tract signs: hyperreflexia in the upper or lower extremities, a positive Babinski sign (upgoing toes); the presence of clonus; the absence of the abdominal or cremasteric reflex indicating cord compression or upper motor neuron disease. See Differential Diagnosis of Upper Back Pain.

Guidelines for Diagnostic Tests

Careful consideration must be given to the value of the diagnostic study when treating the patient. Each study should provide more information and guidance in treatment. The results of the study must be integrated with the history and physical examination. Isolated tests have no benefit and add unnecessary costs. The study ordered should be based on the working diagnosis. All patients presenting with upper back pain will need x-ray evaluation when the study will impact the decision-making process. When indicated, obtain standing thoracic spine films (AP/LAT) during the first visit. Plain spine films distinguish abnormal spinal alignment (scoliosis, Scheuermann's disease). Radiographs help to identify fractures, degenerative processes, infection, and destructive lesions. If there is no improvement in symptoms in 6 weeks, obtain a bone scan. The bone scan may reveal insufficiency fractures, tumors, and infection. If a herniated disc is suspected, magnetic resonance imaging (MRI) or computed tomography (CT) will aid in the diagnosis. These tests are ordered to aid in surgical planning. The sensitivity of the MRI will confirm the clinical diagnosis of tumor and infection earlier than the bone scan. It is the diagnostic study of choice. If the patient is claustrophobic, either oral sedative medications or intravenous conscious sedation can be used to allay anxiety. The newer, open MRI machines can accommodate individuals whose body weight and size prohibit standard MRI testing (Herzog, 1995).

Upper Back Pain in Children

There are many causes of back pain in children (see Causes of Back Pain in Children). Youngsters with a complaint of back pain deserve a thorough history and physical examination to determine the cause. Most often, the cause is found not to be serious.

Predisposing Factors

Constitutional and activity-related factors predispose children to upper back pain. During the adolescent or second growth spurt, there is increased susceptibility of the growth tissues to injury. Increasing the risks for pain are sports, especially skiing, football, rugby, wrestling, competitive swimming (butterfly stroke), and weightlifting.

Etiology

Acute muscle strains (pectoralis minor/major), contusions, or hematomas can result from compression of the chest during contact sports. Treatment consists of ice,

Differential Diagnosis of Upper Back Pain

Ligamentous/muscular Disorder

Costochondritis
Strain/sprain syndrome
Overuse syndrome
Poor posture

Neurologic Disorders

Herpes zoster
Intercostal neuralgias
Nerve root compression

Skeletal Disorders

Scheuermann's disease
Metastatic disease
Thoracic disc herniation
Compression fractures
Metabolic bone disease (osteoporosis, Paget's disease)
Ankylosing spondylitis
Scoliosis
Thoracic spondylosis

Spinal Cord

Intramedullary and extramedullary tumors

Cardiac Disorders

Myocardial infarction
Aortic dissection
Angina pectoris
Mitral valve prolapse
Coronary insufficiency

Pulmonary

Acute pulmonary embolism
Pleurisy

GI

Hiatal hernia
Peptic ulcer
Cholecystitis
Pancreatitis

Renal Disease

analgesics (ibuprofen or acetaminophen), and avoidance of the sport until the pain subsides.

A sudden, catching pain ("stitch") in the side of the competing athlete is attributed to an intercostal muscle spasm. The treatment consists of extension and elevation of both arms above the head.

Localized injury can occur to the thoracic joints at the costovertebral, costosternal, or costochondral junctions. Carefully review the history for the mechanism of

> ### Causes of Back Pain in Children
>
> Tumors
>   Spine
>   Spinal cord
> Herniated nucleus pulposus
> Spondylolysis
> Spondylolisthesis
> Scheuermann's kyphosis
> Postural kyphosis
> Vertebral osteomyelitis
> Diskitis
> Overuse syndromes
> Rheumatologic condition

injury. Athletes are injured during "pile on" in football and during wrestling when the chest is compressed by the opponent. Obtain chest and thoracic spine films to differentiate joint injury from fracture.

Rib fractures occur after blunt trauma. The pain is localized, severe, and increases with inspiration. The treatment is analgesics, rest, and avoidance of sports for 4 to 6 weeks to allow for healing. *Note:* Do not strap the chest. This will restrict respiratory excursion and may result in atelectasis and pneumonia.

Prevention of Sports-Related Pain

A preparticipation sports screening examination identifies physical maturation, skill level, muscular endurance, power and flexibility, and nutritional status. Reduce risks by tailoring educational and body-conditioning regimens to individual need. Coaches and trainers must be in agreement to ensure the best outcome for the athlete. The training techniques must continue for 12 months. Sound nutritional education, especially for wrestlers, is vital. Initiate a rehabilitation exercise program for at-risk athletes.

Common Management Problems

Scheuermann's Disease (Juvenile Kyphosis) or Postural Roundback Deformity

Scheuermann's kyphosis, a structural sagittal plane deformity, is seen most often in the thoracic spine but may occur at the thoracolumbar junction. The cause is unknown. The upper thoracic deformity occurs equally in males and females. It is rarely found in children younger than 10 years of age. There is a suggestion of a familial predilection. It is most often diagnosed during the adolescent growth spurt around puberty. It is the noticeable round back deformity that brings the child to the clinician. Pain, if present, is usually of low intensity. The pain will resolve with cessation of growth. On physical examination, patients may complain of pain on palpation above or below the kyphosis. If the patient has an increased lumbar lordosis, lumbar spine pain may be present. There is often associated hamstring and hip flexor muscle tightness. The neurologic examination is usually normal. An evaluation for scoliosis, which is associated with Scheuermann's kyphosis, is a key component of the physical examination (see Chapter 1). Young people who present with a severe kyphotic thoracic curve and a compensatory increase in the lumbar lordotic curve may have Scheuermann's disease and should be carefully screened for organic roundback deformity. Differentiating postural roundback from Scheuermann's kyphosis may be difficult. The diagnosis of Scheuermann's kyphosis is confirmed by a standing lateral radiograph of the cervical, thoracic and lumbar spine, which demonstrates decreased height of the vertebral bodies, Schmorl nodes, vertebral wedging of at least three adjacent vertebrae, and end plate irregularity. Patients with Scheuermann's disease will have a fixed, sharp, angular kyphosis (gibbus) deformity on forward bending. Patients with postural roundback have a gentle rounding of the back (flexible kyphosis), which is often mild when bending forward. The radiographs show no structural abnormality.

Treatment for postural roundback consists of stretching and a strengthening exercise program designed to increase spinal flexibility, correct the hyperlordosis, and stretch the hamstring and pectoralis muscles. A referral to an orthopedic spine specialist for a complete evaluation is necessary to prevent back pain and severe deformity if Scheuermann's disease is suspected. Exercise alone is not sufficient to treat Scheuermann's kyphosis. Patients may need serial bracing to prevent excessive deformity. The natural history of Scheuermann's kyphosis is unclear. Some believe the pain will subside with the end of growth; others believe it will increase throughout life and the deformity may increase as well. Adults who have Scheuermann's disease have pain described as fatigue around T11-12, which is increased with activity (Winter, 1995; Weinstein, 1994).

Scoliosis

See Chapter 1.

The Adult With Upper Back Pain

Predisposing Factors

1. The aging spine, degenerative changes resulting from prolonged abnormal disc stress that are most noticeable in individuals with kyphosis or scoliosis
2. Menopause
3. Repetitive, work-related movements such as lifting, bending, and reaching
4. Certain recreational activities that require repetitive arm movement, such as swimming the freestyle stroke
5. Poor posture

Etiology

1. At menopause bone mass diminishes, bones become weaker and thinner, and the risks for fracture increase.

2. Acute or chronic muscle or ligament strain from improper posture, failure to warm up before heavy labor or recreational activity, and overuse related to employment activity.

Prevention

1. It is important to increase the person's awareness of the risks. A pre-exercise evaluation should be based on age, the level of competition, and the sport and should include a cardiovascular assessment for all people in a known high-risk group and all those over 40 years of age. A specific exercise prescription to increase muscle strength, flexibility, and overall physical fitness is recommended.
2. For the worker, pay attention to the environment to identify risks and eliminate injury through education, proper stretching before work, and initiation of a regular, weekly exercise regimen.
3. For perimenopausal women, a risk assessment for osteoporosis and the elimination of identified risks is encouraged (see Chapter 10).

Common Management Problems

Rhomboid Strain

Rhomboid strain is common in occupations requiring static postures (eg, secretaries and sewing machine operators). The patient complains of a chronic, aching pain in the middle back.

ETIOLOGY
Static posture (the back is partially flexed while the arm is held forward and downward) and a stooped forward position

SYMPTOMS
1. Burning and aching pain over the rhomboid muscles
2. Shooting or stabbing pains
3. Pain that increases with rest and increased muscle stiffness after rest

SIGNS
1. Tenderness over the muscle
2. Trigger points
3. Reproduction of symptoms when the arm is held in the position of maximum rhomboid strain

TREATMENT
1. Increase the patient's understanding of the positions that cause the strain. Offer suggestions to modify incorrect posture. If necessary, alter the height of work surfaces to relieve rhomboid strain.

2. Ice/heat can be used, as necessary, to relieve symptoms.
3. Anti-inflammatories can be used until symptoms subside.

OUTCOME
1. Complete relief will be hindered if the posture continues.
2. Even with postural changes, recovery is often slow.

Adult Scoliosis

The adult with scoliosis may have been aware of the problem since adolescence. If the scoliosis has existed since childhood, determine the age of onset. Ask female patients if onset occurred before or after the start of menses. It is important to define idiopathic scoliosis versus degenerative scoliosis because the treatment may be different. Determine if the spinal deformity has worsened. Assess for changes in the fit of clothing, either at the waist or leg length. Back pain may or may not be related to the preexisting curvature. Determine the severity of the back pain and whether there is pulmonary impairment. Eliminate other causes of back pain, such as disc syndrome, osteoarthritis, degenerative joint disease, and ankylosing spondylitis.

Obtain a *standing,* single-cassette AP, lateral, and side-bending thoracolumbar scoliosis series and compare with previous films. It is essential that the degrees of curvature are determined. Refer the patient to an orthopedic spine specialist for a complete evaluation and the development of an individualized treatment plan. Conservative management is directed toward relieving the pain with non-narcotic analgesics and anti-inflammatories. If these measures are not successful in reducing the discomfort, alternative treatments, which may include physical therapy modalities, facet joint blocks with steroids, and a body cast/plaster jacket, are instituted. If conservative management fails, surgery to fuse the spine may be recommended. This may or may not correct the deformity and reduce pain, but is likely to prevent further progression of the curve.

Thoracic Disc Disease

Due to the limited motion of the thoracic spine, which is protected by the ribs, sternum, and facet joints, disc herniations are rare and occur less frequently than cervical and lumbar herniations. The incidence of thoracic disc herniations peaks in the fourth decade, usually found from T7-T10. Thoracic disc herniations are rarely found in children and young adults. The sophistication of imaging techniques has made it easier to diagnosis thoracic disc disease. The treatment remains difficult.

ETIOLOGY
Remote or recent trauma is the most common cause.

SYMPTOMS
Symptoms may vary.

1. Localized mild to moderate mid back pain
2. Bandlike anterior chest pain
3. Paresthesia or muscle weakness of the lower extremities, possibly inter-mittent
4. Rare complaints of chronic abdominal pain or epigastric pain
5. Interscapular pain
6. Mild sexual and urinary dysfunction

SIGNS
1. Spasm of the paravertebral muscles
2. Decreased response to pin prick along a sensory dermatome
3. Motor weakness including myelopathy
4. Interscapular tenderness
5. Hyperreflexia possibly present if there is cord compression
6. Absent abdominal reflexes

TREATMENT
1. Obtain standing AP and LAT thoracic spine films.
2. Educate the patient regarding treatment and probable outcome, which will depend on the severity of symptoms and objective clinical and diagnostic findings.
3. Apply ice or heat to the affected area.
4. Prescribe physical therapy for instruction in gentle stretching and progressing to hyperextension strengthening exercises, postural training, and body mechanics education for work and leisure.
5. Prescribe anti-inflammatory medications or non-narcotic analgesics.
6. Recommend therapeutic massage.

REFERRAL (ORTHOPEDIST OR NEUROSURGEON)
1. Immediate for myelopathy or cord compression (long tract signs, bowel/bladder alteration)
2. Signs of extremity weakness
3. Intractable pain
4. If no improvement in 4 to 6 weeks with conservative management

OUTCOME
Nonoperative treatment usually results in resolution of symptoms. Rarely, surgery will be needed.

Thoracic Spine Vertebral Hemangiomas

These benign spinal abnormalities are usually found incidentally on x-ray and are more common in females than males. They occur most often in the lower thoracic spine in asymptomatic people (Fig. 3-3). They can be the cause of localized pain and muscle spasm. Rarely, they are associated with nerve root compression from kyphosis due to vertebral collapse. Treatment is usually not required. If symptoms are related to this phenomenon, treatment may consist of low-dose radiation or embolization.

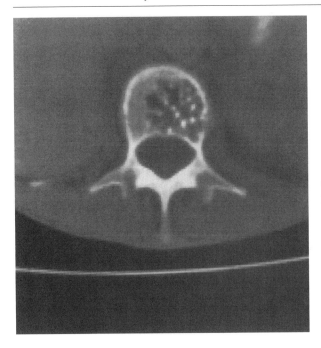

FIGURE 3-3. Computed tomogram of a vertebral hemangioma in the cross section; bony trabeculae produce a polkadot appearance. On plain film hemangiomas of the vertebral body have characteristic vertical striations that have the appearance of corduroy.

The Mature Adult With Upper Back Pain

Predisposing Factors

1. Chronic illness
2. Sedentary lifestyle leading to decreased muscle flexibility and strength
3. Facet joint dysfunction resulting from normal aging
4. Post menopause

Etiology

See The Adult With Upper Back Pain.

Back pain may be caused by spinal stresses that began in adolescence and continue into adulthood. If not addressed at the time of menopause, bone mass loss continues after menopause and the risk for osteoporotic fractures increases.

Prevention

Educate the at-risk group about the importance of remaining physically active. Instruction focuses on decreasing spinal stresses and developing an exercise program for the ambulatory as well as the chair-bound mature adult. A weight-bearing exercise such as walking helps to prevent bone loss and to decrease the risk for fracture. A pre-exercise examination will identify muscle strength and flexibility, chronic illness, and individual goals. The exercise prescription is tailored to individual needs and includes a progressive walking or swimming program and light weight lifting for the ambulatory person, and light weight lifting, stretching, and flexibility for the chair-bound person.

Common Management Problems

Thoracic Spondylosis

Secondary degenerative changes in the aging thoracic spine cause pain and stiffness that is worse upon arising in the morning. This pain may or may not be related to a strain from a sudden and unexpected movement. Patients have limitation of thoracic rotation associated with an increased dorsal curve.

This problem is self-limiting and rarely causes disability. The treatment goals are to decrease pain and increase function. These goals are reached by instructing the patient in the disease process, using aspirin or a nonsteroidal anti-inflammatory drug (NSAID) on a regular basis each day until the symptoms subside, and instituting a regular exercise regimen (swimming is preferred). Spinal manipulation may be beneficial.

Thoracic (Osteoporotic) Compression Fractures

ETIOLOGY. After menopause, whether naturally or by oophorectomy, bone loss in women accelerates and may range from 0.5% to 2% per year. This negative balance occurs because bone formation remains relatively constant but resorption increases (see Chapter 10).

SYMPTOMS
1. Localized thoracic pain, which may be either chronic or acute, that can occur without a direct trauma to the back (simply sitting in a chair may cause a compression fracture in the at-risk older adult)
2. Increase in the thoracic kyphosis, which may or may not be painful
3. Obvious alteration in posture
4. Rest pain
5. Chronic pain in the lumbar region even if fracture occurred from T1-T11

SIGNS
1. Point tenderness on palpation or percussion over the identified vertebral body
2. Obvious pain and difficulty moving from sitting to standing
3. Possible increase in thoracic kyphosis
4. Possible mild to moderate scoliosis

TREATMENT
Treatment consists of referral to an orthopedist.

1. Obtain a standing AP and LAT thoracic spine film. The diagnosis is made on the radiographic evidence of fracture. Most often, vertebral wedging will be seen.
2. Encourage the patient to rest for a couple of days; prolonged bedrest is contraindicated.

3. Prescribe pharmacologic interventions with calcium and vitamin D supplementation, estrogen replacement if not contraindicated, and the biphosphonates such as Fosamax, and/or calcitonin-salmon such as Calcimar (injection) or Miacalcin (nasal spray).
4. Spinal orthoses of lightweight material may help to reduce painful symptoms. If possible, avoid heavy and bulky braces, which are poorly tolerated.
5. Medications such as NSAIDs and, rarely, mild narcotic analgesics may help to reduce symptoms of acute fracture.
6. Prescribe physical therapy with hot/cold packs for the more acute fracture; for chronic pain and prevention of future fractures, prescribe back-strengthening exercises (avoid flexion exercises; they can increase vertebral compressive forces), isometric conditioning of abdominal muscles, and gentle toning exercises.
7. Encourage lifestyle changes (eg, cessation of smoking; see Chapter 10).

OUTCOME
Pain usually subsides over 2 to 6 weeks; however, chronic pain may result.

The Lumbar Spine

The lumbar spine is the most vulnerable to pain and injury. Despite many attempts to determine scientifically the cause of lower back pain, little is known about the exact pathophysiologic mechanisms involved. Lower back pain is ubiquitous. Socioeconomic problems resulting from chronic low back pain disability are very costly. Current treatment is based commonly on experience (what works) rather than science, because few good scientific studies exist. Treatment and assessment guidelines have been established for the management of acute lower back pain. The emphasis is to identify those people with serious conditions and refer them to the appropriate clinician. The majority should be treated with a focus on decreasing pain and early return to normal activities, while avoiding costly, unnecessary diagnostic studies and treatments (Bigos, 1994; Waddell et al, 1996).

The lumbar spine has three functional components: the vertebral bodies, the intervertebral disc, and the zygapophysial (facet) joints. This functional unit provides bony support, flexibility, and protection for the neural structures. The lumbar vertebrae are large and heavy to accommodate the attachment of the lower limb muscles (Fig. 3-4).

History

Meticulous history taking will lead to accurate diagnosis. Have the patient clearly describe the nature of the pain, and determine whether associated pain is present. Use a pain drawing. If leg pain is associated with back pain, determine the nature of the leg pain, the location, and the intensity and compare it to the back pain. Determine which pain is worse. If paresthesias are associated, determine the location, the nature, and the timing. Ask about specific activities that aggravate the pain. Inquire about bowel or bladder problems. Ask if the pain increases or decreases

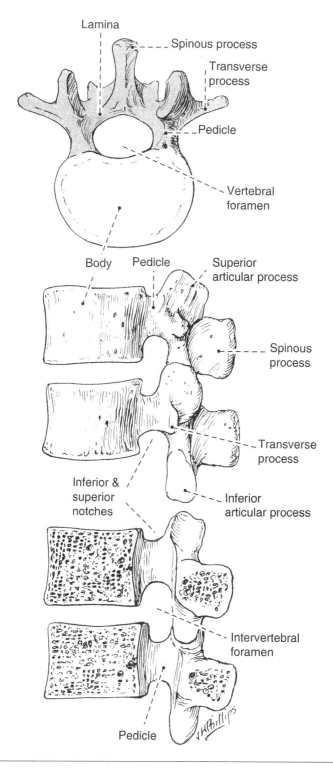

FIGURE 3-4. Parts of a typical vertebra as seen from *above,* from a *lateral view* and on a *sagittal section.* In the *uppermost* figure, the vertebral arch is shaded.

upon lying down. Mechanical back pain is aching in nature, worse toward the end of the day, localized to the lower back or buttocks, does not radiate below the knee, and is better with rest. Discogenic pain is often burning and aching in nature, may be constant, radiates below the knee, may be coupled with numbness and/or pins-and-needles sensation of the leg, and improves with rest. Discogenic pain is aggravated by sitting, sneezing, coughing, climbing stairs, walking, and lifting. The ominous pain of a tumor, which may or may not radiate, is boring in nature, worse at night, unrelieved by bedrest, and relieved by sitting. Pain of infection is characterized by severe muscle spasms of the back. Back pain of lymphoma may be vague, not well localized, and accompanied by intermittent paresthesias and/or weakness of the lower extremities. Inquire about recent weight loss, chills, fever, night sweats, and diarrhea. Intense, unremitting pain across the saddle area accompanied by pins-and-needles sensation, weakness of the lower extremities, and incontinence or constipation of either bowel or bladder is an emergency and requires immediate referral. The diagnosis of cauda equina syndrome is made when a significant neurologic deficit is present on physical examination. Careful symptom analysis will direct the physical examination (Table 3-1).

Physical Examination

Try to develop a standard pattern of examination and evaluation. Subtle clues to diagnosis can be found by examining the patient in different positions. Examine the mechanics of gait and posture when the patient enters the examining room and when he or she stands, walks, and sits. For a thorough examination of the lumbar spine, it is essential that the patient completely disrobe. Observe the mechanics of the lumbar spine as the patient undresses. The patient with significant back trouble avoids painful bending and twisting motions. While the patient is standing, inspect

TABLE 3-1
Physical Examination of the Lumbar Spine

Patient Standing	Patient Sitting	Patient Lying
1. Inspection of skin and spinal curves	1. Evaluate for motor strength	1. Evaluate for sensory function
2. Palpation of soft tissues and bones	2. Evaluate for DTR reflexes, clonus, Babinski	Pin prick
3. Evaluate for ROM	3. Evaluate for vibratory sense	Soft touch
Flexion	4. Evaluate for tension signs	2. Evaluate for tension signs
Extension	Valsalva	Straight leg raising
Lateral bend	Sitting root	Passive dorsiflexion
Rotation		Bowstring
4. Evaluate for motor strength		Femoral nerve stretch
Heel walking		3. Evaluate for muscle atrophy
Toe walking		4. Leg lengths
Hopping on one leg		5. Associated areas
5. Chest expansion (excursion)		Abdominal examination
		Hip and pelvic
		Vascular
		Rectal

the skin for any abnormal markings or tags, such as hairy patches, lipomas, or neurofibromas. Look for symmetry in the spinal musculature. Examine for the normal lumbar lordosis, and look for loss of lumbar lordosis that may indicate paravertebral muscle spasm (Fig. 3-5). An exaggerated lumbar lordosis is characteristic of weak anterior abdominal wall musculature or compression fractures. Palpate bony structures as the patient stands. Palpate the spinous processes for tenderness. Examine for sacral and coccygeal tenderness. Palpate the soft tissues in the midline and over the iliac crests. In the midline, the supraspinous and interspinous ligaments are palpated for tenderness (Fig. 3-6). Only the superficial paraspinal musculature is palpable when examining for spasm. The iliac crest is palpated for tenderness. The sciatic nerve is the largest nerve in the body and runs down the posterior aspect of the thigh. It exits the pelvis through the greater sciatic foramen under the piriformis muscle. The sciatic nerve can be located midway between the greater trochanter and ischial tuberosity; it is palpated with the hip flexed (see Fig. 3-6). Ask the patient to stand and to place one foot on a stool to facilitate palpation.

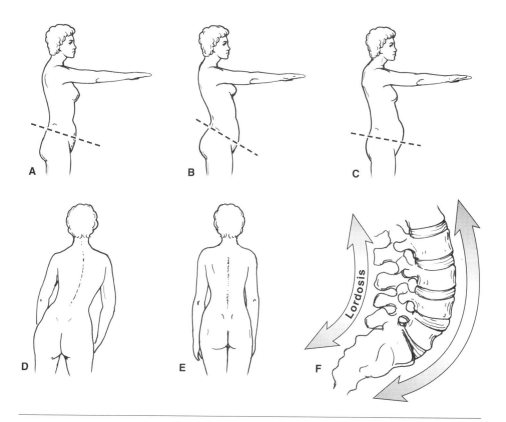

FIGURE 3-5. (**A**) Normal posture with normal lumbar lordosis. (**B**) Exaggerated lumbar lordosis due to pelvic tilting. (**C**) "Paunchy" posture. (**D**) Spastic scoliosis due to muscle spasm. (**E**) Normal posture without scoliosis. (**F**) The normal orientation of the lumbar spine is that of mild lordosis. Exaggerated lordosis may predispose the patient to mechanical back pain. (Reilly, B. M. [1991]. *Practical strategies in outpatient medicine.* Philadelphia: W. B. Saunders.)

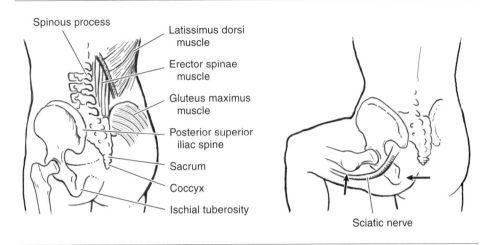

Spinous process
Latissimus dorsi muscle
Erector spinae muscle
Gluteus maximus muscle
Posterior superior iliac spine
Sacrum
Coccyx
Ischial tuberosity
Sciatic nerve

FIGURE 3-6. (**Left**) Bony and muscular landmarks. (**Right**) The *small arrows* point to the two landmarks, the *ischial tuberosity* and the *trochanter,* which help you to identify the location of the sciatic nerve. With the patient resting his foot on a stool, place your thumb on the trochanter and your index finger on the ischial tuberosity. With firm pressure, palpate the sciatic groove between these landmarks.

With the patient's back to you, observe flexion, extension, lateral bending, and rotation (Fig. 3-7). To test flexion, the patient should bend forward as if to touch the toes with the knees straight. If the patient cannot touch the floor, measure the distance from the fingertips to the floor with a tape. This is an accurate reproduction of the limitations of flexion. To assist in testing extension, place your hands on either side of the patient's hips. Support and stabilize the pelvis to allow maximal extension. Spondylolisthesis, spondylolysis, and spinal stenosis cause increased back pain with extension. Using the same technique, stabilize the pelvis during lateral bending. Compare right lateral bending to left lateral bending. Record any limitations by noting restriction of motion, and measure the distance of the fingers in relation to the knee on the same side. Lateral bend is to the knee and is equal on both sides. Test rotation by stabilizing the pelvis and asking the patient to twist around until facing you. Normal rotation is 35 degrees.

The Neurologic Examination

The neurologic examination of the lower extremities as it relates to the lumbar spine consists of examinations of reflexes, motor strength, sensation (light touch or pin prick), vibratory sense, and evidence of tension signs. For each neurologic level, there are specific localizing tests for motor, reflex and sensation. Motor testing is recorded using a five-point scale (see Table 2-1).

For the upper lumbar region—L1, L2, L3—there are no specific reflexes. The sensory examination is an essential component for evaluating for nerve root compression at these levels. While the patient is seated on the edge of the examination table with the legs over the side, test the strength of the iliopsoas (T12, L1, L2, L3) by having the patient flex the knee against resistance. Test quadriceps (L2, L3,

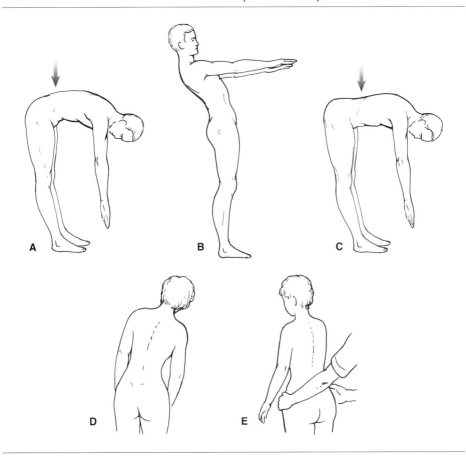

FIGURE 3-7.   Back range of motion. (**A**) Flexion—note the normal reversal of lumbar lordosis during flexion (*arrow*). (**B**) Extension. (**C**) Persistent lordosis during back flexion due to muscle spasm (*arrow*). (**D**) Lateral flexion. (**E**) Lateral torsion (rotation). (Reilly, B. M. [1991]. *Practical strategies in outpatient medicine.* Philadelphia: W. B. Saunders.)

L4) strength by having the patient squat and return to the upright position. Test the strength of the hip adductors (L2, L3, L4). Stabilize the pelvis by placing one hand on the iliac crest and the greater tubercle and have the patient turn on the side and abduct the leg as you offer resistance against the lateral thigh by attempting to force the leg into adduction. All these muscle groups contain multiple in-nervations, so identifying loss of specific muscle strength may be difficult.

At the L4, L5, and S1 levels, the examination is more specific. At the L4 level, the tibialis anterior is examined for motor function (have the patient walk on his or her heels with the feet inverted). The knee jerk is examined for reflex, and the medial side of the leg is examined for sensation. At the L5 level, the extensor hallucis longus is examined for motor function (have the patient walk on his or her heels). At this level, there is no reflex. The dorsal aspect of the foot is tested for sensation. At the S1 level, peroneus, longus, and brevis are examined for motor function (have the patient walk on the medial border of his or her feet). The ankle jerk is examined for reflex; the lateral aspect and the plantar surface of the foot are tested for sensation (Fig. 3-8). The patient with hyperreflexia should be examined

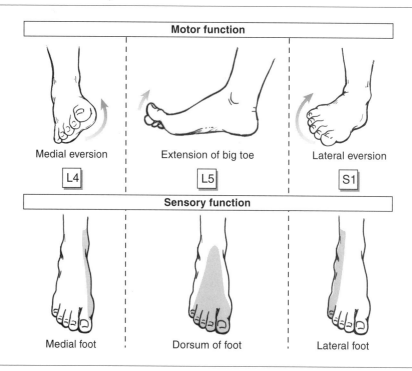

FIGURE 3-8. The neuromuscular control and function of the lower extremity. Disc L3−L4, nerve root L4: motor−anterior tibialis, medial eversion of the foot; sensory−medial leg and foot; reflex−patellar. Disc L4−L5, nerve root L5: motor−extensor hallucis longus, extend big toe; sensory−lateral leg and dorsum of foot; reflex−none. Disc L5−S1, nerve root S1: motor−peroneus longus and brevis, lateral eversion of foot: sensory−lateral foot; reflex−Achilles.

for upper motor neuron pathology. In the normal person, excessive reaction to deep tendon reflex testing is prevented by the higher cerebral centers. With loss of this inhibition, there is an exaggerated deep tendon reflex. Confirmatory tests for upper motor neuron lesions include an absence of the superficial abdominal reflex, the superficial cremasteric reflex, and the superficial anal reflex. The Babinski is the traditional test for upper motor neuron lesions. Dorsiflexion of the great toe with fanning of the other toes upon stroking the outer sole of the foot indicates upper motor neuron disease.

The vibratory threshold is assessed by using a 128-Hz tuning fork, although a 256-Hz tuning fork is more sensitive. Vibratory sensation is lost in peripheral neuropathy and spinal stenosis. The elderly may have diminished vibration sense secondary to spinal stenosis. Tap the tuning fork on the heel of your hand and place the vibrating fork on the patient's great toe or the medial or lateral malleoli of the ankle. Ask the patient what he feels. If he feels the vibration, ask him to let you know when it stops. An important criterion is the ability to feel the fork as vibration slows. If the vibration sense is impaired, move proximally to the tibia or anterior iliac spine. Record as vibration sense absent at the appropriate level.

Examination for Tension Signs

A number of tests are designed to stretch the spinal cord and sciatic nerve to test for nerve root compression. The straight leg test is performed with the patient supine while the leg is lifted upward by the foot and supported by the heel. The knee should be kept straight. The angle between the table and the extended leg at which pain is produced is the measure of positive straight leg raising. The pain of a positive test should extend below the knee. Perform on both the affected and unaffected leg. Test the unaffected leg first. Radicular pain in the affected leg during straight leg raising of the unaffected leg is a positive cross leg test (Fig. 3-9). The test should become negative when the knee is flexed and then become positive again when the knee is extended. Raising the leg to the area of pain, then backing off and dorsiflexing the foot should also produce pain. A variation of this test is

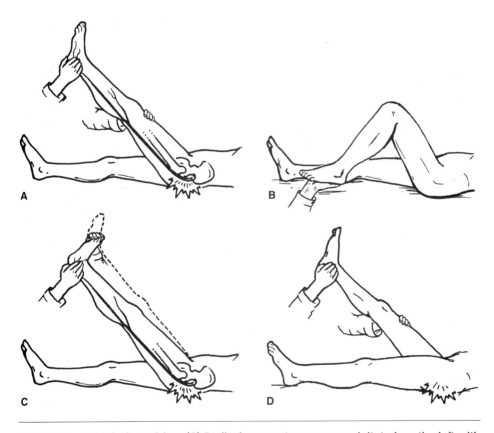

FIGURE 3-9. Straight leg raising. (**A**) Radicular symptoms are precipitated on the left with the straight leg raised 45 degrees. The affected leg is raised with the knee extended, producing pain in a positive test. (**B**) The second confirmatory maneuver, lifting the affected leg with the knee flexed will not cause pain. (**C**) Dorsiflexion of the foot sometimes exaggerates straight leg raising responses. (**D**) Crossed straight leg raising pain on the left side is precipitated by straight leg raising on the right side. (Reilly, B. M. [1991]. *Practical strategies in outpatient medicine.* Philadelphia: W. B. Saunders.)

the sitting root test. With the patient seated, the knee is extended while the patient grips the side of the examination table. The test is positive if the patient leans backward and complains of radicular pain. Evaluation of the fourth lumbar nerve root is performed with the femoral nerve stretch test. With the patient prone, the affected leg is elevated so the hip is extended and the knee is slightly flexed. The test is positive if the patient complains of radiating anterior thigh pain. Remember that lesions above and below can refer pain; therefore, diseases of the hip, rectum, and sacroiliac joints may refer pain to the lumbar region.

Associated Tests

Assess the abdomen for bruits, which may indicate an aortic aneurysm; aortic aneurysms can present as low back pain. Evaluate for costovertebral angle (CVA) tenderness to rule out kidney disease. Rectal and pelvic examinations should be done when there is no mechanical stress associated with the pain or when the patient is elderly. Prostatic or rectal cancer may present as low back pain.

Differential Diagnosis—Low Back Pain

Congenital

Transitional vertebrae
Scoliosis

Traumatic

Lumbar strain/sprain
Fracture
Spondylolisthesis

Neoplastic

Primary bone tumors
Metastatic malignancies
Spinal cord tumors

Metabolic

Osteoporosis
Hyperparathyroidism

Toxic

Chronic radium poisoning

Infectious

Disc-space infection
Osteomyelitis
Spinal epidural/subdural
  abscess

Inflammatory

Ankylosing spondylitis
Psoriatic arthritis
Rheumatoid arthritis

Degenerative

Osteoarthritis
Facet arthropathy
Disc degeneration/protrusion
Spinal stenosis

Vascular

Abdominal aortic aneurysm/
  dissection

Mechanical

Postural
Obesity
Deconditioning
Pregnancy

Visceral

Pancreatitis
Cholecystitis
Pyelonephritis
Ulcer disease
Pelvic disease (ovarian)

Psychogenic

Compensation neurosis
Hysteria

Guidelines for Diagnostic Tests

Several tests will assist in differentiating the several causes of lower back pain (see Differential Diagnosis—Low Back Pain).

Lumbar/sacral spine x-ray (five views—standing AP, LAT, spot [coned down] lumbar sacral and both obliques): Research indicates that spine films provide little information regarding muscle strains and disc herniations. These should be ordered when structural abnormalities (metastatic disease, fracture, scoliosis, spondylolysis, or spondylolisthesis) are of concern. Routine adult films should be limited to standing AP and lateral to avoid unnecessary radiation exposure.

Bone scan: Obtain a full or limited bone scan if there is a suspicion of fracture, Paget's disease, tumor, infection, or with persistent symptoms after 4 to 6 weeks of conservative management.

Laboratory tests: Any time an underlying medical problem is suspected (tumor, infection, or multiple myeloma). Suggested screens: CBC, UA, SMA 12, PSA, SPEP, ESR.

Electromyography (EMG): Distinguishes peripheral nerve deficits (neuropathy) from spinal nerve root compromise (radiculopathy). Changes can be seen 10 days after episode of leg pain. Do not order an EMG before 10 days have elapsed.

CT scan: Obtain after 4 to 6 weeks with persistent symptoms to evaluate the spinal canal and associated structures for the presence of a herniated nucleus pulposus, tumor, or spinal stenosis. Use if the patient is claustrophobic or has a contraindication to an MRI study.

MRI: The gold standard and the test of choice. Obtain after the patient complains of leg and back pain for 4 to 6 weeks or at any time the patient's condition warrants (before surgery and for progressive neurologic deficit). MRI evaluates the spinal canal and associated structures. The sagittal views of this noninvasive study aid in confirming the diagnosis of a disc herniation (Fig. 3-10).

Myelogram: Rarely used since the advent of MRI except for surgical planning, often in conjunction with a CT scan.

Lower Back Pain in Children

Predisposing Factors

1. The adolescent or second growth spurt
2. Increased susceptibility of the growth tissues to injury
3. Participation in contact sports (football, rugby, soccer, basketball, hockey, and lacrosse) and sports that require weight training to maximal effort (bodybuilding, football, and competitive weight lifting

Etiology

1. Acute or chronic muscle, tendon or ligamentous strain, which results from hyperlordotic postures during standing, gymnastics, and football. Occurring during the second growth spurt, it may be accompanied by weak-

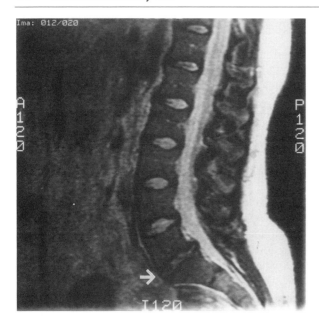

FIGURE 3-10. MRI of lumbar spine illustrating L5-S1 disc protrusion.

ened abdominal muscles, tight hamstrings, and mild roundback posture. Treatment consists of flexibility exercises for the hamstrings and strengthening exercises for the abdominal muscles.

2. A discrete, localized injury to the vertebral end plates, occurring at the thoracolumbar junction in young athletes. These athletes usually have tight lumbar dorsal fascia and are involved in repetitive flexion and extension activities, such as rowing, gymnastics, and diving.

3. Direct blows to the back either during sports or due to a fall can cause pain and spasm (Micheli & Wood, 1995).

Prevention

In this age group, it is important to prevent back pain before it occurs. This can be achieved by the following measures:

1. Preseason screening of the lumbar spine should include postural observation and flexibility and abdominal strength testing.

2. An appropriate training program must be followed for 12 months and should include stretching, flexibility and strengthening exercises, isometrics, and swimming.

3. Proper protective gear must be used (eg, gymnastics: proper thickness and placement of mats, elimination of the board during initial vaulting training, and avoidance of the trampoline [the trampoline should not be used in regular gym classes]; football: proper equipment and careful instruction in techniques).

Common Management Problems

Discogenic Low Back Pain

Herniated discs occur infrequently in children. Seen more often in males and associated with lumbar vertebral congenital abnormalities, they are often associated with trauma.

Discogenic back pain differs in presentation from the adult. *Adolescents can have minimal back pain without radiculopathy.* They may have a thoracolumbar scoliosis, tightness of the lumbar dorsal fascia, and tight hamstrings as the only significant findings on physical examination. Asymmetric hamstring tightness may be the only finding on physical examination, indicating a herniated nucleus pulposus. The correct diagnosis can be determined by CT scan and MRI. The treatment is the same as for the adult (see Discogenic Low Back Pain).

Spondylolysis/Spondylolisthesis

Spondylolysis is an acquired or stress fracture of the pars interarticularis. At risk are female gymnasts as well as football linemen who must assume a hyperlordotic posture before the ball is snapped. Conservative management consists of rest, no sports until the pain subsides, and anti-inflammatories. For very severe pain, a low-profile brace may be used during acute episodes. Spondylolisthesis, a slippage of one vertebra on another, is classified in grades I through IV according to the degree of the slippage. Standing plain radiographs with flexion and extension views may be helpful in aiding diagnosis, but often a single photon emission computerized tomography (SPECT) bone scan or an MRI is needed to differentiate an acute pars interarticularis stress fracture from a developmental spondylolisthesis. Treatment is aimed at relieving the symptoms and preventing further slipping and consists of rest, stretching of the hamstrings, abdominal strengthening exercises, and bracing. Patients may return to sports as long as they are asymptomatic, flexible, and do not progress (slip). A 6-month follow-up that includes standing thoracolumbar x-rays is used for evaluation. If the spondylolisthesis is grade II or greater, participation in skiing, contact sports, and gymnastics is contraindicated. Grades I and II can usually be managed by conditioning exercises, anti-inflammatories, observation, or bracing depending on the amount of pain. If the pain does not respond or the slippage progresses, surgical stabilization with an in situ fusion may be necessary. Grades III and IV will require surgical stabilization with an in situ fusion or, in some cases, with fusion and instrumentation. A low-profile brace is used for 6 months after any surgical intervention (Weinstein, 1994).

The Adult With Low Back Pain

Predisposing Factors

1. Age 30 to 50
2. Repetitive movements such as lifting, pulling, bending, and twisting
3. Job-related activities that involve prolonged sitting (eg, the constant vibration of long-distance driving)

4. Recreational activities (jogging, skiing)
5. Personal behaviors (sedentary lifestyle, cigarette smoking, emotional stress, poor posture, and obesity; Frymoyer, 1986)

Etiology (Unknown)

1. Acute or chronic muscle, tendon, or ligamentous strain resulting from work-related postures or recreational activities
2. Lumbar disc herniation resulting from excessive loading of the spine or from a sudden unexpected force or blow to the spine
3. Degenerative changes that begin after the age of 25
4. Metabolic diseases that weaken the bone and result in mechanical failure
5. Facet joint dysfunction

Prevention

Prevention focuses on education and screening. Educational programs increase the awareness of the problem, provide the necessary facts to identify which people are at greatest risk, and teach the skills that minimize the risks for lower back pain. These programs have the greatest success when participants are actively involved in protective back care. On-site instruction in proper body mechanics (individualized and job specific) followed by employee demonstration with immediate critique and reinforcement aids retention and adaptation of the newly learned skills. Screening programs in the work environment are cost-effective. They identify people with a history of previous injury (past injury increases the risks for future injury) and those personal behaviors that are associated with back pain. Classes in stress management, weight control, and modification of the work and home environment to alleviate spinal stressors provide the opportunity for employees to change at-risk behavior.

Common Management Problems

Acute Mechanical Low Back Pain (Strain/Sprain)

Refer to Table 3-2 for the etiology, symptoms, and signs of low back pain.

TREATMENT (ACUTE)
1. Most patients do well with avoidance of activities that increase the pain. Bedrest for acute low back pain is usually not necessary. If bedrest is recommended, 1 to 3 days is adequate. Avoid prolonged bedrest because it increases muscle stiffness, lengthens healing time, promotes the sick role, and increases dependence.
   Bed position (on a firm mattress):
   a. On the back with knees flexed on a pillow
   b. On the side with a pillow between the knees
   c. On the stomach with a small pillow placed under the lower abdomen to prevent hyperextension of the back (avoid prone lying)
2. For the first 72 hours, avoid heat (initially, heat increases the inflammatory response), then apply ice as a pack or massage to the painful area for 15 to 20 minutes several times each day. For the ice massage, position the

TABLE 3-2

Overview: Low Back Pain

Mechanical Back Pain Age 30 to 55	Discogenic Back Pain Age 30 to 55	Spinal Stenosis Above Age 50
Etiology		
Improper posture Trauma Lifting Bending Twisting Prolonged standing	Repeated minor stresses Discrete injury (may sense a snapping in the back) Trauma after bending Degeneration of the disc as part of aging	Constriction and bony compression of nerve roots as osteophytes form on disc margins or facet joints.
Symptoms		
Aching pain in the lower back that may or may not radiate Radiation into the thigh but never below the knee Restriction of spinal motion Sudden onset Increased pain with walking, bending, and sitting Decreased pain with rest	Similar to those reported with low back pain Leg pain that radiates below the knee, dull or burning in nature with pins-and-needles quality Altered sensation in the lower extremities described as numbness or tingling Leg pain may be worse with coughing, sneezing, or bearing down during defecation Weakness or giving way sensation of the knee	Backache radiating leg pain below the knee Leg pain without back pain Bilateral leg pain "claudicant" in nature Increased with walking and associated with pins-and-needles sensation and a sense of weakness in the calf and foot Claudicant pain relieved with lying down
Signs		
Spasm and tenderness of paravertebral muscles Restricted spinal movement Local tenderness over the spinous process may be present Abnormal gait with hips flexed Sciatic list (listing away from the pain) may be present Difficulty with sitting (sits on the edge of the chair with legs extended)	Limitation of spinal movement may be present Increased pain during spinal flexion Antalgic gait Sciatic list Hip and knee flexed while standing Absent or diminished reflexes Motor weakness Decreased sensation along a dermatome Positive straight leg raising test Positive tension signs may be present	Full range of motion may be present Increased pain during spinal extension May have normal examination
Treatment		
Bedrest 2–5 days Ice massage Anti-inflammatories Education Exercise/fitness	Bedrest 2–5 days (acute) Ice massage Anti-inflammatories Education Exercise/fitness	Bedrest rarely employed Ice/heat Anti-inflammatories Education Exercise/fitness

patient prone, supporting the abdomen with a small pillow (see Treatment, p. 65, and adapt application to painful lower back area).

3. After 72 hours, heat may be applied using a moist heating pad for 20 minutes in each hour; avoid lying on the pad.
4. Avoid sitting during the acute period.
5. Gentle stretching exercises several times a day (after the acute pain subsides) promote flexibility and decrease stiffness (see Appendix E).
6. Prescribe medications (see Appendix A).
    a. Non-narcotic analgesics (Ultram)
    b. NSAIDs
    c. Muscle relaxants (Flexeril 10 mg at hs) or low-dose tricyclic antidepressants (Elavil 10 mg at hs). Muscle spasm is a result of the inflammatory process; once the inflammation has subsided, the spasms stop (most muscle relaxants are centrally acting and tend to produce unpleasant side effects).
7. Abdominal supports are particularly helpful for short-term use for those who do heavy lifting or have weakened abdominal muscles, or for those who need reinforcement of good body mechanics. Supports provide a sense of security and diminish pain through a placebo effect.
8. Provide education (instruction/evaluation):
    a. Teach form and function of the spine using a three-dimensional model (this will make the back more understandable to the patient).
    b. Teach the rationale for treatments. The well-informed patient experiences less anxiety, is able to formulate realistic goals, and complies more often with the recommended regimen.
    c. Teach the expected outcome. Discussing the short-term limitations of the disability and the undulating nature of the disease reduces the fear that the treatment will fail. Use positive reinforcement, reassurance, and active listening.
    d. Teach the side effects of medications, appropriate dosages, and potential adverse reactions.
    e. Counsel on injury prevention, the use of proper body mechanics, and the importance of general fitness programs.

GOALS OF THE EDUCATIONAL PROGRAM
1. Foster active participation in addressing own health problem.
2. Promote independence.
3. Reduce chances of long-term disability.
4. Preserve self-esteem.
5. Promote early mobility.
6. Promote return to work/home responsibilities in a shortened period of time.

RETRAINING/REHABILITATION
1. Graduated mobility program (3 to 10 days after episode)
    a. Stretching/flexibility exercises
    b. Strengthening exercises (see Appendix E)
2. Establishment of aerobic exercises routine five times per week for 40 minutes (2 to 6 weeks after episode)

a. Swimming
b. Walking
c. Bicycling
3. Back School (classroom education for patients with back pain)

REFERRAL TO ORTHOPEDIST OR NEUROSURGEON
1. Failure to respond to therapy (after 6 weeks)
2. Lack of specific diagnosis
3. Associated gastrointestinal (GI) or genitourinary (GU) symptoms
4. Neurologic symptoms
5. Litigation pending
6. Suspected disc herniation
7. Fever
8. Suspicion of a tumor

OUTCOME (BASED ON THE NATURAL HISTORY OF LOW BACK PAIN)
1. Resolution should occur within 3 to 21 days (with or without treatment based on the natural evolution of the disease process).
2. The patient may return to work as soon as the acute phase subsides (2 days); return to work with light-duty restriction is helpful. Light-duty restriction may consist of an alteration in job tasks to eliminate spinal stress and/or restricted hours.
3. The patient may take 4 to 6 weeks for return to full work/home responsibilities.
4. The patient may have intermittent aches during the 2- to 6-week period after the initial bout. These aches can be relieved by brief rest periods (after work) and NSAIDs.
5. Occasionally, patients fail to respond to therapy and the pain persists. They are reluctant to resume activities of daily living or to return to work. If there is no response to treatment after 3 to 6 months, consider a chronic pain syndrome. The etiology is complex and may be related to compensation claims, pending litigation (or other secondary gains), depression, lack of compliance with recommended regimen, or undetected disease process. All require appropriate intervention and investigation. Refer the patient to a primary care provider for complete medical workup if one has not already been done (see section entitled Chronic Low Back Pain).

Discogenic Low Back Pain

This is low back pain that is associated with unilateral leg pain radiating below the knee. The leg pain is significantly more bothersome than the back pain. Occasionally, no back pain is reported. Ten percent of all backaches are related to some form of nerve root irritation; of those 10%, only 2% to 3% require surgical intervention.

PATHOLOGY
Nuclear material either bulges, protrudes, or extrudes, causing pressure on the ligaments and the nerve roots. In disc bulging there is circumferential symmetric disc extension beyond the end plates in a outwardly convex fashion, whereas in disc herniation there is focal asymmetric disc extension beyond the interspace

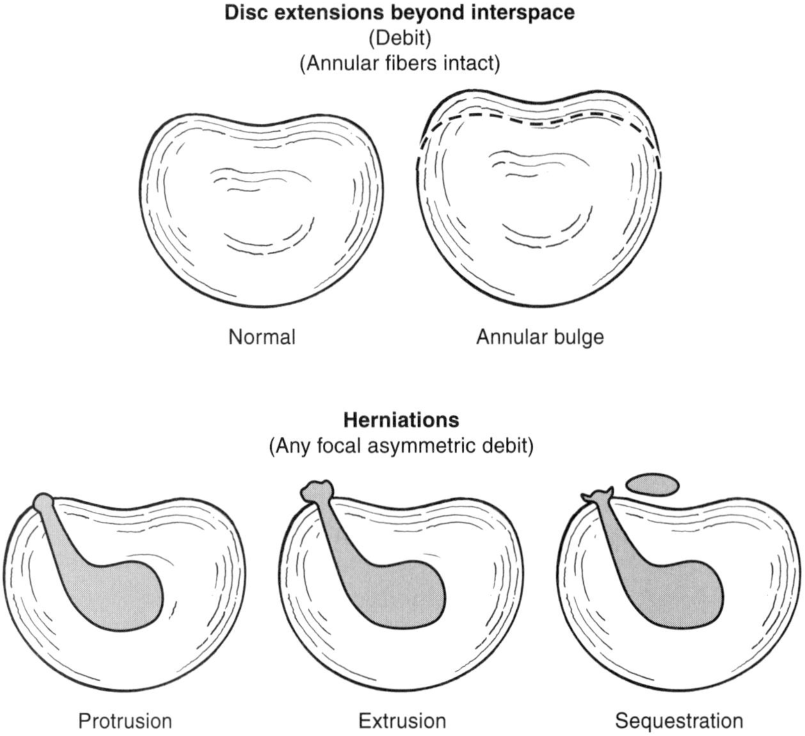

Disc extensions beyond interspace
(Debit)
(Annular fibers intact)

Normal　　　　　　　Annular bulge

Herniations
(Any focal asymmetric debit)

Protrusion　　　　　Extrusion　　　　　Sequestration

FIGURE 3-11. (**Top**) In disc bulging the annular fibers are not disrupted. (**Bottom**) In herniations the annular fibers are disrupted. Under such circumstances the nucleus pulposus may be confined solely by the outermost fibers of the annulus (protrusion); the nucleus may break through the outermost fibers of the annulus and come to lie underneath the posterior longitudinal ligament (extrusion); or a free fragment of the nuclear material may break through the posterior longitudinal and lie free in the spinal canal (sequestration).

(Brant-Zawadzki et al, 1995; Fig. 3-11). Both protrusion and extrusions can cause alteration in neurologic status and pain (Fig. 3-12).

ETIOLOGY
The molecular changes of the aging disc alter both the nucleus and annulus. The disc becomes dry, cracks, and is unable to withstand physical stressors.

SYMPTOMS
1. Initially, similar to those reported with acute low back strain
2. Leg pain of a lancinating or pins-and-needles quality (sciatica), which is dull or burning in nature
3. Altered sensation in the lower extremities described as either "numbness" or "tingling"
4. Pain worse with maneuvers such as coughing, sneezing, or bearing down during defecation
5. Weakness or giving way at the knee

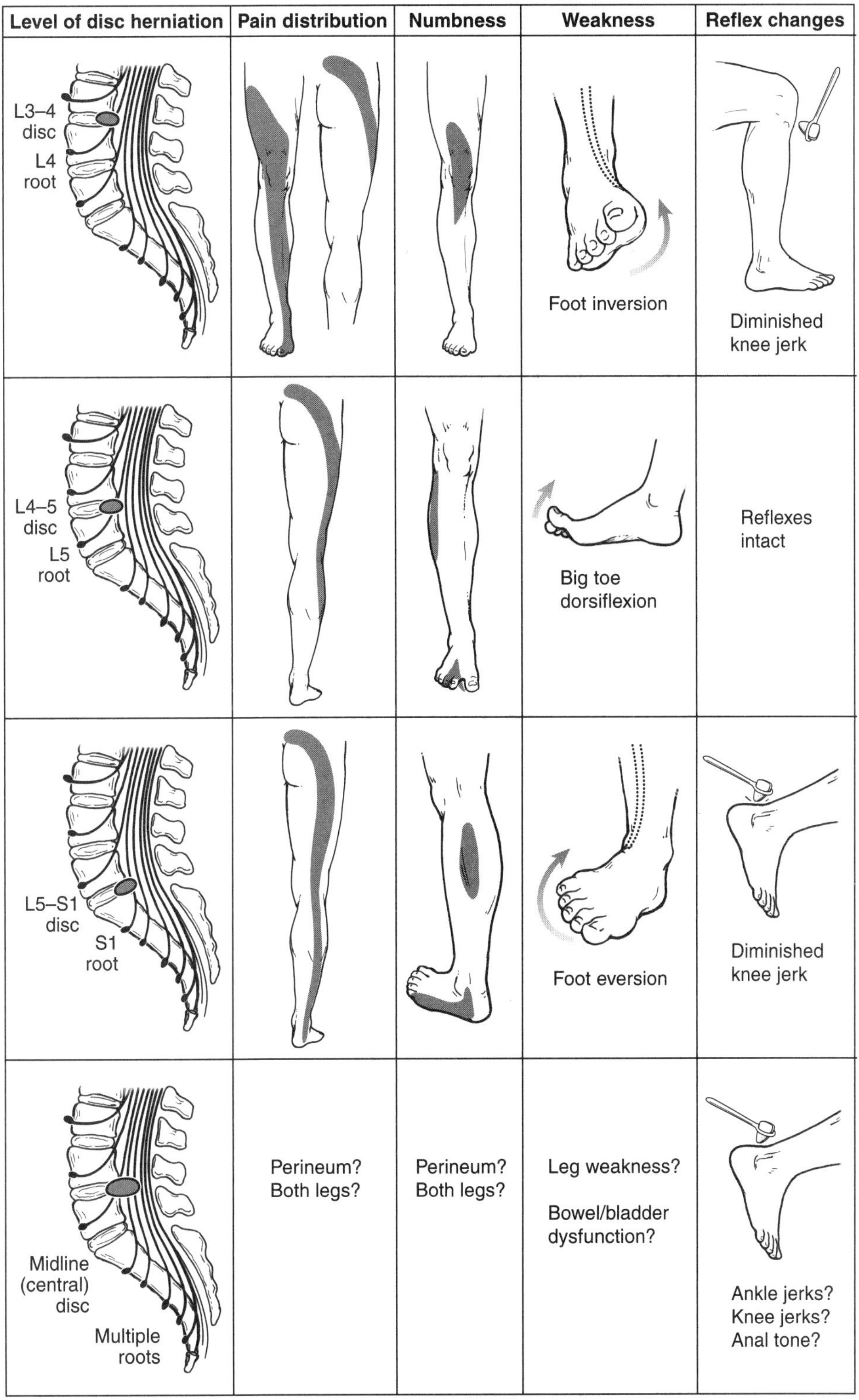

Level of disc herniation	Pain distribution	Numbness	Weakness	Reflex changes
L3–4 disc L4 root			Foot inversion	Diminished knee jerk
L4–5 disc L5 root			Big toe dorsiflexion	Reflexes intact
L5–S1 disc S1 root			Foot eversion	Diminished knee jerk
Midline (central) disc Multiple roots	Perineum? Both legs?	Perineum? Both legs?	Leg weakness? Bowel/bladder dysfunction?	Ankle jerks? Knee jerks? Anal tone?

FIGURE 3-12. Common disc syndromes: neurologic findings. (Reilly, B. M. [1991]. *Practical strategies in outpatient medicine.* Philadelphia: W. B. Saunders.)

6. *Note:* Central disc herniations can present as back pain without leg pain, especially in people under 30 years of age. Other patients with a central disc herniation may complain of bilateral leg pain and paresthesias.

SIGNS
1. Possible limitation of spinal motion
2. Antalgic gait
3. Sciatic list (functional scoliosis secondary to a unilateral muscle spasm)
4. Hip and knee flexed while standing
5. Reproduction of radicular symptoms during flexion
6. Absent or diminished reflexes
7. Motor weakness
8. Decreased sensation along a sensory dermatome
9. Positive straight leg raising test
10. Reproduction of sciatic symptoms during forced passive ankle dorsiflexion
11. Positive sitting root test

TREATMENT
1. In the early stages of management, it is sometimes difficult to differentiate a herniated intervertebral disc from degenerative disease (including spinal stenosis, displacement of facet joints related to disc degeneration, foraminal narrowing caused by osteoarthritic spurring) and other causes (eg, diabetes and other neuropathies, spinal neoplasms, or psychogenic back pain). Diagnostic testing aids diagnostic decision making. Obtain as previously indicated if positive tension signs, loss of a reflex, a sensory loss that follows a dermatome pattern, motor weakness, or progressive neurologic deficits are present, or if surgery is contemplated.

   Explicit instructions and explanations of treatments increase understanding and reassurance; they also promote patient participation in self-care and encourage transfer of control to the patient. Refer to the treatment section entitled Acute Mechanical Low Back Pain for specific interventions.

   Treatment of disc herniation may be either conservative or surgical. Conservative treatments consists of the following:
   a. Bedrest, usually for brief periods (2 to 5 days; see section entitled Acute Mechanical Low Back Pain). For every 3 hours of daytime bedrest, a 20-minute walk is recommended (except in the very acute). Prolonged bedrest deconditions the body and fosters calcium loss. This increases the risk for osteoporosis. *Avoid sitting.*
   b. Medications (see section entitled Acute Mechanical Low Back Pain)
   c. Epidural steroid injection
   d. Back education
   e. Encourage decision making
   f. Encourage the patient to participate actively in management
   g. Gradually return to normal activities with planned rest periods

Patients may return to work in 2 to 4 weeks if able and if the job does not require heavy lifting. If recovery is complete, they may return to normal work activities. However, even in this case, frequent lifting should be evaluated on an individual basis. Generally, frequent lifting should be limited for 3 to 6 weeks.

REFERRAL
1. Persistent symptoms after 4 to 6 weeks of conservative management
2. Progressive neurologic deficits
3. Litigation pending
4. Lack of a specific diagnosis
5. Associated GI or GU symptoms

OUTCOME
1. Generally accepted time frame for relief of sciatica:
   a. 60% in 4 weeks
   b. 90% in 3 months
   c. 96% in 6 months
2. Persistence of low back pain
3. Intermittent relief of pain
4. Preservation of family role
5. Increased understanding of the nature of the problem and the need for personal control
6. Surgical intervention with progression of neurologic deficits, positive objective findings, and unrelenting lower extremity pain
7. Occasionally, symptoms persist regardless of treatment; consider chronic pain syndrome

Cauda Equina Syndrome

Cauda equina syndrome is a rare condition in which a large midline disc herniation can compress several nerve roots of the cauda equina. This usually occurs at the L4 and L5 level. Symptoms can vary, back or perianal pain predominates, and the patient may or may not complain of bowel or bladder dysfunction. The dysfunction can be either the loss of bowel or bladder control (incontinence) or the inability either to defecate or urinate (males may report a recent onset of impotence). This may be followed by leg pain, numbness of the legs or feet, and difficulty with walking. This is an emergency requiring immediate referral (Rothman et al, 1992).

Chronic Low Back Pain

Chronic low back pain is traditionally defined as pain that has continued for more than 6 months. More recently, chronic back pain has been defined as pain that has continued for more than 3 months.

ETIOLOGY
1. History of mechanical stress that has failed to respond to traditional regimens
2. Lack of compliance with therapeutic recommendations
3. Depression
4. Environmental reinforcement that provides either psychological or monetary secondary gains

SYMPTOMS
1. Back pain described as knifelike and unbearable
2. Leg pain, if present, always less than back pain

SIGNS
1. Abuse of medications (suspect if the patient shows familiarity with many drugs, requests special medications, or develops drug allergies, slurred speech, hostility, or defensiveness)
2. Obvious depression (flat affect, "blue moods," inappropriate crying, lack of sexual desire, appetite changes, disturbance in sleep patterns, or expressed attitude that the patient "never has fun")
3. Amplification of symptoms
4. Excessive dependence on others
5. Manipulative behavior
6. Lack of motivation or interest in own management of symptoms
7. Lack of objective findings

TREATMENT
1. Therapeutic drug regimens are best directed by the comprehensive pain team management approach. Therapeutics may consist of NSAIDS, tricyclic antidepressants, antiepileptics, and nonaddictive analgesics. Narcotics should be avoided when treating chronic nonmalignant pain. Efficacy is short term.
2. If the patient describes disproportionate pain, pain that disturbs sleep, or migratory pain, rule out underlying causes with the following diagnostic tests: blood and urine laboratory studies, TB skin tests, bone scan, CT scan, or MRI.
3. Retraining/rehabilitation includes goals for chronic low back pain that are the same as those for acute low back pain. The patient needs a therapeutic regimen that is directed toward maintaining normal relationships and activities of daily living.

    However, the patient with chronic low back pain has special needs. Referral to an aggressive functional restoration program may offer the best outcome. This multidimensional program focuses on behavioral support that includes psychological treatment (stress management), which reduces subjective feelings of disability; aggressive physical therapy (floor stretching and strengthening exercises, progressive weight training, and general endurance exercises [ie, arm and leg cycling, swimming, and walking]); occupational therapy with work simulation; and didactic programs to explain the anatomy and function of the spine and the rationale for treatments (Hildebrandt et al, 1997).
4. Prevention consists of developing strategies during the initial management phase of acute low back pain that reduce long-term disability.
    a. Allow time during the visit for the patient to express concerns.
    b. Help the patient to formulate reachable goals.
    c. Help the patient to identify past coping skills and strengths; review existing abilities and help the patient use them.
    d. Have the patient plan daily rest periods; adequate rest/sleep increases

coping skills and lessens frustration. Try nontraditional methods for pain control (acupuncture, progressive relaxation, therapeutic touch, or creative imagery).

e. A transcutaneous electrical nerve stimulation (TENS) unit for pain control may be indicated. TENS units are small, battery-operated electrical pulse generators used to help control pain. An electrical current is applied to the skin via electrodes attached to the generator. This current stimulates peripheral nerves, thereby modulating pain sensation. The generator controls electrical output, frequency, and duration. Although TENS units are used for many different chronic pain problems and occasionally for acute pain, the most common use is for controlling chronic low back pain, There are two methods of delivering the stimulation: conventional high frequency with continuous stimulation or low frequency with the TENS delivered in bursts. The mode used is determined by which mode works more successfully for the patient. The conventional mode is tried first. Pain relief may be immediate or may occur after a few weeks of use. The relief may last only when the unit is turned on, or it may last for hours and even days after using the unit.

f. Provide an atmosphere that maintains independence and accustomed family roles.

g. Initiate steps that modify the work environment. If necessary, contact the patient's employer or supervisor.

h. Recognize that prevention might not be possible.

REFERRAL
1. Psychologist
2. Exercise physiologist
3. Occupational rehabilitation specialist
4. Chronic pain program

OUTCOME
1. Improvement
2. Withdrawal, loss of family and friends
3. Social isolation
4. Chronic pain syndrome that is refractory to all treatments
5. Severe depression/suicide

The Mature Adult with Low Back Pain

In this age group, the most common cause of low back pain is the degenerative changes that occur as the spine ages. However, back pain in this age group can be a clue to an underlying disease that may or may not be intrinsic. Careful screening is essential to rule out the extrinsic causes.

Degenerative Back Pain (Lumbar Spondylosis)

Etiology is a result of either facet joint dysfunction or arthritis, repeated episodes of acute low back sprain/strain, osteoarthritic spurring, or chronic disc degeneration.

Symptoms

1. Aching pain in lower back or buttock, which may or may not radiate
2. Radiation into the thigh, but never below the knee
3. Possible restriction of spinal motion
4. Gradual onset
5. Increased pain with walking and bending
6. Decreased pain with bedrest

Signs

See section entitled Acute Mechanical Low Back Pain.

Treatment

1. Education to increase knowledge and to decrease fear and pain
2. Patient identification of stressors that increase pain
3. Reduction of activities that increase the symptoms
4. Involvement in a protective back regimen, which includes back flexibility and strengthening exercises, aerobic exercises, and progressive relaxation
5. Planned periods of rest each day; an understanding of the need to get adequate rest and sleep
6. Short course of NSAIDs
7. Office visits scheduled at 6-week intervals to reinforce treatment plan and modify if necessary
8. Back School

Referral

1. Failure to respond to therapy
2. Lack of a specific diagnosis
3. Neurologic symptoms
4. Suspicion of a tumor
5. Suspicion of infection

Outcome (Chronic)

The goal is to maintain functional ability and to offer modification of treatment to increase the patient's comfort.

Degenerative Spondylolysis/Spondylolisthesis

Etiology

Disc degeneration, facet arthropathy, joint laxity and subluxation allow for changes that cause anterior displacement of a vertebra in relation to the vertebrae below. Usually seen over the age of 50, with a higher incidence in female diabetics.

Symptoms

1. Radicular symptoms often of more than one level, usually at L4-5
2. Subtle urinary changes, which may indicate a neurogenic bladder and must be evaluated by a urologist

Signs

1. Patients must be examined for hip osteoarthritis and peripheral vascular disease.
2. Signs are similar to disc herniation (ie, at L4-5 extensor hallucis longus [EHL] weakness, numbness of the dorsum of the foot).

Treatment

1. Lumbar corset
2. Physical therapy soft tissue modalities (heat, ultrasound, massage)
3. Epidural steroid injections to reduce inflammatory component

Referral

Referral should be made to an orthopedic spine surgeon for persistent pain and/ or motor weakness.

Spinal Stenosis

Etiology

This condition may be congenital or acquired (degenerative), resulting in one or all of the following: osteophytes forming on the disc margins and facet joints, causing bony overgrowth that constricts the nerve roots; ligamentous thickening and discogenic protrusion.

Symptoms

1. Claudication that is worse with walking (typically, patients are unable to walk 100 yards before having leg pain and/or back pain). If walking continues, the patient may experience pins-and-needles sensation and a sense of weakness in the calf and foot (Macnab & McCulloch, 1990).
2. Leg pain relieved by either sitting or lying down (stopping does not relieve the pain as it does with vascular claudication)
3. Possible sensory changes that, if present, are described as a feeling of water or candle wax dripping down the leg
4. Back pain with or without leg pain; if leg pain is present, it may or may not radiate below the knee
5. Possible increase in back pain with climbing stairs
6. Sense of imbalance

Signs

1. May have normal examination except for loss of vibratory sense (bilateral or unilateral)
2. May have increased pain during back extension
3. If permitted to walk to the point of claudicant leg pain, the patient may present with neurologic deficits on examination
4. May have unsteady gait performing heel-to-toe maneuvers
5. May have positive Romberg

Treatment

Differentiate neurogenic claudication from vascular claudication. Patients with vascular claudication cannot swim or ride a bike without leg pain.

1. Anti-inflammatories
2. Education
3. Ice/heat
4. Exercise (aerobic conditioning)
5. Surgery to decompress the nerve root

Tumor

Most tumors in this age group result from metastases. Primary spinal tumors are rare. Tumors are either intraspinal or extraspinal and may present like a herniated disc (Unni, 1996).

Symptoms

1. Progressive low back pain
2. Inability to relieve the pain with rest
3. Night pain that awakens the patient from sleep; relief is achieved by either sitting upright or pacing the floor

Signs (Dependent on the Location of the Tumor)

1. Neurologic deficit may be present.
2. Increased back pain on percussion of the spinous processes may be present.

Treatment

1. Referral to an orthopedic surgeon, neurosurgeon, or vascular surgeon
2. Plain films at first office visit
3. Immediate bone scan or MRI if patient presents with night pain, a history of previous carcinoma, or progressive unrelenting pain that is out of proportion or if the patient fails 4 to 6 weeks of conservative treatment
4. Patient and family education
5. Support and reassurance

Infection (Disc Space, Osteomyelitis, Spinal Epidural Abscess)

Most infections occur after spinal surgery and are iatrogenic. They also can occur in people of any age who are intravenous drug abusers or have immune deficiencies. Antecedent respiratory or urinary infections and trauma can predispose the individual to an infectious process.

Symptoms

1. Dull, unrelenting back pain
2. Severe low back pain with leg pain
3. Pain increased by any jarring motion
4. Possible increased pain at night

Signs

1. Low-grade fever
2. Spasm of the paraspinal muscles
3. Tenderness to percussion over the involved vertebral body

Treatment

1. Immediate referral
2. Diagnostic tests at the initial visit: ESR (elevated), CBC with differential (usually normal), plain spine films (changes may not be seen for 3 to 6 weeks, and x-rays then will reveal disc destruction with early bony erosion of the end plates). MRI is most sensitive.
3. Identification through needle biopsy of the vertebral body of the specific organism
4. Antibiotics
5. Immobilization (bedrest until pain subsides)
6. Treat nerve/cord compression and, if necessary, treat spinal instability

Referral

Immediate.

Outcome

Dependent on timeliness of the correct diagnosis followed by the appropriate treatment.

References and Recommended Readings

Bigos, S., Bowyer, O., Braen, G., et al. (1994). *Acute low back problems in adults.* Clinical Practice Guideline, Quick Reference Guide Number 14. AHCPR Pub. No. 95-0643. Rockville, MD: Agency for Health Care Policy and Research.

Borenstein, D. A. (1997). A clinician's approach to acute low backpain. *American Journal of Medicine, 102*(a), 16S.

Boyd, R. R. (1995). Evaluation of back pain. In Goroll, A. H., May, L. A., & Mulley, A. G. (Eds.). *Primary care medicine* (3rd ed.). Philadelphia: J. B. Lippincott.

Bradford D. A., Moe, J. H., & Winter, R. B. (1992). Scoliosis and kyphosis. In Rothman, R. H., & Simeone, F. A. (Eds.). *The spine* (3rd ed.). Philadelphia: W. B. Saunders.

Brant-Zawadzki, M. N., Jensen, M. C., Obuchowski, N., Ross, J. S., & Modic, M. T. (1995). Interobserver and intra observer variability in interpretation of lumbar disc abnormalities: a comparison of two nomenclatures. *Spine, 20,* 1257.

Brown, C. W., Deffer, P. A., Akmakjian, J., Donaldson, D. H., & Brugman, J. L. (1992). The natural history of thoracic disc herniation. *Spine, 17*(Suppl 6), 97.

Deen, H. G. (1996). Diagnosis and management of lumbar disc disease. *Mayo Clinic Proceedings, 71,* 283.

Deyo, R. A., Diehel, A. K., & Rosenthal, M. (1986). How many days of bed rest for acute low back pain? *New England Journal of Medicine, 315*(17), 1064.

Frymoyer, J. W. (1996). Magnitude of the problem. In Wiesel, S. W., Weinstein, J. N., Herkowitz, H. N., et al. (Eds.). *The lumbar spine* (2nd ed.). Philadelphia: W. B. Saunders.

Frymoyer, J. W., Pope, M. H., Clements, J. H., Wilder, D. G., MacPherson, B., & Ashikaga, T. (1986). Risk factors in low-back pain: an epidemiological survey. *Journal of Bone and Joint Surgery, 65-A*(2), 213.

Hardy, R. W., Jr. (Ed.). (1993). *Lumbar disc disease* (2nd ed.). New York: Raven.

Herzog, R. J. (1995). Radiologic imaging of the spine. In Weinstein, J. N., Rydevik, B. L., & Sonntag, V. K. H. (Eds.). *Essentials of the spine* (pp. 111-138). New York: Raven.

Hildebrandt, J., Pfingsten, M., Saur, P., & Jansen, J. (1997). Prediction of success from a multidisciplinary treatment program for chronic low back pain. *Spine, 22,* 990.

Hoppenfeld, S. (1976). *Physical examination of the spine and extremities.* East Norwalk, CT: Appleton-Century-Croft.

Kendall, F. P., & McCreary, E. K. (1993). *Muscle testing and function* (4th ed.). Baltimore: Williams & Wilkins.

MacNab, I., & McCulloch, J. (1990). *Backache* (2nd ed.). Baltimore: Williams & Wilkins.

Markey, B. T., & Graham, M. (1997). Management of chronic pain with epidural steroids. *AORN Journal, 65,* 791-2.

Micheli, L. J., & Klein, J. D. (1991). Sports injuries in children & adolescents. *British Journal of Sports Medicine, 25,* 6.

Micheli, L. J., & Wood, R. (1995). Back pain in young athletes. Significant differences from adults in causes and patterns. *Circ. Pediatric Adolescents Medicine, 149,* 8.

Mooney, V., Saal, J. A., & Sall, J. S. (1996). Evaluation and treatment of low back pain. *Clinical Symposia, 48,* 1.

Patel, R. P., & Lauerman, W. C. (1997). The use of magnetic resonance imaging in the diagnosis of lumbar disc disease. *Orthopaedic Nursing, 16,* 59.

Rothman, R. H., Simeone, F. A., & Bernini, P. M. (1992). Lumbar disc disease. In Rothman, R. H., & Simeone, F. A. (Eds.). *The spine* (3rd ed.). Philadelphia: W. B. Saunders.

Sheon, R. P., Moskowitz, R. W., & Goldberg, V. A. (Eds.). (1996). *Soft tissue rheumatic pain* (3rd ed.). Baltimore: Williams & Wilkins.

Spitzer, W. O., LeBlanc, F. E., & DuPuis, M. (1987). Scientific approach to the assessment and management of activity-related spinal disorders. A monograph for clinicians. Report of the Quebec Task Force on Spinal Disorders. *Spine, 12*(7S), 59.

Travell, J. G., Simons, D. G. (1995). *Myofascial pain dysfunction: The trigger point manual* (Vols. I & II). Baltimore: Williams & Wilkins.

Unni, K. K. (1996). *Dahlin's bone tumors* (5th ed.). Philadelphia: Lippincott-Raven.

Waddell, G., Feder, G., McIntosh, A., et al. (1996). *Low back pain evidence review.* Royal College of General Practitioners Guide. London, England: Royal College of General Practitioners.

Waddell, G., McCulloch, J. A., Kummel, E., & Venner, R. M. (1986). Nonorganic physical signs in low-back pain. *Spine, 5*(2), 117.

Weinstein, S. L. (1994). The thoracolumbar spine. In Weinstein, S. L., & Buckwalter, J. A. (Eds.). *Turek's orthopaedics* (5th ed.). Philadelphia: J. B. Lippincott.

Weinstein, S. L., & Buckwalter, J. A. (Eds.). (1994). *Turek's orthopaedics* (5th ed.). Philadelphia: J. B. Lippincott.

Weinstein, J. N., Rydevik, B. L., & Sonntag, V. K. (1995). *Essentials of the spine.* New York: Raven.

Winter, R. B. (1995). Spinal deformity. In Pang, D. (Ed.). *Disorders of the pediatric spine.* New York: Raven.

Chapter 4

The Shoulder

William H. Simon, MD, FACS

The normal function of the shoulder joint represents a triumph of motion over stability. Instability is a common consequence of injury, and pain and limitation of normal motion are the sequelae.

The prominent role that athletics (baseball, basketball, football, ice hockey) play in the adolescent's life predisposes him or her to significant traumatic problems (most unavoidable) with the shoulder joint. Other problems that occur are due to overuse syndromes that result from too-vigorous training techniques. Patients presenting with the latter syndrome require follow-up with school athletic departments and/or athletic trainers to prevent repeated problems.

Adults also suffer from overuse syndrome, particularly in industry where repetitive motions in an overhead position place undue strain on shoulder structures. These patients also deserve follow-up in the workplace to prevent the recurrence of problems.

Degenerative changes in the shoulder are common in the elderly. These changes produce pain and limited motion. Frozen shoulder syndrome, the opposite of instability, may be the result of painful, restricted motion, caused by pain syndromes originating outside of the shoulder joint (ie, the cervical spine or the cardiovascular system).

In an outpatient setting, the primary care provider must have knowledge of the anatomy and function of the shoulder joint to diagnose and properly treat shoulder problems or to refer patients for treatment. This chapter provides such knowledge. Treatment recommendations are those expected of a primary care provider, including first aid before referral for definitive treatment, either nonsurgical or surgical.

Anatomy and Function of the Shoulder Joint

The shoulder joint (*glenohumeral joint*) literally hangs from the axial skeleton. It is suspended by muscular attachments and articulates with the body by means of a strut bone known as the *clavicle*. At either end of the clavicle is a joint. The more stable joint, the *sternoclavicular joint*, is the only direct connection between the shoulder and the axial skeleton. The less stable joint, the *acromioclavicular joint*, is at the distal end of the clavicle, is palpable subcutaneously, and is a major bony landmark about the shoulder.

The *clavicle* is an S-shaped bone and is subcutaneous throughout its length. It rotates during flexion and extension of the shoulder, and it aids in the stability of the joint. The clavicle is not necessary for shoulder motion. People who are born without this bone (a condition known as cleidocranial dysostosis) have shoulders that function perfectly well (Fig. 4-1).

The *scapula* is a complex bone. The major portion of the scapula is the blade, a triangular structure to or from which major muscles that control the strength, stability, and function of the shoulder mechanism attach or originate. It is divided by the spine into a smaller upper supraspinatus portion and a larger infraspinatus segment.

The *supraspinatus muscle*, the major component of the so-called rotator cuff, originates above the spine and attaches to the greater tuberosity of the humerus. It is a major stabilizer of the glenohumeral joint. The infraspinatus and teres

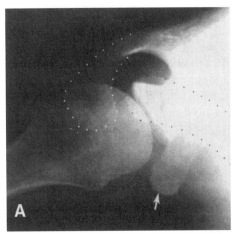
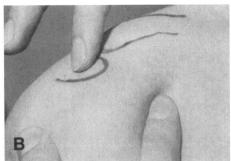

FIGURE 4-1. Bony points of the shoulder region. **(A)** A transaxillary radiograph of the shoulder region. The x-ray film is placed above the acromion and the x-rays travel through the axilla. The acromion (*white dots*) overhangs the humeral head and is separated from the lateral end of the clavicle (*black dots*) by a radiolucent gap, which is occupied chiefly by articular cartilage and an articular disk in the acromioclavicular joint. The clavicle is superimposed over the glenoid cavity, which is separated from the humeral head by radiolucent articular cartilage. The coracoid projects forward, its tip (*arrow*) being level with the lesser tubercle of the humerus. The coracoacromial ligament (invisible) bridges the gap between the coracoid and acromion. **(B)** The relation of the acromion, lesser tubercle, and coracoid process. The index finger of one hand is on the tip of the acromion, that of the other hand on the coracoid, and the middle finger of the same hand is on the lesser tubercle. The three bony points outline a regular triangle. This relation is disturbed when the humerus is dislocated. (A, courtesy of Dr. Rosalind H. Troupin.)

minor muscles, two more components of the rotator cuff, originate below the spine. Both stabilize and externally rotate the humeral head in the glenoid cavity.

The *teres major muscle,* an internal rotator, also originates on the scapula and attaches to the humerus at the lesser tuberosity. Also attaching to the scapula and acting as stabilizers and rotators of this bone are the rhomboids, the levator scapulae, and the trapezius muscles.

The *latissimus dorsi muscle* covers the tip of the scapula as it swings from the mid-back to attach on the lesser tuberosity of the humerus to depress and internally rotate the humerus.

The undersurface, or thoracic surface, of the scapula is the site of origin of the *subscapularis muscle*—the fourth and final component of the rotator cuff—a depressor and internal rotator of the shoulder. In addition, the *serratus anterior muscle* comes off of the thorax and attaches to the undersurface of the scapula, thereby stabilizing the scapula against "winging" out away from the thorax. All of the muscles attaching to the scapular blade aid in the complex coordinated movements of this bone including elevation, depression, rotation, abduction, and adduction (motion in the plane of the thorax). Many of these movements will occur in any complete motion of the shoulder joint, such as elevation of the arm from the side of the body to the overhead position (Fig. 4-2).

The *deltoid muscle,* the major elevator of the shoulder, and the *rotator cuff muscles,* the major muscles stabilizing the humeral head against the glenoid, form what is known in biomechanics as a *force couple.* The normal function of one set of muscles depends on the normal function of the other. The rotator cuff muscles stabilize the humeral head in the glenoid, and the deltoid acts to rotate the arm in an upward direction. Failure of one part of this force couple disturbs the entire function of the shoulder joint.

Other portions of the scapula, the *acromion,* the *glenoid,* and the *coracoid process,* each play a major role in the shoulder function (Fig. 4-3).

The *glenoid,* the portion of the scapula that articulates with the *head of the humerus,* extends forward from the blade on a short neck of bone. It has a shallow, concave surface covered by articular cartilage and is deepened for stability by a fibrous ring known as the *labrum* or lip. Attached to the glenoid is the *fibrous capsule* of the shoulder, which also attaches to the neck of the humerus to contain the glenohumeral joint.

The *capsule* is lax with the arm at the side and is taut in the overhead position. The capsule is reinforced anteriorly by three ligaments: superior, middle, and inferior. A relatively small gap between the middle and inferior ligaments acts as a locus minoris resistentiae (place of least resistance) with the arm overhead; this gap is the place through which anterior dislocations of the glenohumeral joint most typically occur.

The *biceps tendon (long head)* attaches to the superior surface of the glenoid. It travels inside the shoulder capsule over the head of the humerus, into the bicipital groove, and then down the shaft of the humerus. The long head of the triceps tendon attaches extracapsularly to the inferior surface of the glenoid.

The *acromion* is the outrigger of the scapula. It is the main subcutaneous landmark of the lateral aspect of the shoulder. It acts as the "roof" of the shoulder, and the strong deltoid muscle (the major overhead rotator of the humerus) is also

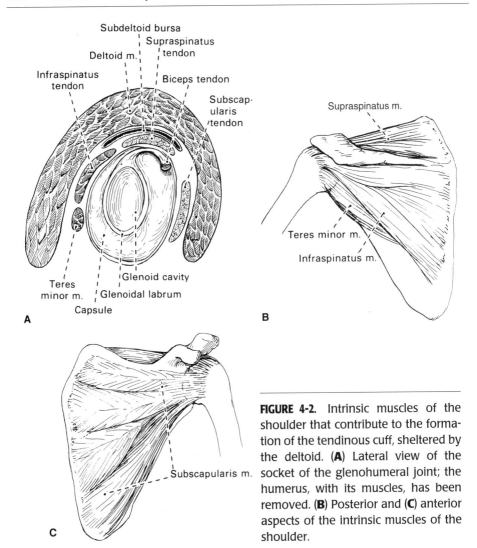

FIGURE 4-2. Intrinsic muscles of the shoulder that contribute to the formation of the tendinous cuff, sheltered by the deltoid. **(A)** Lateral view of the socket of the glenohumeral joint; the humerus, with its muscles, has been removed. **(B)** Posterior and **(C)** anterior aspects of the intrinsic muscles of the shoulder.

attached to it. Beneath the *acromion*, the *rotator cuff tendons* function, separated from the *deltoid muscle* by the *subacromial bursa* (an envelope of synovial tissue that allows one tendon to glide over the other). Extending from the anterior tip of the acromion to the coracoid process is a tough fibrous ligament (the *coracoacromial ligament*) that forms an arcade over the anterior aspect of the rotator cuff and the biceps tendon (see Fig. 4-3).

The *coracoid process* is a finger-like anterior protuberance off of the scapular blade to which is attached the conjoined tendons of the short head of the *biceps,* the *pectoralis minor,* and the *coracobrachialis muscles.* In addition, the major stabilizing ligaments of the clavicle—the *trapezoid* and *conoid ligaments*—attach to the coracoid process. The *humeral head* (a spherical structure) is covered with articular cartilage and moves unimpeded on the glenoid surface. Its movements are tethered only by the capsular attachment at the anatomic neck, the biceps tendon, and the

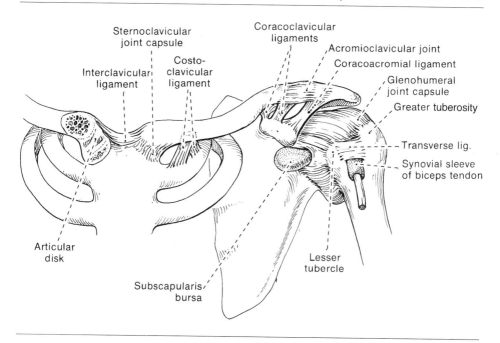

FIGURE 4-3. The sternoclavicular, acromioclavicular, and glenohumeral joints, with associated ligaments seen from the *front.*

tendons of the rotator cuff. The bony prominence lateral to the head (the *greater tuberosity*) is another shoulder landmark covered by the thick deltoid muscle (Fig. 4-4).

The complex neurovascular supply of the shoulder will not be described here in detail. The major nerves and blood vessels enter the axilla just medial to the coracoid process and inferior to the glenohumeral joint.

The *musculocutaneous nerve* runs under the coracoid process beneath the conjoined tendon. The *axillary nerve* runs from back to front about 1 inch below the acromion in the deltoid muscle, which it innervates. It is subject to injury in shoulder dislocations and by direct blows to the shoulder. The *suprascapular nerve,* supplying the rotator cuff muscles, runs in the supraspinatus portion of the scapula. It is subject to injury by blows to the top of the shoulder. The *long thoracic nerve* runs down the side of the thorax. An injury to this nerve, which supplies the serratus anterior muscles, produces winging of the scapula (Fig. 4-5).

The extreme mobility of the shoulder joint allows for 180 degrees of motion in flexion and abduction away from the side of the body, 180 degrees of rotation internal to external, 70 to 90 degrees of backward extension, and 45 degrees of adduction across the body. When viewed from behind, the synchronous function of the shoulder structures produces a smooth "scapulohumeral rhythm" when the arm is raised overhead. After the first few degrees of motion, the glenohumeral joint moves 2 degrees for every 1 degree of scapulothoracic motion, in a coordinated effort. Any significant dysfunction in a major shoulder structure will disturb this rhythm, and dysfunction can be detected by comparing the appearance of shoulder

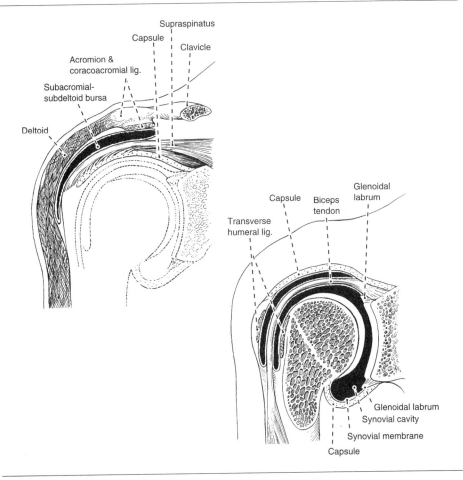

FIGURE 4-4. Schematic diagram of a coronal section of the shoulder region to show anatomic relations. (**A**) The position of the deltoid and supraspinatus in relation to the subacromial bursa and the shoulder joint capsule. (**B**) Relations of the glenoidal cavity, labrum, capsule, and biceps tendon.

elevation right to left. This is the simplest test of normal shoulder function. The gross observation of swelling, muscle atrophy, pain on motion, and point tenderness is the mainstay of a basic shoulder examination.

History

The most important aspect of the medical history as it relates to the shoulder is to obtain a clear and concise chief complaint. Questions to ask include: Is there pain on any movement of the shoulder? Pain on a particular motion of the shoulder? Intermittent pain in the shoulder without relation to movement? Weakness in the shoulder? Limitation of the range of motion of the shoulder? A feeling of shoulder

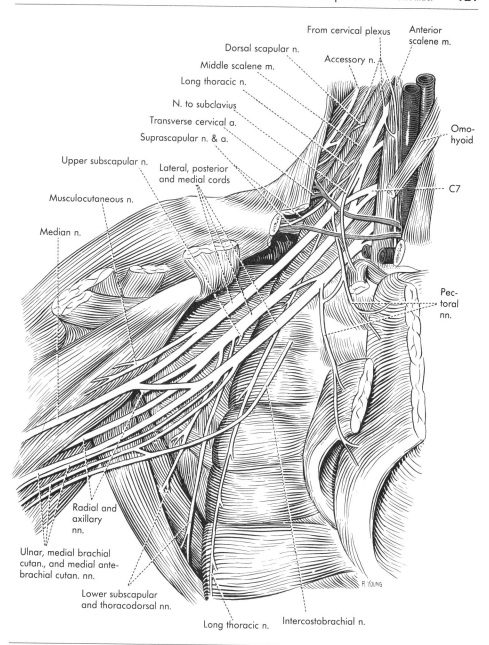

FIGURE 4-5. The brachial plexus and its branches in a dissection of the axilla and neck. In this specimen, the lateral pectoral nerve arises higher than usual, above the clavicle instead of from the lateral cord of the axilla.

instability ("dead arm" sensation, or a feeling of the joint "coming out of its socket")?

Once the chief complaint is established, the history then delves into the how, where, and when. In determining how the problem began, it is important to determine whether it was a *traumatic* or *nontraumatic* onset. If traumatic, a description of the trauma (in simple terms) is important. Questions to ask include: Did the patient fall on the point of the shoulder or on an outstretched arm? Was there a blow to a specific part of the shoulder? Was there a specific activity connected with the onset of shoulder pain such as the difficult opening of a stuck window frame or garage door?

In nontraumatic problems, one should ask if there was a certain activity that brought about the awareness of the problem, such as repetitive use of the shoulder in an overhead position either at work or at play. Can the patient determine exactly where he or she feels the problem is in the shoulder? Can the patient put one finger on the area of the pain? Is the problem generalized in and about the shoulder? Does pain radiate from the shoulder upward to the neck or downward to the arm and hand? Does the patient feel something going on inside the shoulder, such as clicking or a sensation that the shoulder is going out of place? Can the patient demonstrate one particular position where the pain is most acute? Is it reaching overhead at 90 degrees of elevation, in reaching behind the back, in reaching out to the side, or in placing the arm overhead in a throwing position? When did the problem begin? Is it an old, recurrent problem or something entirely new? Has it been going on for hours, days, weeks, or months? Does it occur at any particular time of the day or night? Has it been a persistent problem, intermittent, gradually increasing in severity, or changing in severity from time to time? The answers to all of these questions should be recorded precisely and concisely.

Each patient should have a basic past medical history taken and a statement of any present systemic illnesses recorded, including the presence or absence of fever, chills, loss of appetite, or weight loss. The names and dosages of any medications being taken at the time of the examination should be recorded.

Physical Examination

It is most important that the examination of the shoulder joint be made with the patient properly exposed to the examiner. Men must clearly expose their bodies to the waist. Women must remove undergarments, and they should be gowned, covered from the breasts in front to below the shoulder blades in back. This can be done with either a sheet that is pinned behind the patient or with a standard cloth or paper gown wrapped around the patient (keeping their arms free) tied in the back.

The patient must be *observed* from front and back for any significant shoulder asymmetry including the presence of unilateral swelling, skin temperature or color changes, prominence of a particular part of the shoulder, such as the sternoclavicular joint, acromioclavicular joint, or anterior or posterior prominence of the humeral head area. Atrophy or flattening of the deltoid muscles, trapezius muscle, supraspinatus or infraspinatus muscle groups, or pectoral muscles must be noted and recorded. It is also important to observe if winging of the scapula away from the thoracic cage is present.

Palpation

Before initiating any movement of the shoulder, *palpation* of the shoulder structures is carried out using the fingertips of one hand. This examination begins at the sternoclavicular joint, moves along the subcutaneous border of the clavicle, directly to the acromioclavicular joint, and then to the acromion. Pressure is exerted below the acromion anteriorly, laterally, and posteriorly to detect the presence of any point tenderness. Pressure is exerted on the trapezius muscle from the occiput to the point of the shoulder. The supraspinous and infraspinous portions of the scapula are palpated. Finally, pressure is exerted over the biceps tendon in the bicipital groove of the proximal humerus.

Frequently, it is just as easy to examine the nonaffected shoulder with one hand and the symptomatic shoulder with the other hand. The examination is performed to elicit tenderness or to feel any abnormalities, such as swelling, muscle spasm, or increased mobility of the affected shoulder compared with the normal shoulder.

Range of Motion

The examination for range of motion of the shoulder joint is performed both actively and passively. The patient is asked to perform the movements initially; if the patient cannot complete a normal range of motion, gentle active assistance is provided by the examiner to determine if the problem is one of restriction by pain, restriction by weakness, or actual physical block to movement. The movements of the symptomatic shoulder are compared with the movements of the normal shoulder (Fig. 4-6).

The patient is placed with his or her arm at the side, with the palm facing the body. The first movement tested is *flexion*, moving the arm forward into the overhead position (a straight overhead position measuring 180 degrees of flexion). Be sure to record the point in this arc of motion at which the patient complains of any pain. *Extension* of the shoulder begins with the arm at the side. The patient is asked to move the arm directly backward; the normal range is approximately 70 degrees.

Rotation of the shoulder is tested in two positions. The first position is with the arm at the side and the elbow bent to 90 degrees so the thumb points upward. The shoulder is then externally and internally rotated, and the range of motion is recorded. A normal range of motion is approximately 70 degrees of *external rotation* and 70 degrees of *internal rotation.* Care must be taken to keep the elbow directly against the side of the body. Testing internal rotation in this position may be difficult in obese patients. The second position to test shoulder rotation is done with the arm abducted to 90 degrees. (This, of course, is impossible if the patient is unable to perform this maneuver because of pain.) The elbow is bent 90 degrees and the palm is facing downward. In this position, normal *external rotation* is 90 degrees and normal *internal rotation* is 90 degrees.

Abduction of the shoulder is tested in two positions. In the first position the arm is at the side with the palm facing the body, and the patient is asked to lift the arm away from the side and overhead. This can normally be accomplished to 180 degrees.

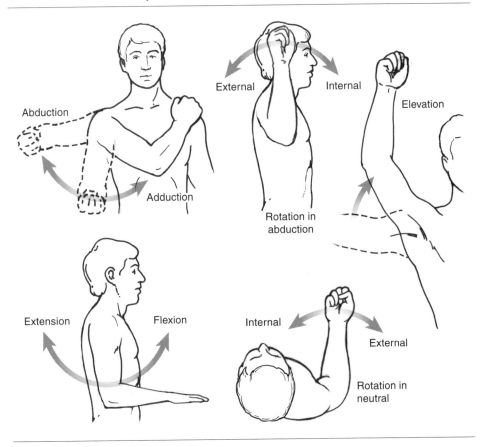

FIGURE 4-6. Normal shoulder range of motion.

If the patient resists this movement at some point in the arc of motion, the hand is returned to the side of the body and the palm is turned outward. This maneuver places the greater tuberosity of the shoulder behind the acromion process and therefore reduces any impingement of soft tissues between the greater tuberosity and the acromion. In the second position the patient is asked to elevate the arm away from the body. If the patient can elevate to 180 degrees with the palm turned outward, but not with the palm turned inward, it is likely that there is a rotator cuff problem, caused by an *impingement* in the narrow space between the acromion and the acromioclavicular joint and the underlying rotator cuff tendons (painful inflammation in the form of a subacromial bursitis, or tendinitis).

While the patient is performing these activities, the scapulohumeral rhythm should be observed. Ordinarily, this is a smooth coordination between the motion of the glenohumeral joint and the scapula and thorax. If this rhythm is disturbed so that the coordinated motion appears jerky or awkward, this is an indicator of major shoulder dysfunction.

Adduction of the shoulder is carried out with the elbow extended and the arm moved across the chest. This function can also be tested from the position of 90 degrees of elevation with the arm directly in front of the patient, then moved across the chest in this fashion. Adduction normally goes to approximately 45 degrees.

Muscle Strength

A general sense of strength of these major muscle groups can be obtained by the examiner resisting the specific movements as the patient performs the range-of-motion maneuvers and comparing how well the patient counters this resistance on the affected side with the normal side. In testing the strength of the abductor muscles, it is important to apply resistance immediately as the arm leaves the side of the body, rather than in the overhead position. Specific testing of the strength of the shoulder elevators is accomplished by asking the patient to shrug while the examiner gently but firmly resists the shrug with the palms on the top of each shoulder. A specific test for the serratus anterior muscle can be carried out by asking the patient to push forward against the examiner's hand with the elbow at 90 degrees. Winging of the scapula frequently can be detected by this maneuver. Weakness of a specific muscle or muscle group may represent a voluntary response because of pain; a loss of function due to muscle trauma or disease; or a specific neurologic lesion, either in the peripheral nerve supplying the muscle, the cervical nerve roots contributing to the peripheral innervation, or the central nervous system. It is not important for the primary care provider to determine the specific cause of the weakness; this should be left to medical specialists. It is important to accurately record the specific weakness, however.

Joint Stability

A sense of the stability of the glenohumeral joint can be obtained by grasping the humeral head with the examining hand and moving it forward and backward to detect any unusual laxity. This may be difficult to perform or assess in a markedly obese or very muscular individual. Another test for joint instability may be performed with the patient in a relaxed position on the examining table, lying on the back with the arm elevated directly overhead. Pressure is then exerted on the back of the humeral head, thereby pushing it forward. Often the patient with instability in the shoulder joint will resist this movement, stating that it feels as if the shoulder is about to go out of place. Additional physical tests are described with specific pathologic entities in the following sections.

Neurologic Testing

There are no motor reflexes about the shoulder joint. However, a sensory examination should be carried out over the entire shoulder, including the area of the anterior and posterior chest, upper arm, and lateral chest wall. The simplest way to do this is to use a pin or pinwheel type of sensory testing device.

In general, the cervical nerve roots supplying sensation to the shoulder cap include the C4 root on the top of the shoulder, extending in a capelike fashion anteriorly and posteriorly to include the C5 root, and more distally (pectoral area in front and the scapular area behind) the C6 root (see Fig. 2-4).

The only peripheral nerve with its own area of innervation in the shoulder area is the axillary nerve. Because this nerve may be injured in shoulder dislocations, it is very important to examine for this autonomous zone before reducing the dislocation.

The small autonomous zone of sensory innervation from the axillary nerve is found in a band about 2 inches wide, beginning about an inch below the acromion, running from posterolateral to anterolateral (Fig. 4-7).

Diagnostic Guidelines

The examiner should obtain an A/P shoulder x-ray at the initial visit to rule out tumor, infection, or arthritis of the acromioclavicular joints. Additional x-rays should include external and internal views to exclude calcification and, if dislocation is suspected, an axillary view. If neck motion produces shoulder pain, the examiner should obtain cervical spine films.

Shoulder Problems in the Newborn and Early Childhood

Shoulder problems in the newborn usually relate to the delivery process or to congenital abnormalities. *Fracture of the clavicle* is seen at times after a difficult delivery when, either coincidentally, or intentionally, the clavicle is fractured. There may be swelling over the fracture or pain on motion of the extremity. The neonate may actually splint the arm, giving the appearance of a "pseudoparalysis."

The rapid healing potential of the newborn stabilizes this fracture within a matter of 10 days. Before that time, gentle handling of the extremity is all that is necessary in terms of treatment. The clavicle remodels quickly, and there should be no residual deformity.

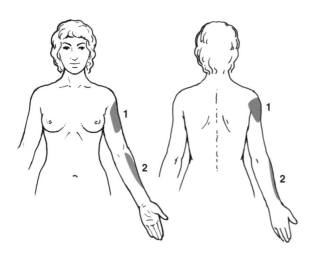

FIGURE 4-7. Area of sensory loss following injury to (**1**) axillary nerve, (**2**) musculocutaneous nerve.

Brachial Plexus Injury (Obstetric Brachial Palsy)

Another shoulder problem related to a difficult delivery is an injury to the brachial plexus of nerves that forms from the cervical nerve roots. These injuries are of two basic types, depending on which elements of the brachial plexus are injured. The *upper arm paralysis* is known as *Erb-Duchenne paralysis.* In this paralysis, the large muscles around the shoulder and upper arm are often paralyzed, due to involvement of the fifth and sixth cervical nerve roots or their derivatives. *Klumpke paralysis* involves the lower portion of the brachial plexus. In this type of paralysis, the hand and finger muscles are paralyzed, leaving the shoulder and elbow muscles intact.

Occasionally, the entire brachial plexus is involved in the birth injury, leaving a flaccid paralysis of the entire upper extremity. The treatment involves first diagnosing the condition and differentiating it from the "pseudoparalysis" produced by a clavicular fracture. At that point, attention should be paid to making sure no harm comes to the upper extremity in handling the child because of the motor paralysis (ie, inadvertent fractures or dislocations). After that, daily passive stretching exercises and splinting at times (for hand deformities) are necessary.

The prognosis, of course, depends on the severity of the injury. Occasionally, the patient will completely recover. More likely, however, there will be some residual weakness that will persist into later childhood. It is at this latter stage that definitive treatment in the form of muscle transfer operations can be carried out.

Sprengel's Deformity

A congenital deformity of the shoulder, known as Sprengel's deformity, occurs rarely. In this deformity the scapula does not descend into its normal position, and the patient has an abnormally small, elevated scapula with some limitation of motion of the shoulder. There is an associated congenital abnormality of the cervical spine at times.

This deformity is often difficult to diagnose in the neonatal period. Therefore, the most likely time that the primary care provider will see this deformity is in early childhood, when the parents realize that there is something wrong with the appearance of the child's shoulder.

The diagnosis is apparent on observation and confirmed by x-ray (a small, elevated scapula on one side compared with a normal-sized scapula in proper position on the opposite side). There is no immediate treatment necessary. The child should be referred to an orthopedic surgeon for definitive operative care.

The Adolescent With Shoulder Pain

The main difference between the adolescent and the adult shoulder is the presence of growth centers in the former. The three growth centers in the proximal humerus—humeral head, greater tuberosity, and lesser tuberosity—do not fuse until approximately age 20. Therefore, in any traumatic injury to the adolescent shoulder, consideration must be given to fracture or avulsion through these cartilaginous plates; comparative x-ray views of both shoulders are mandatory. Common nontraumatic and traumatic conditions of the shoulder are listed in Table 4-1.

TABLE 4-1
Shoulder Problems Across the Ages

Traumatic	Nontraumatic
Adolescents	
Shoulder separation (acromioclavicular joint)	Overuse syndrome (tendinitis)
Shoulder dislocation (glenohumeral joint)	Infection (septic arthritis and osteo-
Fracture of clavicle	myelitis)
Fracture of proximal humeral epiphysis	Monoarticular arthritis (juvenile
	rheumatoid arthritis)
	Malignant tumor
Adults	
Rotator cuff tear	Impingement syndrome
Avulsion greater tuberosity	Calcific tendinitis
Rupture biceps tendon	Bicipital tendinitis
Comminuted fracture of proximal humerus	Frozen shoulder syndrome
Mature Adults	
Impacted fracture (proximal humerus)	Cervical radiculopathy
Hand-shoulder syndrome	Degenerative arthritis
	Degenerative tendinitis

Nontraumatic Conditions

Overuse Syndrome (Tendinitis)

Overuse syndrome is seen in sports-minded adolescents, particularly those requiring vigorous training conditions such as high school baseball (pitching), tennis, and swimming. Typically, the shoulder ache or pain is only produced on elevation beyond 90 degrees. Point tenderness is common over the biceps tendon and rotator cuff immediately beneath the acromion anteriorly.

Treatment is rest, ice after use, and gradual return to sports participation with observation by a coach or trainer who has been alerted to the adolescent's problem. The child should not return to sports activities until he or she has a full range of motion of the shoulder joint, without pain. This may take several weeks. Treatment and rehabilitation entail stretching exercises after the inflammation has settled down and certainly requires a warm-up period before each participation in sports activities, once the child is ready to resume these activities.

Infection

Signs of shoulder infection are severe pain (particularly on any motion of the shoulder joint), increased local temperature, systemic fever, and, occasionally, swelling. Diagnosis is made by physical examination and aspiration of the joint with Gram's stain and culture of the aspirate. If there is suspicion of infection, the patient should be immediately referred to an orthopedic specialist.

The early differentiation between septic arthritis and osteomyelitis of the proximal humerus with a secondary effusion of the shoulder capsule may be impossible. An early sterile shoulder aspirate and, after several days, elevation of the proximal humeral periosteum on x-ray, indicating osteomyelitis, may help to separate the conditions. Treatment is the use of appropriate antibiotics (determined by culture and usually given intravenously, at least in the early stages of treatment). Drainage of pus from the joint and surgical drainage of pus from the medullary canal are secondary treatment modalities.

Aspiration of the Shoulder Joint

The shoulder joint can be aspirated, either from an anterior or posterior approach. In addition, it may be necessary to aspirate the region of the subacromial bursa. This is done laterally by palpating the edge of the acromion, which is subcutaneous, and placing the needle just under this edge. This is the area where calcific tendinitis is often aspirated and injected. In addition, it is the area where corticosteroid injections and local anesthetic injections may be placed, either for diagnosis or treatment of rotator cuff tendinitis.

Anterior aspiration of the shoulder joint is performed just below and lateral to the palpable coracoid process. First, palpate the tip of the coracoid; drop one fingerbreadth below and lateral to the coracoid and place the needle at this point. The needle should penetrate the capsule of the shoulder joint, between the humeral head and the glenoid. When the capsule is distended by fluid (pus, in the case of septic arthritis, or sterile effusion, in the case of osteomyelitis), the aspiration is fairly easy. When there is no excess fluid, it often requires a certain amount of skill and dexterity to place the needle into the shoulder capsule without striking either the humeral head or the glenoid.

The posterior approach to the shoulder joint for aspiration is performed a fingerbreadth below the acromion posteriorly, where there is a natural indentation in the muscle. This spot is just below the point of the acromion posterolaterally. Again, some skill is needed to place the needle between the glenoid and the humeral head if the joint is not distended with fluid.

Another area where injections are often made into the shoulder area is just below the acromion, anteriorly, between the humeral head and the acromion. This is the area where the biceps tendon and the rotator cuff come together and is often the site of painful tendinitis. An injection in this area of a combination of local anesthetic and steroid compound can act as both a diagnostic and a therapeutic injection (Fig. 4-8).

Monoarticular arthritis (juvenile rheumatoid arthritis) involving the shoulder presents with less pain and fever than septic arthritis. An elevated sedimentation rate may be the only positive laboratory finding. Referral to a pediatrician or rheumatologist is necessary for long-term treatment.

Malignant Tumor

Malignant tumor (osteosarcoma) is usually considered after a shoulder x-ray reveals either a lytic lesion in the proximal humeral bone or periosteal new bone in a young person who complains of a vague pain for some time (weeks or several months).

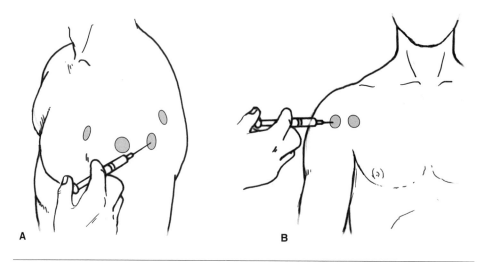

FIGURE 4-8. Sites used for injection of the shoulder (corticosteroid and local anesthetic). (**A**) Front to back—biceps tendon, supraspinatous (rotator cuff), subacromial bursa, joint capsule posteriorly. (**B**) Long and short head of biceps tendon—inject parallel to the tendon after penetrating the skin and subcutaneous tissue.

There may be a history of relative minor trauma. The physical examination may not be revealing, or it may find localized swelling and tenderness. Immediate referral to a specialist (orthopedic surgeon or oncologist) is mandatory. These malignancies spread rapidly and are often fatal.

Benign Tumor

Many benign tumorous conditions may appear on routine x-ray and cause concern. These conditions may often be recognized on routine chest x-rays. Benign bone cysts, enchondromas, bone islands, and fibrous cysts all give an abnormal appearance on x-ray but are symptom free. These findings, of course, should be referred to an orthopedic surgeon who specializes in bone tumors or a pediatric orthopedic surgeon.

Pain associated with any of these benign lesions often means that a fracture has occurred through the lesion. Under ordinary circumstances, unless the fracture involves a major portion of the proximal humerus, simple splinting is all that is needed for healing and return of normal function.

Rarely, a benign tumor will cause a painful condition without fracture. An *osteoid osteoma* is such a tumor. This unusual tumorous condition causes severe night pain, which is specifically relieved by aspirin or aspirin-containing substances. The typical appearance of a osteoid osteoma is that of a hole in the bone with a dense bull's-eye in the center of the hole, as seen on x-ray. Any such finding, of course, requires referral to an orthopedic surgeon because surgical ablation is the only known cure for this condition.

Traumatic Conditions

Most traumatic injuries in the adolescent are related to sports or recreational activities. Such injuries are usually treated on an emergency basis with x-ray facilities and referral services immediately available.

Shoulder Separation

A shoulder separation is an injury to the acromioclavicular joint produced by a downward force on the point of the shoulder. This injury occurs from a fall or a direct blow to the shoulder. The damage to the joint that results depends on the force of the blow and ranges from a sprain to a complete dislocation. Physical findings range from moderate point tenderness over the acromioclavicular joint to an elevated unstable distal clavicle. The injuries are classified as grades I through IV: grade I is a partial tear of the acromioclavicular ligament, grade II is a complete ligament tear, grade III includes the addition of a coracoclavicular ligament tear, and grade IV is an unstable, irreducible grade III injury. The grade III acromioclavicular joint separation with ligament rupture represents 90% to 95% of all dislocations. X-ray evaluation is performed with and without the patient holding hand weights in the upright position. Both shoulders are examined and compared; the subluxing or dislocated joint will be obvious when compared with the uninjured shoulder (Figs. 4-9 and 4-10).

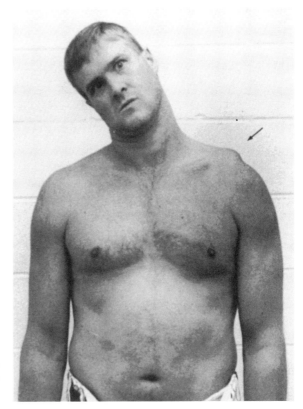

FIGURE 4-9. Grade III sprain of the acromioclavicular joint.

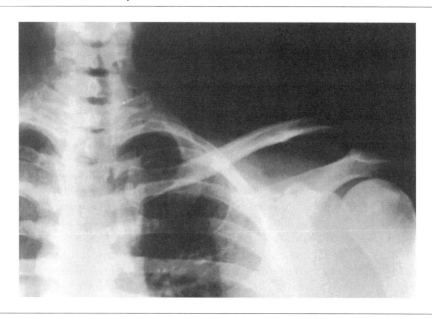

FIGURE 4-10.   Radiographic view of grade III sprain of acromioclavicular joint. (From Marone, P. J. [1992]. *Shoulder injuries in sports* [p. 82]. Rockville, MD: Aspen.)

Treatment

For all except the grade IV injury, treatment is conservative: ice, sling immobilization, and mild analgesia. Surgery rarely is necessary for these injuries. The patient, however, should be referred to an orthopedic surgeon. There is controversy as to whether open surgery, pinning the dislocated joint in place, gives better results than the natural course of conservative care. The surgeon and patient will have to decide this for each individual case.

The grade IV injury, or irreducible dislocation, requires surgery to avoid skin breakdown over the distal clavicle. In conservative care, immobilization is necessary for approximately 3 weeks, with an additional 3 weeks of range-of-motion and strengthening exercises.

Shoulder Dislocation

Anterior shoulder dislocation (glenohumeral joint) represents 90% to 95% of all dislocations that result from a strong blow to the back of the joint with the arm elevated. The humeral head ruptures the anterior capsule and comes to rest anterior and inferior to the glenoid, producing an abnormal anterior prominence and flattening the posterior shoulder contour. The patient initially is in severe pain, but with the arm at the side the pain is reduced, only to be reactivated by any movement of the shoulder. X-ray evaluation is done primarily to rule out a fracture and confirm the diagnosis. To determine if the axillary nerve has been damaged, it is important to perform a sensory test over the shoulder before any attempt at reduction. Stimson's reduction maneuver may be attempted with relative safety. The patient is placed prone on an examining table with the affected limb hanging over the side with 5- to 10-lb weights strapped to the involved hand. Reduction should occur within 15 to 20 minutes. If reduction cannot be achieved even with light analgesia or muscle relaxation, the arm should be replaced in a sling and immediate consultation obtained with an orthopedic surgeon for possible reduction and general anesthesia. If reduction is successful, the arm may be immobilized in a sling or shoulder immobilizer for 3 weeks with an additional 3 weeks for protected use of the arm and range-of-motion exercises.

Often, the anterior shoulder dislocation produces a tear in the glenoid labrum anteriorly, where the middle humeral ligament attaches. Recent studies utilizing arthroscopy have shown that up to 50% of these lesions (*Bankart lesions*) do not heal completely after the shoulder dislocation is reduced in young athletes. This leads to recurrent subluxation and dislocation in later life. Therefore, there is some controversy as to whether this lesion should be repaired if it is detected arthroscopically in these individuals. This repair usually requires two operative procedures: (1) an arthroscopic diagnostic procedure and (2) an open repair of the Bankart lesion. (Arthroscopic repairs of the Bankart lesion are possible to perform, but do not give as good a result as the open repair.) Obviously, this is a decision for the treating orthopedic surgeon to make after referral from the acute care setting.

Recurrent Shoulder Dislocation or Subluxation

THE SLAP LESION

In addition to the anterior glenoid tear (Bankart lesion), arthroscopic surgery has identified a series of tears involving the superior glenoid labrum at the attachment of the biceps tendon. This has been called the SLAP lesion (superior labrum anterioposterior). This lesion is often seen in adolescent or adult baseball pitchers or after a traumatic episode in which the patient falls on an outstretched arm, or falls and grabs hold of an object, and then supports the body weight with one arm. The injury creates an element of tendinitis and synovitis and a slight tendency toward instability of the humeral head in the glenoid.

Smaller lesions can be treated by rest, anti-inflammatory drugs, and stretching exercises. Larger lesions, or those that are not relieved by conservative care, need arthroscopic surgery. There is literally no way to diagnose this condition without an arthroscopic evaluation.

Occasionally, a child or young adult with a history of prior shoulder dislocation will complain that the shoulder redislocates with the arm elevated and externally rotated (sleeping position or throwing position). Usually, individuals learn to relocate the humeral head themselves, but if they complain of this problem, they should be referred to an orthopedic surgeon for consideration of an open repair of the torn capsule and glenoid labrum.

Even more rare is the young person who demonstrates the voluntary ability to sublux or even dislocate the humeral head. These individuals sometimes need psychological support, but they too should be referred to the orthopedic surgeon for definitive care.

Clavicle Fracture

A fracture of the clavicle may result from a direct blow to, or a fall on, the shoulder. Often the injury is sustained by "piling on" in athletic endeavors such as football and rugby. The physical findings are local pain, swelling, and painful shoulder motion. X-rays confirm the injury and determine the degree of displacement, angulation, and possible comminution. If the fracture occurs distal to the coracoid process and the coracoclavicular ligament, the fracture is unstable and orthopedic consultation should be obtained immediately. Cyanosis of the upper extremity indicates vascular compromise and demonstrates the necessity for emergency reduction, possibly by open means.

Treatment of the simple fracture is by means of the figure-of-eight clavicular strap that maintains the shoulder in extension for 6 to 8 weeks. Frequent adjustment of the strap must be made during the treatment period to avoid skin breakdown and to maintain reduction (Fig. 4-11).

Proximal Humeral Fracture

A *fracture of the proximal humerus* in an adolescent may result from a fall on the outstretched arm (either forward or behind the body axis) or on the point of the elbow. It often causes injury to, or displacement through, the epiphyseal growth plate at the base of the humeral head. Pain, swelling, and limitation of motion are the physical findings. X-ray evaluation of both shoulders should be performed to determine any change in the position of the ossified bone on either side of the growth plate. If no fracture is identified but the pain is severe, consider a crush injury to the growth plate and immobilize the limb in a sling for 3 to 4 weeks. Follow-up x-rays may reveal callus about the growth plate injury.

Displaced epiphyseal injuries require reduction only if they are severe. Closed reduction with moderate prolonged downward traction may be successful in restoring satisfactory alignment. Open reduction and internal fixation are rarely necessary.

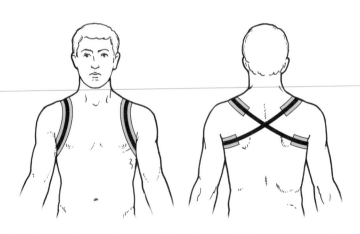

FIGURE 4-11. Figure-of-eight harness for clavicular fracture.

The Adult With Shoulder Pain

Nontraumatic Conditions

Impingement Syndrome

The impingement syndrome presents as tenderness over the anterior shoulder, beneath the acromion, on elevation of the shoulder beyond 90 degrees. The patient usually seeks help only after the condition has been present for several weeks. X-rays are negative. The patient usually describes some repetitive work or sports activity that aggravates the condition.

The etiopathology of the condition may be complex, containing elements of one or more local inflammatory or degenerative conditions within the confined space beneath the acromioclavicular arch. Bicipital and rotator cuff tendinitis and acromioclavicular joint synovitis may be present in varying degrees, causing local swelling and painful compression of inflamed tissues on reaching overhead (Fig. 4-12).

Treatment is rest and sling immobilization with the use of salicylates or nonsteroidal anti-inflammatory agents. If these measures do not alleviate the problem, referral is indicated for possible steroid injection. A single injection of corticosteroids into the anterior subacromial space may be helpful. Gradual rehabilitation over several weeks, including gentle stretching and strengthening exercises and instructions in avoiding frequent repetitive overhead activities, is usually efficacious in preventing a recurrence. Instruct athletes to warm up before overhead sports.

Calcific Tendinitis

Calcific tendinitis is a degenerative condition in which a "calcium boil" develops acutely in the rotator cuff (with a preexisting asymptomatic degenerative calcified tendinitis). The symptoms are severe, localized pain occurring virtually with any

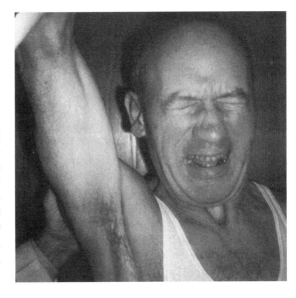

FIGURE 4-12. A positive impingement sign. The examiner's hand is on the superior scapula, and the affected arm is elevated in the overhead position. As the rotator cuff area contacts the coracoacromial arch, a reproduction of the pain is evident. Elimination of this pain with a subacromial injection of lidocaine solidifies the diagnosis.

movement of the shoulder. X-rays show a radiodense deposit, usually several milli-meters in diameter, just above the humeral head (Fig. 4-13). Treatment is rest, sling immobilization, and anti-inflammatory drugs. Often the use of a large-bore needle to puncture the boil and at times to aspirate some of the calcium-containing material, with the concomitant injection of a local anesthetic and corticosteroid compound, immediately relieves the patient.

Bicipital Tendinitis

Bicipital tendinitis is a local synovitis about the proximal portion of the long head of the biceps tendon in the bicipital groove of the humerus immediately proximal to the point where the tendon enters the glenohumeral joint, beneath the rotator cuff tendons. The clinical findings consist of local tenderness in the bicipital groove, pain in the shoulder on resisted elbow flexion and forearm supination, and pain on shoulder elevation.

Pathologic changes include degenerative tears of the tendon and overlying rotator cuff and at times an overly mobile tendon that easily subluxes in and out of the bicipital groove. Rest and anti- inflammatory drugs are the mainstays of treatment. A single injection of a steroid compound and a local anesthetic into the bicipital groove may give immediate and long-lasting relief.

Frozen Shoulder

The "frozen shoulder syndrome" is a complex phenomenon in which capsular thickening and adhesive capsulitis develop in response to a painful stimulus that causes the patient to limit shoulder motion for a prolonged period of time. Condi-tions such as cervical radiculopathy, diabetes mellitus, and angina pectoris may be associated with the onset of the problem. The patient presents with a history of gradually increasing pain and limitation of motion of the shoulder joint. Clinical findings include generalized shoulder pain on movement with restricted passive motion in several or all directions that are not present in the opposite shoulder.

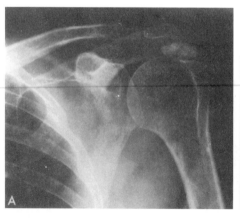
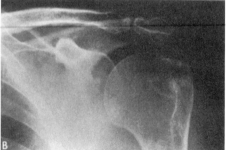

FIGURE 4-13. Calcific tendinitis.

Pathologic changes include a collagenous proliferation of the shoulder capsule, causing it to become thickened, adherent to the humeral head, and reduced in its intra-articular volume.

In most cases, the syndrome is self-limiting; with rest and gradual gentle rehabilitation, the condition will go through the phases of "freezing, frozen, and thawing" so that a normal painless range of motion is restored within a period of weeks or perhaps a few months. Often, however, the problem is of several months' duration when the patient presents and the continuing painful stimulus persists. In this case a full range of motion cannot be restored, even after careful rehabilitation. Under these circumstances the patient should be referred to an orthopedic surgeon for an "infiltration brisement" under general anesthesia. This procedure involves stretching the capsule with hydrostatic pressure from an intra-articular injection of saline, local anesthetic, and steroid compound and gently placing the shoulder through a full range of motion to restore capsular length. The procedure may be done on an outpatient basis.

Traumatic Conditions

Rotator Cuff Tear

Tear of the rotator cuff tendons is more likely to occur in an adult, secondary to the early degenerative changes that may be found—just proximal to the tendinous insertion to the greater tuberosity. The injury is produced during a fall if the patient puts out a hand to break the fall and the weight of the body causes the arm to collapse while the tendon is under tension. The tear may be incomplete through the tendon, complete but small (a few millimeters in length), or large (several centimeters in length). The supraspinatus tendon is frequently involved. The immediate symptoms are pain that may get worse as swelling occurs and an inability to raise the arm, particularly away from the side of the body (abduction).

X-rays may be negative or may show a humeral head resting lower in the glenoid than in the opposite shoulder. Pain on motion and point tenderness over the anterolateral humeral head are the early physical findings. Several days or weeks later, loss of scapulohumeral rhythm, pain on elevation beyond 45 degrees, and weakness in abduction against resistance are prominent findings. Usually, the patient's arm can be elevated passively to 180 degrees, but upon lowering the arm to 90 degrees the patient loses control and the arm falls painfully to the side. If the tear is small, treatment with rest, immobilization, and anti-inflammatory agents, with gradual rehabilitation to full functional use over a period of several weeks to several months, can be prescribed. Larger tears result in permanent pain and weakness. The extent of the tear may be determined by several diagnostic procedures, some noninvasive, some invasive. When properly done, *ultrasonography* compares the normal and injured shoulder, often diagnosing a tear and giving some idea as to its size (Fig. 4-14). *Computed tomography (CT)* and magnetic resonance imaging (MRI; Fig. 4-15) are two additional noninvasive diagnostic studies. Invasive studies include *shoulder arthrography* and *arthroscopy*. Arthrography is performed by a radiologist and involves injecting dye into the shoulder joint. The leakage of the radiopaque dye into the subdeltoid bursa is demonstrated on an x-ray and is diagnostic of a tear. Arthroscopy is performed by an orthopedic surgeon under general anesthesia

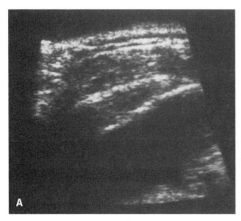
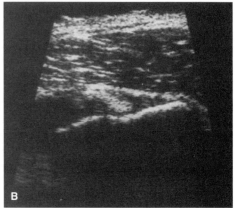

FIGURE 4-14. (**A**) A normal shoulder ultrasound. The rotator cuff layer is seen adjacent to the dark bone of the humeral head. The supraspinatus is seen to taper toward its insertion on the greater tuberosity. (**B**) With a torn rotator cuff, the layer of supraspinatus tapering toward the greater tuberosity is absent. There is an echogenic focus, which is the torn edge of tendon. In addition, the deltoid sags to fill in the area left vacant by the torn rotator cuff.

and allows for direct observation and surgical debridement of the tear. Surgical repair of larger tears requires an open operation, followed by several months of rehabilitation.

Greater Tuberosity Avulsion Injury

An avulsion injury to the greater tuberosity occurs through the same mechanism as the rotator cuff tear. Instead of the tendon giving way, however, a piece of the

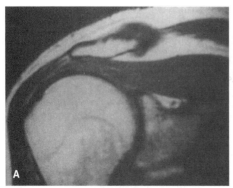
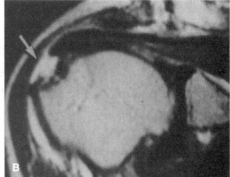

FIGURE 4-15.   Magnetic resonance image of (**A**) normal shoulder rotator cuff and (**B**) a complete rotator cuff tear (*arrow*).

bony attachment of the tendon is pulled away. If the avulsed fragment on x-ray is large and with minimal displacement, it may be allowed to heal in place. If the fragment is significantly elevated out of its normal bed or a small fragment is pulled into an intra-articular position, the fragment will permanently affect shoulder joint function; therefore, an open operation for repair is required.

Ruptured Biceps Tendon

Rupture or a complete tear of the long head of the biceps tendon may occur upon rapid overuse of this partially degenerated tendon, such as in a failed attempt to raise a stuck window or an overhead door. The tendon may rupture intra-articularly or, more typically, extra-articularly, producing immediate pain and swelling. A deformity of the shortened biceps muscle is immediately noticeable. Treatment can be conservative or operative. Conservative care results in almost normal function with a slightly weakened and permanently deformed biceps muscle. Operative repair may produce an excellent result in terms of function, but surgical complications may mar the result and the final outcome may be worse than if the injury had been treated nonoperatively.

Comminuted Fracture of the Proximal Humerus

The comminuted fracture, or four-part fracture of the proximal humerus, may be one of the most difficult injuries to treat about the shoulder joint. After x-ray evaluation, the injury must be referred to an orthopedic surgeon. The problem with this injury is that the fracture line at the base of the humeral head may cut off all vascular supply. Therefore, no matter what the treatment, closed or open, the result may be avascular necrosis of the head of the humerus, requiring prosthetic joint replacement.

Recurrent Shoulder Dislocation or Subluxation

Dislocation of the glenohumeral joint may produce a tear in the glenoid labrum—the so-called Bankart lesion. This lesion causes instability and recurrent anterior dislocation or subluxation, the latter causing a sudden feeling of loss of function ("dead arm syndrome").

The physical examination demonstrates a sudden click or clunk on elevation and external rotation of the shoulder. Even if a click is not significant, the patient develops an "apprehension sign" with the arm overhead, complaining that the shoulder feels like it is about to dislocate.

The x-ray is an important diagnostic feature in the condition. The view of the humeral head in internal rotation often reveals a posterolateral V-shaped or "hatchet" defect, the so-called *Hill-Sachs lesion*. Treatment requires strengthening of the shoulder internal rotator muscles, particularly the subscapularis. This can be accomplished with a simple loop of rubber tubing. The patient should be counseled to avoid overhead activities. If conservative treatment fails, the patient should be referred for operative treatment.

Posterior Dislocation of the Glenohumeral Joint

A rare (less than 2% of glenohumeral dislocations) and often difficult-to-diagnose traumatic condition is the posterior glenohumeral dislocation. The most common etiology is a seizure state or the use of electroshock therapy. Occasionally, the patient sustains a strong blow to the front of the shoulder with the humeral head in maximum internal rotation. The humeral head ruptures the posterior joint capsule and dislocates posteriorly.

The physical examination shows a patient in obvious pain holding the arm at the side. External rotation is particularly painful. In contrast to the examination in the anterior dislocation, in this examination a bulge (the dislocated humeral head) is palpated posteriorly and a loss of shoulder contour is noted anteriorly.

X-ray evaluation is critical. The anteroposterior view may be interpreted as normal. Only the axillary view can demonstrate the position of the humeral head posterior to the glenoid. There may also be an impaction-type fracture of the humeral head as the posterior lip of the glenoid creates a V-shaped defect in the anterior aspect of the head (reverse Hill-Sachs lesion; Fig. 4-16).

Treatment requires traction and an external rotation maneuver (as opposed to internal rotation in the anterior dislocation). This maneuver should be carried out by an orthopedic surgeon and often requires general anesthesia.

Immobilization and rehabilitation are similar to that required for an anterior dislocation except that the arm is immobilized at the side (holster position) and strengthening of the shoulder external rotators is stressed, rather than the internal rotator muscles.

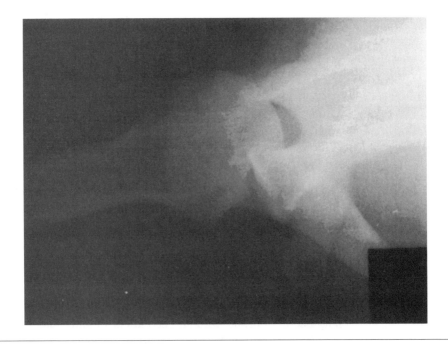

FIGURE 4-16. Radiographic view of posterior shoulder dislocation.

The Mature Adult With Shoulder Pain

Nontraumatic shoulder problems in the elderly are usually caused by degenerative conditions. Degenerative disc and joint disease of the cervical spine may refer pain to the shoulder (a manifestation of cervical radiculopathy). The pain may be produced by the elevation of the shoulder and may be associated with a tendinitis-type syndrome of the rotator cuff (Fig. 4-17). In addition, there is a strong association between cervical radiculopathy and the frozen shoulder syndrome. It may be extremely difficult to differentiate referred cervical radicular pain to the shoulder from primary tendinitis. If the pain radiates from the shoulder upward into the neck, or if it radiates from the shoulder downward toward the elbow, the examiner should consider the possibility that it is radicular pain rather than primary pain from the shoulder joint. A cervical spine x-ray and a shoulder x-ray should be taken (Fig. 4-18). A complete neurologic examination of the upper extremity should be performed, and a range-of-motion examination of the cervical spine and shoulder should be performed to make this diagnosis.

Treatment must be directed toward both the shoulder and the cervical spine (range-of-motion exercises, cervical traction, and anti-inflammatory drugs). Often an electromyogram (EMG) will confirm the presence of cervical radiculopathy.

Osteoarthritic degeneration of the acromioclavicular and glenohumeral joints and degenerative tendinitis are common ailments that cause shoulder pain (Fig. 4-19). Palpation of areas of point tenderness can detect the areas of involvement. Treatment is rest, anti-inflammatory drugs, and gradual rehabilitation with active assisted exercises and then stretching exercises.

Occasionally, a well-placed injection of local anesthetic and a steroid compound will act as both a diagnostic test (immediate pain relief) and a therapeutic treatment for this condition. Longstanding and disabling conditions should be referred to an orthopedic surgeon.

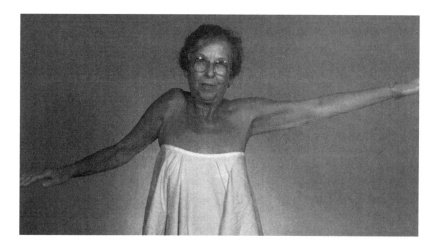

FIGURE 4-17. A patient with cuff tear arthropathy of the right shoulder. The patient has little ability to elevate the arm above shoulder level because of a severe massive rotator cuff tear.

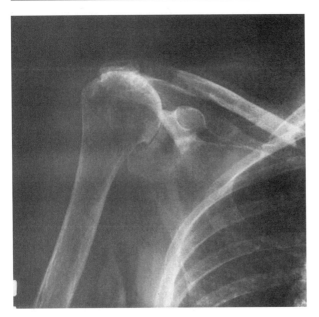

FIGURE 4-18. Radiographic appearance of cuff tear arthropathy. Because of the loss of the depressor activity of the rotator cuff (due to a massive rotator cuff tear), there is high riding of the humeral head, which directly articulates with the undersurface of the acromion. There is narrowing of the glenohumeral joint as well.

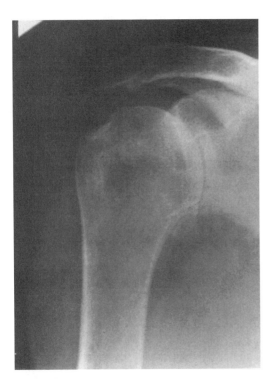

FIGURE 4-19. Primary osteoarthritis of the shoulder. There is joint space narrowing, sclerosis of the humeral head, and a large inferior osteophyte, which is a classic radiographic finding. The osteophyte is, in fact, circumferential.

Rarely, a malignant pulmonary tumor in the apex of the lung (Pancoast tumor) is the source of shoulder pain. A normal chest x-ray usually rules out this condition. If any questions concerning the chest film arise, the patient should be immediately referred to a pulmonary specialist or thoracic surgeon.

Traumatic Conditions

Falls on the shoulder or elbow often cause impacted fractures in the osteoporotic bone of the proximal humerus. These injuries, diagnosed by x-ray, cause severe pain and limitation of motion. Treatment requires a brief 10-day immobilization and gradual remobilization of the shoulder. If complete immobilization is maintained too long, full range of motion may never be restored.

At times, after an injury to the upper extremity, such as a Colles' fracture, the patient will complain of shoulder pain. In addition, the rehabilitation of the injured part (wrist, hand, or forearm) becomes complicated by pain, stiffness, and persistent swelling. This is the "hand-shoulder syndrome." The etiology of this problem is related to a reflex sympathetic dystrophy involving cervical nerve root irritation and peripheral autonomic neurovascular responses. There is often an underlying cervical radiculopathy that is unrecognized by the patient before the trauma. Treatment must be gentle, prolonged, and directed at all involved areas—neck, shoulder, and peripheral joints. Hand-shoulder syndrome is extremely difficult to treat. It requires a great deal of patience in therapy, along with psychotropic drugs and, often, psychological couseling because of the severe pain.

Rehabilitation of the Injured Shoulder

Three words describe the major goal of a rehabilitation program for the injured shoulder: motion! motion! and motion! Only after a full, or nearly full, range of motion is restored should the patient begin to rehabilitate the shoulder musculature for strength.

An appreciation of the capsular structure of the shoulder joint (lax and redundant with the arm at the side, and taut in the overhead position) is pivotal to successful rehabilitation. With injury comes post-traumatic synovitis and capsular fibrosis and shortening. This ruinous triad must be overcome to restore shoulder function to normal.

However, the problem is less critical in children and teenagers. Their tissues are flexible, heal rapidly, and patients are well motivated to return shoulder motion to normal to rejoin their playmates and athletic teams. On the other hand, adults and older individuals have a more difficult recovery. Their tissues are not flexible; they are usually not as well motivated to recover as children, and pain (involved to some extent in all rehabilitation programs) is not well tolerated.

Early Range-of-Motion Exercises

The program to restore normal shoulder motion should begin as soon as possible after the injury (or surgery). The onset of treatment depends on the stability of the joint tissues (fractures, dislocations, and surgical reconstruction). It also depends on the motivation of the patient, and factors such as fear and anxiety often need to be overcome by personal contact and encouragement.

In most cases, the injured shoulder, usually supported by a sling, can be moved within 24 to 72 hours of the injury. Immediately after the injury, the patient should be instructed to use the hand, wrist, and forearm as a "helping hand" in performing activities of daily living. Early shoulder motion begins in the sling with the so-called Codman exercises. These are performed by having the patient lean forward to allow the arm to hang free (with the elbow bent at 90 degrees). Gravity allows the shoulder to assume a position of 90 degrees of elevation (relative to the trunk of the body). This position eliminates the lax and redundant axillary pouch of the shoulder capsule.

From this relaxed "hung out" position, the patient is asked to begin making increasingly larger circles with the point of the elbow, first in one direction and then in the other. These exercises continue daily, at least temporarily, until the sling can be removed.

Without the sling, motion from 90 degrees to 180 degrees may be restored by two simple maneuvers. The patient is asked to stand at a door frame with both palms at shoulder height resting on the door frame. Then, using the fingertips, the patient climbs up and down the frame, allowing the friction between the fingertips and the frame to move the shoulder joint.

Gradually, the patient is encouraged to move closer to the door frame and stretch the shoulder structures to 180 degrees overhead. This maneuver must be carried out with both the injured and uninjured extremities to prevent the patient from "cheating" by tilting the trunk away from the door frame, thereby reducing effective capsular stretch.

The second maneuver is carried out with the patient lying flat on the back without a pillow. There must be enough overhead room to allow the noninjured limb to be raised 180 degrees to touch the resting surface. The patient then grasps the wrist of the injured limb with the noninjured hand and, using only the power of the noninjured extremity, lifts the injured arm upward. After 90 degrees of elevation is obtained, gravity aids the maneuver in bringing the arm from 90 degrees to 180 degrees. The arm is *always* brought back to the side by the normal extremity (see Appendix E).

Strengthening Exercises

After 180 degrees of elevation is achieved and stability of the joint or bone is assured (at approximately 3 to 4 weeks), more strenuous exercises may begin to rehabilitate tendons and muscles. Active, assisted range-of-motion exercises begin in flexion-extension, internal and external rotation, and adduction-abduction. Strengthening exercises using light (1- to 2-lb) weights, isometric strengthening, and the use of rubber tubing exercises are next in the rehabilitation program. Active stretching of a small (2-ft) loop of rubber tubing is an excellent strengthening exercise. The patient may hold the tubing in front of the body with the opposite hand or in back of the trunk while stretching, thereby strengthening the shoulder rotators. Attaching the loop to a hook or doorknob or looping it around the foot allows the patient to control strengthening of most of the shoulder muscles.

The patient should use weighted or hydraulic gymnastic equipment in the final stage of strengthening and rehabilitation.

Length of the Rehabilitation Program

As long as the program proceeds gradually and progressively, there is no time limit. Some patients may be completely rehabilitated in 3 to 6 weeks. Others, due to the complexity of the injury or surgical reconstruction or due to patient factors (low pain threshold, high-anxiety level, or poor motivation), may require 3 to 6 months or longer. In general, after 1 year of an adequate rehabilitation program, very little further improvement can be expected.

Conclusion

The shoulder conditions described in this chapter constitute the major shoulder problems seen by medical and nursing personnel in an outpatient setting. This chapter is not meant to be an exhaustive discourse on all shoulder conditions. The practitioner must know when to treat and when to refer the patient; the information provided in this chapter should aid in making this decision. The interested reader should refer to texts mentioned in the bibliography for further information.

Recommended Readings

Bateman, J. E. (1987). *The shoulder and neck.* Philadelphia W. B. Saunders.

DePalma, A. F. (1973). *Surgery of the shoulder.* Philadelphia: J. B. Lippincott.

Gloussemen, R. E. (1993). Instability versus impingement syndrome in the throwing athlete. *Orthopedic Clinics of North America, 24*(1), 29.

Hertling, D., & Kessler, R. M. (1996). *Management of common musculoskeletal disorders* (3rd ed.). Philadelphia: Lippincott-Raven.

Marone, P. J. (1992). *Shoulder injuries in sports.* Rockville, MD: Aspen.

Simon, W. H. (1989). The shoulder. In Gates, S. J., & Mooar, P. A. (Eds.). *Orthopaedics and sports medicine for nurses.* Baltimore: Williams & Wilkins.

Simon, W. H. (1975). Soft tissue disorders of the shoulder: frozen shoulder, calcific tendinitis, and bicipital tendinitis. *Orthopedic Clinics of North America, 6*(2), 521.

Snyder, S. J., Karzel, R. P., Del Pizzo, W., Ferkel, R. D., & Friedman, M. J. (1990). S.L.A.P. lesions of the shoulder. *Arthroscopy, 6*(4), 274.

Weinstein, S. L., & Buckwalter, J. A. (Eds.). (1994). *Turek's orthopaedics* (5th ed.). Philadelphia: J. B. Lippincott.

Yamaguchi, K., & Flatow, E. W. (1995). Arthroscopic evaluation and treatment of the rotator cuff. *Orthopedic Clinics of North America, 26*(4), 643.

Chapter 5

The Elbow and Forearm

Jeffrey L. Zilberfarb, MD

Functional Anatomy

Elbow

The elbow is a double hinge joint consisting of the humerus, ulna, and radius (Fig. 5-1). The spool-shaped trochlea of the humerus articulates with the trochlear notch of the ulna, and the capitellum of the humerus articulates with the head of the radius, thus allowing flexion and extension of the elbow and pronation and supination of the forearm. The elbow is enclosed by a relatively thin articular capsule.

The main stabilizer of the elbow is the triangular medial (ulna) collateral ligament attaching from the medial epicondyle of the humerus to the medial side of the olecranon of the ulna (Fig. 5-2). The lateral (radial) collateral ligament attaches from the lateral epicondyle of the humerus to the annular ligament of the ulna. The annular ligament surrounds the proximal radius, stabilizing the proximal radioulnar joint and allowing pronation and supination of the forearm. Three elbow bursa surround the elbow (Fig. 5-3). These bursa allow gliding between tissue planes. The posterior bursa over the olecranon may become infected after trauma to the posterior elbow (eg, a puncture wound or abrasion).

Forearm

The brachial artery crosses anterior to the elbow joint between the biceps tendon and the medial nerve to supply vascularity to the forearm and hand. After crossing the elbow, the brachial artery divides into the radial artery and, a short distance later, bifurcates into the ulnar artery and the common interosseous artery (Fig. 5-4).

The ulnar nerve passes through the cubital tunnel posterior to the medial humeral epicondyle as it enters the flexor carpi ulnaris. It then continues distally into the forearm deep to the flexor carpi ulnaris lying on the flexor digitorum profundus.

146

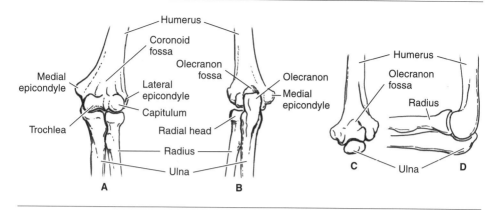

FIGURE 5-1.   The elbow joint. (**A**) Anterior view. (**B**) Posterior view. (**C**) Posterior view, 90 degrees flexion. (**D**) Lateral view.

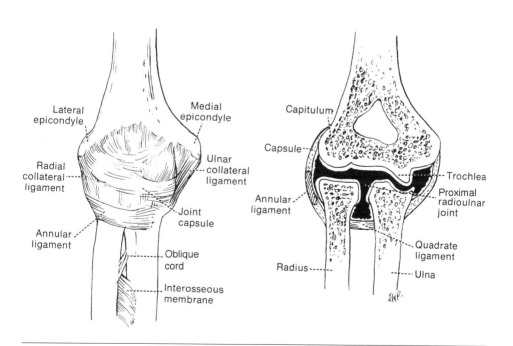

FIGURE 5-2.   The elbow joint: On the left, the joint capsule is shown with its associated ligaments. The coronal section of the joint on the right shows the relation of the proximal radioulnar joint to the elbow. Articular cartilage is shown as an *even white line;* synovial membrane as a *ruffled white line;* synovial fluid is *black.*

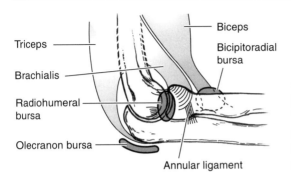

Triceps

Brachialis

Radiohumeral
bursa

Olecranon bursa

Biceps

Bicipitoradial
bursa

Annular ligament

FIGURE 5-3. Three elbow bursae. The lateral collateral ligament, and common extensor tendon have been reflected away to expose the radiohumeral bursa.

The median nerve leaves the upper arm through the antecubital fossa by passing between the two heads of the pronator teres to lie deep to the flexor digitorum superficialis. This nerve then continues distally between this muscle and the flexor digitorum profundus. In the forearm, it innervates the pronator teres, pronator quadratus, and all the finger and wrist flexors, except the flexor carpi ulnaris and the ulnar half of the flexor digitorum profundus, which are innervated by the ulnar nerve (see Fig. 5-4).

The flexor muscles of the forearm are divided into superficial and deep groups. The superficial group includes the pronator teres, flexor carpi radialis, and palmaris longus innervated by the median nerve, as well as the flexor carpi ulnaris innervated by the ulnar nerve. The superficial group originates from the medial epicondyle of the humerus. The deep group consists of the flexor pollicis longus, flexor digitorum profundus, and the pronator quadratus, all innervated by the median nerve except the ulnar half of the flexor digitorum profundus (ulnar nerve; see Fig. 5-4).

The flexors are separated from the extensors by the interosseous membrane, which passes between the radius and ulna. The extensor compartment (the dorsum of the forearm) contains the brachioradialis, extensor carpi radialis longus, extensor carpi radialis brevis, extensor digitorum communis, extensor digiti minimi, and extensor carpi ulnaris (Fig. 5-5). The deep extensor group is made up of the abductor pollicis longus, the extensor pollicis brevis and longus, and the extensor indicis proprius. All extensor muscles are supplied by the radial nerve (Table 5-1).

History and Physical Examination

A good diagnostician asks "Where, what, when, and how?" *Where* does it hurt—is the pain diffuse or localized, stationary or migratory? *What* caused the pain and what makes it better? *What* was the patient doing when the pain started or the injury occurred? *When* does it hurt? Tumors often ache at night, whereas arthritis is associated with early morning stiffness. Is the pain related to a particular activity such as pitching, or a particular position, or twisting motion? *When* did the injury occur? Was it at play, at home, or at work? Finally, *how* did the injury occur? Was the patient involved in an unusual or new activity?

Physical examination includes inspection, palpation, active and passive range of motion, ligament evaluation, manual muscle testing, sensory evaluation and vascular evaluation.

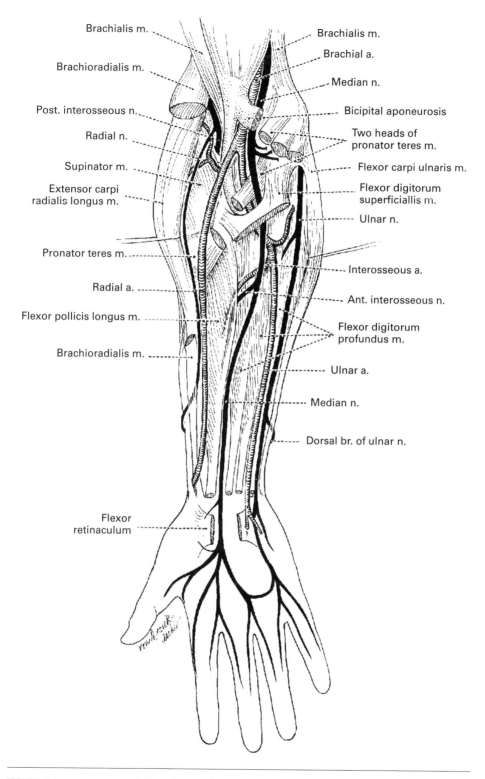

FIGURE 5-4. Anatomic relations in the forearm, showing the chief nerves and vessels in the anterior compartment.

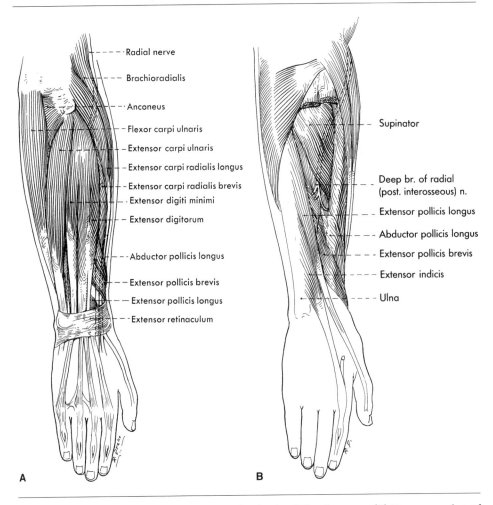

Radial nerve

Brachioradialis

Anconeus

Flexor carpi ulnaris

Extensor carpi ulnaris

Extensor carpi radialis longus

Extensor carpi radialis brevis

Extensor digiti minimi

Extensor digitorum

Abductor pollicis longus

Extensor pollicis brevis

Extensor pollicis longus

Extensor retinaculum

Supinator

Deep br. of radial
(post. interosseous) n.

Extensor pollicis longus

Abductor pollicis longus

Extensor pollicis brevis

Extensor indicis

Ulna

A   B

FIGURE 5-5. **(A)** The extensor muscles in the back of the forearm. **(B)** Deep muscles of the extensor group in the forearm.

INSPECTION. With the patient sitting or standing, begin with observation of the carrying angle. The normal arm should have a valgus (lateral) carrying angle of 5 to 15 degrees. More than 15 degrees valgus is called cubitus valgus, and a decrease in the angle to less than 5 degrees is called cubitus varus. Abnormalities in the carrying angle are usually the result of a supracondylar or other elbow fracture in early childhood. Inspect the skin for bruises, needle tracks, abrasions, scars, and swelling. Swelling occurs with inflammation, with joint effusions, and after trauma. A comparison with the opposite arm is useful for subtle cases. With an elbow effusion, there is loss of soft tissue contours. Bursae may also be swollen and appear as discrete soft tissue swelling; this is particularly true with the olecranon bursa. Ecchymosis with swelling is suggestive of fracture or dislocation. Loss of symmetry and soft tissue contours may be secondary to dislocation. This presents as a deformity with loss of motion.

TABLE 5-1

Summary of Movements of the Forearm, Wrist, and Hand, and Their Chief Controllers

Movement	Muscles	Nerves
Pronation of the forearm	Pronator teres Pronator quadratus	Median nerve Median nerve
Supination of the forearm	Supinator Biceps	Radial nerve Musculocutaneous nerve
Wrist flexion	Flexor carpi radialis Flexor carpi ulnaris Palmaris longus	Median nerve Ulnar nerve Median nerve
Wrist extension	Extensor carpi radialis longus Extensor carpi radialis brevis Extensor carpi ulnaris	Radial nerve Radial nerve Radial nerve
Radial deviation of the wrist	Abductor pollicis longus Extensor pollicis brevis Extensor carpi radialis longus and brevis	Radial nerve Radial nerve Radial nerve
Ulnar deviation of the wrist	Extensor carpi ulnaris Flexor carpi ulnaris	Radial nerve Ulnar nerve

Flexors of the thumb
  Interphalangeal joint
  Metacarpophalangeal joint
	Flexor pollicis longus
	Flexor pollicis brevis
		Median nerve
		Median nerve

Abduction of the thumb	Abductor pollicis longus Abductor pollicis brevis	Radial nerve Median nerve
Opposition of the thumb	Opponens pollicis	Median nerve
Adduction of the thumb	Adductor pollicis	Ulnar nerve

Extension of the thumb
  Interphalangeal joint
  Metacarpophalangeal joint
	Extensor pollicis longus
	Extensor pollicis brevis
		Radial nerve
		Radial nerve

Flexion of the fingers
  Distal interphalangeal joints
  Proximal interphalangeal joints
  Metacarpophalangeal joints
	Flexor digitorum profundus
	
	Flexor digitorum sublimis
	
	Interosseous muscles
	
	Lumbricals 1 and 2
	Lumbricals 3 and 4
	Flexor digiti minimi
		Median nerve and ulnar nerve
		Median nerve
		
		Ulnar nerve
		
		Median nerve
		Ulnar nerve
		Ulnar nerve

Abduction of the fingers	Dorsal interosseous muscles Abductor digiti minimi	Ulnar nerve Ulnar nerve
Adduction of the fingers	Palmar interosseous muscles	Ulnar nerve
Opposition of the 5th finger	Opponens digiti minimi	Ulnar nerve
Extension of the fingers	Extensor digitorum Extensor indicis Extensor digiti minimi	Radial nerve Radial nerve Radial nerve
Extension of interphalangeal joint while metacarpophalangeal joint is flexed	Lumbricals and palmar interosseous muscles	Median and ulnar nerves

From Ramamurti, C. P. (1979). In Tinker, R. V. (Ed.). *Orthopaedics in primary care*, p. 91. Baltimore: Williams & Wilkins.

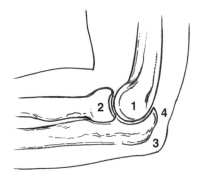

FIGURE 5-6. Common points of elbow tenderness: *1,* lateral epicondylitis; *2,* radial head fracture; *3,* olecranon bursitis; *4,* triceps tendinitis.

PALPATION. Palpate the entire elbow, attempting to localize any masses, swelling or warmth, or tenderness. Common points of lateral elbow tenderness and their associated conditions are shown in Figure 5-6. On the medial side, palpate the medial epicondyle, which is tender in medial epicondylitis (golfer's elbow). Palpate above the elbow to look for an enlarged epitrochlear node, present in infections and other inflammatory conditions. Posteriorly, palpate the olecranon, which may be tender if fractured, and the olecranon bursa, which is enlarged in bursitis. The triceps tendon insertion will be tender in triceps tendinitis.

RANGE OF MOTION. The elbow is moved actively and passively through a normal range of motion. Normal active range of motion of the elbow should be between 0 and 5 degrees extension to 135 degrees flexion, with approximately 90 degrees of pronation and supination (Fig. 5-7). Synovitis, an effusion, or a bony block (eg, a loose body) may cause a limitation of normal flexion or extension.

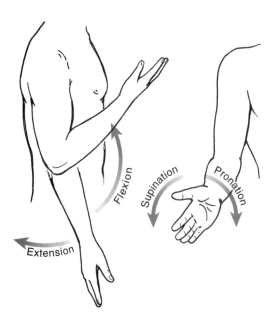

FIGURE 5-7. Range of motion of the elbow.

LIGAMENTOUS STABILITY. Evaluate the stability of the medial and lateral collateral ligaments. Cup one hand over the posterior aspect of the patient's elbow and hold the patient's wrist with the other. Instruct the patient to slightly flex the elbow. With the elbow flexed, force the forearm laterally. Note any "opening up" of the medial side, signifying medial collateral ligament instability. Always compare with the opposite arm (Fig. 5-8). Stress the elbow in the opposite direction to test for lateral collateral ligament instability.

MUSCLE TESTING. Apply resistance at the wrist as the patient flexes the elbow, testing biceps and brachioradialis muscle strength. Apply resistance on the dorsal aspect of the wrist as the patient extends the elbow, thus testing triceps muscle strength. Resisted supination assesses the biceps and supinator muscles, whereas resisted pronation assesses pronator teres and pronator quadratus strength. Muscle testing of the wrist and hand will be covered in the sections on the wrist and hand.

SENSORY EXAMINATION. Evaluation of the sensory portion of the radial, median, and ulnar nerves is shown in Figure 5-9.

VASCULAR EXAMINATION. Evaluate the distal pulses, capillary refill, and skin temperature.

Special Tests

TINEL'S SIGN. Tinel's sign is a sensation of electric shocks radiating into the hand when there is tapping over a nerve. In the elbow, this may occur at the ulnar nerve where it passes through the groove between the olecranon and the medial epicondyle (cubital tunnel). It may be due to neuroma formation or compression of the ulnar nerve as it passes around the elbow. Tinel's sign may also occur overlying the median nerve in the anterior elbow and forearm.

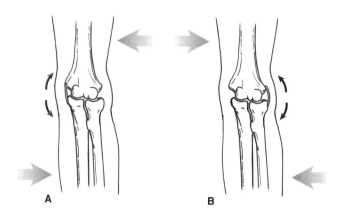

FIGURE 5-8. Test the integrity of ligaments by exerting medially and laterally directed pressure as shown. If the ligaments are ruptured, abnormal opening of the joint space will occur. (**A**) Medial collateral ligament stress test. (**B**) Lateral collateral ligament stress test.

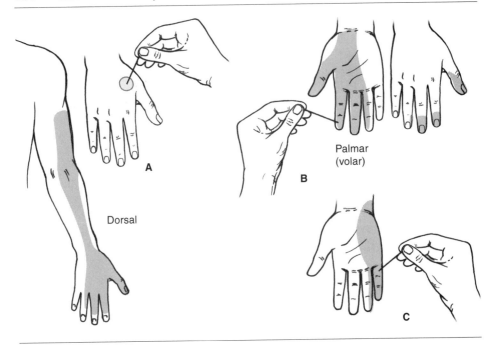

FIGURE 5-9.   Sensation radial (**A**), median (**B**), and ulnar (**C**) nerves.

TENNIS ELBOW TEST. Have the patient vigorously dorsiflex his or her wrist against your hand. If the patient has lateral epicondylitis (tennis elbow), there will be pain over the origin of the wrist extensor muscles at the lateral epicondyle of the humerus.

GOLFER'S ELBOW TEST. This is the opposite of the tennis elbow test. Have the patient vigorously palmar flex his or her wrist against your hand. If the patient has golfer's elbow, there will be pain at the origin of the wrist flexors at the medial epicondyle.

Diagnostic Guidelines

An AP and lateral elbow x-ray should be performed whenever a fracture, dislocation, loose body, or arthritis is suspected. Oblique views may be helpful if a small osteochondral fracture is suspected. Additionally, radiographs may detect an occult tumor that, although rare, otherwise might be missed.

Joint or bursal aspiration is helpful in diagnosing inflammatory conditions, such as infections, gout, or rheumatoid arthritis. Bursal aspiration technique is shown in Figure 5-10.

Children With Elbow Pain

Pain in the elbow of the throwing arm in young athletes is a common problem best exemplified by the baseball pitcher. A detailed history includes the precise location of the pain and exactly when the pain occurs (At rest? During the "cocking" phase

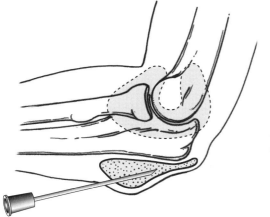

Enter at the base of the bursa, securing the needle in the subcutaneous tissue; advance the needle into the center of the bursa.

Needle: 1 1/2", 18 gauge

Depth: 3/8" to 1/2"

FIGURE 5-10.   Olecranon bursa aspiration. (Anderson, B. C. [1995]. *Office orthopedics for primary care.* Philadelphia: W. B. Saunders.)

of throwing? During the deceleration phase?). Referred pain to the forearm may indicate soft tissue inflammation or peripheral nerve irritation. Locking or catching may indicate loose bodies in the anterior or posterior compartment of the elbow. After exercise, recurrent swelling and stiffness of the elbow joint may indicate osteochondritis dissecans. A history of loss of range of motion is common and nonspecific. Stability should be checked with the elbow both in full extension and 45 degrees flexion. As was previously mentioned, medial stability is tested by applying a valgus stress to the forearm and comparing this with the opposite elbow. An abnormal amount of opening (laxity) to the elbow joint or an increase in pain should make one suspicious of an injury to the medial collateral ligament, which can occur in pitchers due to the extremely high valgus loads placed across the elbow in the acceleration phase of the throwing motion (Fig. 5-11).

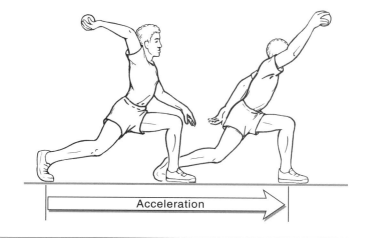

Acceleration

FIGURE 5-11.   Acceleration phase of the throwing motion.

If instability of the elbow is present, either acute or chronic, a referral should be made to an orthopedic surgeon for further evaluation and treatment. If left untreated, instability can result in the development of premature degenerative arthritis of the elbow joint. If the injury is acute, a long-arm posterior splint should be applied and an immediate referral made; if the injury is chronic, a splint may not be necessary, but the patient should still be referred for further evaluation.

Little Leaguer's Elbow (Panner's Disease)

Little leaguer's elbow is a lateral compression injury of the throwing elbow in young pitchers, often resulting in osteochondrosis of the capitellum. Ninety-eight percent of the patients are male. These injuries usually occur in the youngest, least experienced pitchers. The predisposing factors that increase the risk for injury are the unfused lateral humeral epiphysis and immature bones. The lateral epiphysis is the last to close in the elbow.

Patients usually complain of dull, achy elbow pain, often aggravated by throwing. Physical examination may reveal decreased range of motion and lateral elbow tenderness and swelling. X-rays may reveal sclerosis in the capitellum (Fig. 5-12). Initial treatment should consist of rest and anti-inflammatory medications. Patients should be referred to an orthopedic surgeon for follow-up.

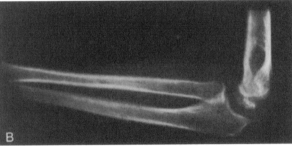
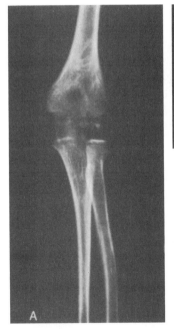

FIGURE 5-12. (**A**) AP view of the right elbow of a 9-year-old boy showing involvement of the entire capitellum in alternating irregular areas of sclerosis and patchy rarefaction. (**B**) Lateral view: osteochondrosis.

Prevention of elbow injuries is possible if weaknesses found in the preseason examination are corrected. Proper strengthening and flexibility exercises along with aerobic conditioning will decrease fatigue and build endurance. The young athlete must understand that the best protection for the pitching arm is a 12-month conditioning program. Proper warm-up before playing followed by gentle stretching and ice applied directly to the elbow after a game or practice are vital. Coaching techniques now limit the number of throws during practice and the number of curve balls during a game, and stress correct throwing mechanics. Instruct the athlete to do the same with pick-up games.

Osteochondritis Dissecans

In adolescents, osteochondritis dissecans, an inflammation of both bone and cartilage, may occur (Fig. 5-13).

Symptoms of dull, achy elbow pain aggravated by use are similar to those seen in younger patients with osteochondrosis of the capitellum. Loss of motion may also occur, along with tenderness and swelling along the lateral elbow. A computed

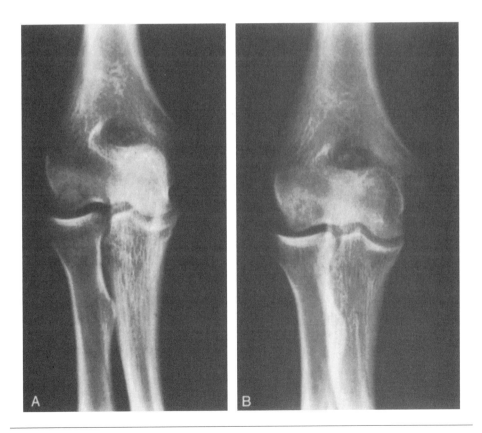

FIGURE 5-13. (**A**) AP view, type I lesion in a 14-year-old boy with osteochondritis dissecans. (**B**) AP view 1½ years later. The zone of rarefaction surrounding the lesion is becoming less distinct, and the patient is asymptomatic.

tomography (CT) scan, and possibly CT/arthrography, may provide additional diagnostic information.

Arthroscopic surgery may be indicated in those patients with partially or completely detached osteochondral lesions who do not respond to conservative treatment.

The Adult With Elbow Pain

Tennis Elbow (Lateral Epicondylitis)

This is the most common etiology of lateral elbow pain. It is an overuse injury of the origin of the wrist extensor tendons. Patients commonly complain of pain when lifting heavy objects against gravity, especially with the forearm pronated. They may also complain of pain when shaking hands. They are tender along the lateral epicondyle and have pain in this area with resisted wrist dorsiflexion. Radiographs are usually normal.

Treatment consists of decreasing the inflammation with rest, icing, and nonsteroidal medications, along with gentle wrist-stretching exercise. It is important to attempt to determine what activities may have led to the development of the syndrome (eg, carrying a heavy briefcase, using an improper tennis backhand, and so forth) so the patient can change this behavior. A tennis elbow brace is sometimes helpful. Iontophoresis or phonophoresis may help decrease inflammation. Once the inflammation has resolved, a gentle wrist extensor strengthening exercise program is begun (see Appendix E). Most patients improve after 4 to 6 weeks of treatment. One or two corticosteroid injections overlying the lateral epicondyle may be beneficial in those patients who fail this initial treatment. Inject 1 to 1.5 cc of 1% lidocaine with 0.5 cc corticosteroid (betamethasone is frequently used because of its high potency and long duration) superficial to, but not into, the tendon origin, so as not to risk tendon rupture (Fig. 5-14).

Surgical treatment is reserved for the rare, chronic patients (less than 5%) who

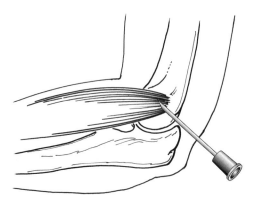

Enter directly over the prominence of the lateral epicondyle.

Needle: 1", 20 gauge

Depth: 1/4 to 3/8" subcutaneously

Volume: 1 to 1.5 ml of anesthetic; 0.5 ml corticosteroid

Note: NEVER inject under forced pressure or if the patient has a sharp pain (too deep); stretch the skin back and forth to ensure that the needle is above the tendon.

FIGURE 5-14. Lateral epicondylitis injection. (Anderson, B. C. [1995]. *Office orthopedics for primary care.* Philadelphia: W. B. Saunders.)

do not respond to this program. Surgical treatment consists of releasing the extensor carpus radialis brevis at its origin, removing damaged tissue, and repairing the lateral extensor origin. Success rates after surgery are greater than 90%.

Golfer's Elbow (Medial Epicondylitis)

This is a similar, but much less frequent, cause of elbow pain. In golfer's elbow, the pain is located at the medial aspect of the elbow, along the medial epicondyle. This is the origin of the wrist flexor musculature. It may occur in golfers who "snap their wrists" during their golf swing. As with tennis elbow, however, it is more commonly an overuse injury from some other activity, more often seen in nongolfers than golfers.

Treatment is similar to that for tennis elbow: modifying activities, decreasing inflammation, bracing, wrist flexor strengthening, and so forth. Golfers may want to have a golf professional observe their swing and make corrections as needed.

Olecranon Bursitis

Patients complain of pain and swelling along the posterior elbow. It is important to differentiate nonseptic versus septic bursitis. In nonseptic bursitis, patients are not febrile and present with olecranon bursa swelling without erythema. There is minimal tenderness to palpation. Range of motion is usually normal. In septic bursitis, patients usually are febrile and the elbow is swollen and extremely tender to palpation. Erythema overlies the bursa, and range of motion is usually restricted.

Bursal fluid aspiration should be performed and the fluid sent to the laboratory for Gram's stain and culture. Crystal examination should be performed if gout or pseudogout is suspected.

Treatment consists of splinting the elbow for comfort. A nonsteroidal anti-inflammatory drug (NSAID), and occasionally a corticosteroid injection, may be helpful for nonseptic bursitis. In chronic cases, bursal excision may be done. If septic bursitis is suspected, empiric oral antibiotics should be started with an anti-staphylococcal medication (eg, cephalosporin or dicloxacillin). A corticosteroid injection should never be performed if infection is suspected. In advanced cases, intravenous (IV) antibiotics, and occasionally surgical debridement, may be required to eradicate the infection.

Gout/Pseudogout

Gout and pseudogout are inflammatory conditions of the elbow joint, although seen less commonly here than in the big toe or knee. Patients complain of severe pain, with decreased range of motion, an effusion, and increased warmth. Diagnosis is made with joint aspiration demonstrating crystals. X-rays may show intra-articular calcium deposition. Treatment consists of immobilization, NSAIDs, and occasionally colchicine and allopurinol.

Arthritis

The most common forms of arthritis in the elbow include osteoarthritis (degenerative joint disease [DJD]) and rheumatoid arthritis (RA). In both forms, patients complain of pain with elbow motion and may have decreased range of motion.

With DJD there may be a history of trauma, and there is usually minimal swelling and warmth. If loose bodies are present, patients may complain of elbow clicking or locking. RA typically presents with increased warmth and swelling, along with symmetric, multiple joint involvement.

X-rays may be diagnostic. In DJD osteophyte formation and subchondral sclerosis are seen, whereas in RA an erosive process with juxta-articular osteopenia is seen. Joint aspiration may be helpful in diagnosing RA, because the characteristics of the synovial aspirate differ (see Laboratory Tests in Chapter 10). Treatment depends on the severity of the patient's symptoms, physical findings, and radiographs. Modifying activities and NSAIDs are usually helpful. In DJD with loose bodies, arthroscopic debridement may provide pain relief. If RA is suspected, referral to a rheumatologist is indicated. Patients not responding to conservative management may benefit from surgical synovectomy and, possibly, radial head excision.

Ulnar Nerve Entrapment at the Elbow (Cubital Tunnel Syndrome)

Ulnar nerve entrapment, with its frequent accompaniment of small muscle wasting and sensory impairment in the hand, may occur as a complication of local trauma at the elbow but is most often idiopathic. Inflammation of the ulnar nerve commonly occurs at the elbow where the nerve is abnormally mobile. In these circumstances, the nerve is exposed to frictional damage as it slips repeatedly in front of and behind the medial epicondyle. The nerve is also subject to pressure as it passes between the two heads of the flexor carpi ulnaris below the elbow. This is a common area of compression in weight lifters. Frequent symptoms of ulnar nerve compression at the elbow are paresthesias and possibly numbness in the little and ring fingers, tenderness of the nerve at the elbow, a positive Tinel's sign on percussion of the nerve as it passes through the cubital tunnel, and wasting of the small muscles of the hand. The differential diagnosis of ulnar nerve symptoms at the elbow should include metabolic abnormalities such as diabetes or rheumatoid arthritis and infectious diseases such as lepromatous leprosy, which often presents with ulnar nerve palsy. Cubitus valgus at the elbow can result in a tardy ulnar palsy, usually appearing between the ages of 30 and 50 years.

Physical examination includes grip strength measurement, sensory testing of the small and ring fingers, motor examination of the ulnar innervated wrist and finger flexors, examination of the small muscles of the hand for wasting, and palpation of the ulnar nerve at the elbow. If on initial presentation there is no evidence of muscle wasting in the hand (compare the involved and uninvolved hands) and the sensory examination of the palmar pulp of the small finger is normal (two-point discrimination is less than or equal to 6 mm), initial treatment is conservative, with night-time splinting of the elbow in extension for 4 weeks to rest the nerve and anti-inflammatory medications.

If conservative management is unsuccessful or if at the time of initial presentation muscle wasting is present or sensory testing is abnormal, the patient should be referred for evaluation for surgical release of the nerve. Before surgical release, electromyography and nerve conduction testing are necessary to localize the lesion to the elbow and to ensure that there is no proximal or distal evidence of nerve compression (eg, cervical radiculopathy).

Median Nerve Entrapment in the Forearm (Pronator Syndrome)

A much less common nerve entrapment syndrome is pronator syndrome, which is median nerve entrapment in the proximal forearm. Most commonly, this presents as pain in the volar forearm and paresthesias in the thumb, index, and middle fingers (and occasionally the ring finger). It may be mistakenly diagnosed as carpal tunnel syndrome because of the similar distribution of pain in the hand. Often patients are found to be excessively pronating the forearm under loads at work or home.

Physical examination may reveal a positive Tinel's sign in the proximal volar forearm (with a negative Tinel's at the wrist), along with numbness in the median innervated digits. Provocative testing, such as pronating the forearm against resistance, may elicit symptoms in the office. Electrodiagnostic studies should be performed to confirm the diagnosis.

Treatment initially should consist of rest and modification of provocative activities. Occasionally, splinting may be helpful. Surgical decompression is indicated if patients fail to respond to conservative treatment.

Traumatic Elbow Problems

Elbow Dislocation

Dislocations of the elbow are frequent, surpassed in frequency only by shoulder dislocations (Fig. 5-15).

As with other types of dislocations, the patient should be referred immediately to an orthopedist for further evaluation, and the reduction should be done as soon as possible. This is especially important in elbow dislocations because the rapid onset of swelling can result in compression of the neurovascular structures that

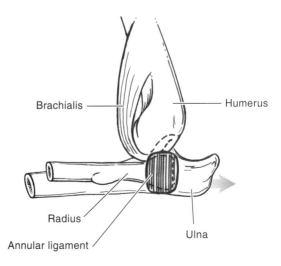

FIGURE 5-15. Dislocation of the elbow.

Brachialis

Humerus

Radius

Annular ligament

Ulna

pass in front of the elbow joint. The immediate danger with persistent swelling at the elbow joint is that circulation to the forearm is decreased, resulting in a possible Volkmann's ischemic contracture of the forearm and hand. Dislocations are named according to the position of the proximal radius and ulna (olecranon) relative to the distal humerus.

Posterior dislocations of the radius and ulna are the most frequent primary elbow dislocation. The deformity is usually obvious, and the patient presents with pain and restriction of motion. The most common mechanism is direct trauma from a fall on the outstretched forearm held in extension. Many patients have a concomitant wrist injury, and the examiner must look for this. A significant amount of soft tissue injury, including tearing of one or both collateral ligaments about the elbow, is necessary to allow the elbow to dislocate.

Physical examination includes documentation of the distal neurovascular status. If this documentation is not performed, it will be difficult to tell when a nerve injury happened if it is noticed only after reduction; that is, at the time of dislocation or during the reduction maneuver. Median nerve function is checked by testing sensation to the volar pulp of the thumb and index fingers. Although a pinprick will give a gross indication that median nerve function is present, a two-point discrimination test gives a much better evaluation of the status of the nerve at the time of the test. Normal two-point discrimination should be 6 mm or less. The test can be performed easily by bending the prongs of a small paper clip and setting the distance between the prongs to measure 6 mm. Two points of the paper clip are then lightly applied to the volar pulp of the index finger and thumb to test the median nerve, and then to the small finger to test the ulnar nerve. The autonomous sensory zone of the radial nerve is on the dorsum of the hand in the web space between the thumb and index fingers. Pinprick and soft touch evaluation are usually sufficient. Muscle function should also be tested: thumb and index finger flexion and thumb opposition test the median nerve; flexion of the tip (DIP joint) of the small finger and the ability to abduct the small finger away from the ring finger test ulnar nerve function; the ability to extend the fingers at the MCP joints and extension of the thumb test the posterior (deep) branch of the radial nerve. The ability to extend the wrist, but not the fingers, points to a lesion of the radial nerve after it has crossed the elbow and become the posterior (deep) interosseous branch of the radial nerve. If the radial nerve is injured above the elbow (as with a displaced humeral shaft fracture), the patient will also be unable to extend the wrist. AP, lateral, and oblique radiographs should be obtained before reduction is attempted and examined for possible fractures. If the elbow is reduced before obtaining radiographs, they are essential after reduction to rule out other associated fractures.

Reduction should only be attempted by experienced personnel who have been trained in the evaluation and management of bony injuries, fractures, and dislocations. An attempted reduction of an elbow dislocation by an inexperienced person can result in accidental fracture of the humerus or ulna or accidental tearing of the brachial artery or one of the nerves crossing the elbow joint. In most cases, splinting the patient in a comfortable position and immediate referral are all that is necessary. In some cases, closed relocation of the joint may not be possible due to intervening soft tissues of bony fragments; if so, surgical reduction and exploration may be necessary. After reduction, radiographs are again taken to assess the adequacy of reduction. A repeat neurovascular examination should also be performed. The patient is placed into a well-padded posterior splint holding the elbow in 90 degrees of flexion and slight pronation. Patients with stable joints after reduction are allowed active flexion after 1 week and may remove the splint for range-of-motion exercise. In some cases, a hinged range-of-motion brace may be used for an additional 5 weeks to allow the collateral ligaments to heal. Patients whose elbows have a limited stable range of motion are splinted in flexion for 2 to 3 weeks and then begin an active physical therapy exercise program in a protective hinged elbow orthosis in the stable range of motion. Radiographs should be taken during this 2- to 3-week period to be sure the elbow remains reduced. Surgical repair of the collateral ligaments or open reduction and internal fixation of fractures, with possible external fixator application, may be required if the elbow joint is not stable in any position. Many of these patients will lose some range of motion, but most are functional. If contractures are severe, they may require open contracture release.

Fractures Around the Elbow

These fractures are usually signaled by the patient's complaint of pain and deformity. A long-arm posterior splint should be applied, and referral to an appropriate facility should be made. If there is a history of a fall and point tenderness is found on examination, a posterior splint should be applied and referral should be made even if no obvious deformity is observed. The most common elbow fracture is of the head of the radius. Most of these fractures will be nondisplaced at the time of initial presentation and may be treated with a splint and early range-of-motion exercises within a few days. Displaced fractures may require surgical treatment. Supracondylar elbow fractures need to be carefully evaluated, because many of these will have displacement at the articular surface requiring operative reduction and fixation.

Distal Biceps Tendon Rupture

Patients complain of pain and weakness in the elbow after lifting a heavy object (eg, a television set). Physical examination reveals tenderness and swelling, and often ecchymosis in the antecubital fossa. The distal biceps tendon is not palpable in its normal location. Although elbow flexion strength testing may be normal (due to the intact brachioradialis muscle), supination strength is always decreased.

Surgical treatment is required to repair the tendon to its normal insertion on the proximal radius. Some elderly patients may not elect to have surgical repair if they are not bothered by the expected loss of supination strength.

Ligamentous Injuries

Both the medial and lateral collateral elbow ligaments may be injured, often from athletic injuries and occasionally from a fall or motor vehicle accident. There will be tenderness and usually ecchymosis and soft tissue swelling overlying the ligament. Radiographs should be obtained. Stress testing of each side of the elbow should be performed (see the section entitled History and Physical Examination above). The elbow should be splinted and referral made to an orthopedic surgeon. Conservative treatment will suffice if the ligament is only partially torn, but surgery is indicated for a completely ruptured ligament to prevent elbow instability.

Forearm Injuries

Crush Injuries

A common industrial injury is a crushing injury to the forearm. Patients should be observed for the development of a compartment syndrome. Obtain anteroposterior and lateral radiographs of the forearm (elbow to wrist) to rule out fracture or dislocation. Physical examination should focus on the neurovascular examination and signs of impending compartment syndrome. *Pain with passive stretch of the fingers and decreased sensibility of the fingers are the early signs of compartment syndrome.* Pulselessness is *not* a reliable sign of compartment syndrome because the pulse is not usually lost. For minor injuries with no evidence of impending compartment syndrome, ice packs that decrease the swelling, along with elevation, splinting, and follow-up by an orthopedist, usually will be all that is required. For severe injuries, patients should be referred to an emergency facility. Patients may be hospitalized and compartment pressures may be monitored with a slit catheter or other compartment pressure monitoring device. Fasciotomies are performed if pressures are abnormal to prevent permanent muscle and nerve damage.

Tumors

Bone and soft tissue tumors about the elbow and forearm are less commonly seen than about the knee. As in other areas of the bony skeleton, metastatic bone tumors are much more common than primary bone tumors. Any patient with chronic elbow or forearm pain should have a radiograph of the painful area to exclude a tumor. Lipomas are soft subcutaneous fat masses, usually nontender and very slow growing. Ganglion cysts may occur about the elbow, although much less commonly than in the wrist and hand. Rarely, an elbow ganglion cyst may cause a cubital tunnel syndrome due to compression of the ulnar nerve. All soft tissue masses should be radiographed to rule out bony involvement. Magnetic resonance imaging (MRI) should be considered if the mass is larger than 2.5 cm or if it is enlarging or fixed to underlying tissues.

Infections

A painful, warm, swollen elbow with markedly restricted range of motion should lead one to suspect a septic elbow. An aspirate of the joint should be performed, with fluid sent to the laboratory for Gram's stain, culture, white blood cell count, and crystals. Radiographs should be obtained to look for bony erosions. Immediate referral to an orthopedic surgeon is required. Treatment consists of IV antibiotics and possibly surgical washout. Osteomyelitis may occur in longstanding cases if untreated.

Recommended Readings

Andrews, J. R., & Whiteside, J. A. (1993). Common elbow problems in the athlete. *Journal of Orthopaedic and Sports Physical Therapy, 17*(6), 289.

Conway, J. E., et al. (1992). Medial instability of the elbow in throwing athletes. *Journal of Bone and Joint Surgery, 74A,* 67.

D'Alessandro, D. F., et al. (1993). Repair of distal biceps tendon ruptures in athletes. *American Journal of Sports Medicine, 21*(1), 114.

Ellenbecker, T. S. (1995). Rehabilitation of shoulder and elbow injuries in tennis players. *Clinical Sports Medicine, 14*(1), 87.

Morrey, B. F. (1997). Complex instability of the elbow. *Journal of Bone and Joint Surgery, 79A,* 460.

Morrey, B. F. (1993). *The elbow and its disorders.* Philadelphia: W. B. Saunders.

Safran, M. R. (1995). Elbow injuries in athletes: a review. *Clinical Orthopaedics, 1*(310), 257.

Wilk, K. E., Arrigo, C., & Andrews, J. E. (1993). Rehabilitation of the elbow in the throwing athlete. *Journal of Orthopaedic and Sports Physical Therapy, 17*(6), 305.

Chapter 6

The Wrist and Hand

Harris Gellman, MD

Anatomy

Joints

The wrist joint is composed of the distal radius, ulna, and the proximal row of carpal bones (the scaphoid, lunate, and triquetrum). The distal radius articulates both with the ulna at the sigmoid notch of the distal radius to form the radioulnar joint, and with the carpus to form the radiocarpal joint.

The triangular fibrocartilage complex is an articular disc of fibrocartilage attached to the medial edge of the radius and the styloid process of the ulna. The articular capsule enclosing the joint is strengthened by the dorsal and palmar radiocarpal ligaments and the radial and ulnar collateral ligaments. There are eight carpal bones (scaphoid, lunate, triquetrum, pisiform, trapezium, trapezoid, hamate, capitate) aligned in two transverse rows, with dorsal and palmar intercarpal ligaments passing between these bones. The intercarpal ligaments link the proximal carpal row and the distal carpal row providing intercarpal stability. The midcarpal joint lies between the proximal and distal rows of carpal bones. Wrist movement occurs both at the radiocarpal and the midcarpal joint, with a contribution to wrist flexion and extension from both joints. The scaphoid is contained in both the proximal and distal rows, thereby linking them.

The hand includes five metacarpals, five proximal phalanges, four middle phalanges, and five distal phalanges. The thumb (first) metacarpal articulates with the trapezium in a saddle-shaped joint known as the trapeziometacarpal joint or the basilar joint. The metacarpophalangeal joints are formed by the rounded head of the metacarpals articulating with the bases of the proximal phalanges. Joint capsules are reinforced dorsally by the extensor tendons, and palmarly by the volar plates which are continuous with the collateral ligaments. The interphalangeal joints of the fingers are hinge-type joints that are structurally the same as the metacarpophalangeal (Fig. 6-1).

Muscles and Tendons

The tendons of the flexor and extensor muscles pass from the forearm to the hand and fingers. The flexor digitorum sublimus is innervated by the median nerve in the forearm and flexes the proximal interphalangeal (PIP) joints of the fingers, whereas the flexor digitorum profundus tendons flex the distal interphalangeal (DIP) joints of the fingers. The flexor profundus is dual innervated: the index and long finger portion is innervated by the median nerve and the ring and small finger

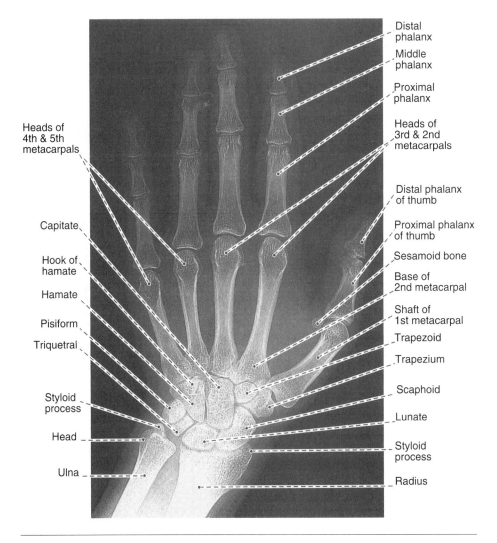

FIGURE 6-1. Bones of the wrist and hand seen on radiograph from the palmar aspect. (Courtesy of Dr. Thurman Gillespy III.)

half of the muscle is innervated by the ulnar nerve. The flexor pollicis longus flexes the thumb interphalangeal joint and is also innervated by the median nerve. The small intrinsic muscles in the hand flex the metacarpophalangeal (MCP) joints of the fingers. The flexor pollicis brevis flexes the MCP joint of the thumb.

The extensor digitorum communis muscle, innervated by the deep branch of the radial nerve, is responsible for extension of the fingers at the MCP joints (Fig. 6-2). The index and small fingers can also be independently extended by the extensor indicis proprius and extensor digiti quinti minimi, respectively. The extensor pollicis longus extends the interphalangeal joint of the thumb. Extension at the MCP joint of the thumb is by the extensor pollicis brevis, and thumb abduction is performed by the abductor pollicis longus. The tendons of the extensor pollicis brevis and the abductor pollicis longus cross from the forearm to the hand through the first dorsal compartment. This is a common area for tenosynovitis (de Quervain's syndrome). The intrinsic muscles of the hand are divided into three groups. There are three thenar muscles: the abductor pollicis brevis, flexor pollicis brevis, and opponens pollicis. The abductor pollicis brevis and the opponens pollicis are innervated by the median nerve, whereas the flexor pollicis brevis usually has dual innervation, with the superficial head being innervated by the median nerve and the deep head of the flexor pollicis brevis as well as the adductor pollicis are innervated by the ulnar nerve. The hypothenar muscles (abductor digiti minimi, flexor digiti minimi brevis, and opponens digiti minimi) are innervated by the ulnar nerve. The interossei and lumbricals have a very important function in the hand allowing finger abduction, adduction, extension of the PIP joints in the fingers, and flexion of the MCP joints. The lumbricals to the index and long fingers are innervated by the median nerve, whereas the remainder of the lumbrical and interosseous muscles are innervated by the ulnar nerve. The intrinsic muscles have been called "the workhorse of the hand" and contribute approximately 50% of our grip strength. Loss of ulnar nerve

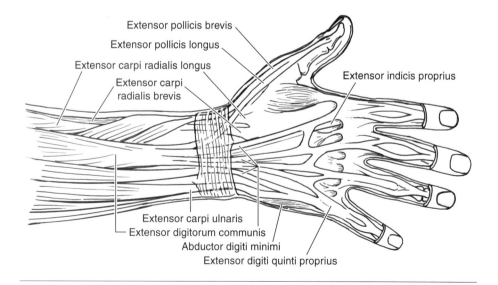

FIGURE 6-2. The hand—deep fascia removed, exposing tendons and muscles.

function can be very disabling and can result in clawing of the ring and small fingers (hyperextension of the MCP joints and flexion of the PIP joints).

Arteries and Nerves

After leaving the forearm, the ulnar artery enters the hand by passing through Guyon's canal (between the radial side of the pisiform bone and the hook of the hamate just distal to the wrist flexion crease). The artery terminates by dividing into a deep branch that joins a deep branch of the radial artery to form the deep palmar arch as well as a superficial branch that joins the radial artery to form the superficial palmar arch (Fig. 6-3). The latter, predominantly from the ulnar artery, lies transversely in the palm immediately under the palmar aponeurosis in line with the fully extended thumb. The common palmar digital branches come off the superficial palmar arch to become the proper digital arteries to the contiguous sides of the fingers. The radial artery enters the hand by passing through the anatomic snuff box deep to the tendons of the abductor pollicis longus and the extensor pollicis longus and brevis. The princeps pollicis and the indicis proprius branches arise as the radial artery pierces the first dorsal interosseous muscle. They supply, respectively, both sides of the thumb and the radial side of the index finger. The deep arch lies on the carpal bones at a level 2 cm proximal to the superficial arch. Branches of the deep arch become the palmar metacarpal arteries. These join with the common palmar digital arteries of the superficial arch to enter the fingers.

Nerves of the Wrist and Hand

The median nerve enters the hand by passing through the carpal tunnel under the flexor retinaculum and transverse carpal ligament at the wrist along with the nine flexor tendons (FDS-4, FDP-4, and FPL; Fig. 6-4). The median nerve innervates

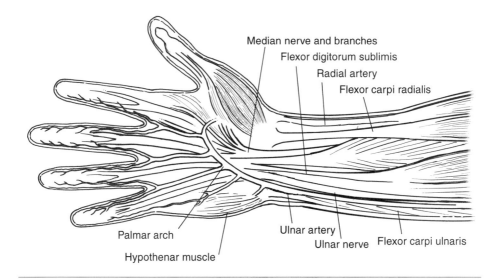

Median nerve and branches
Flexor digitorum sublimis
Radial artery
Flexor carpi radialis
Palmar arch
Hypothenar muscle
Ulnar artery
Ulnar nerve
Flexor carpi ulnaris

FIGURE 6-3. Hand—transverse carpal ligament cut and deep fascia of the forearm, palmaris longus and palmar fascia removed, exposing superficial tendons, ulnar nerve and median nerve.

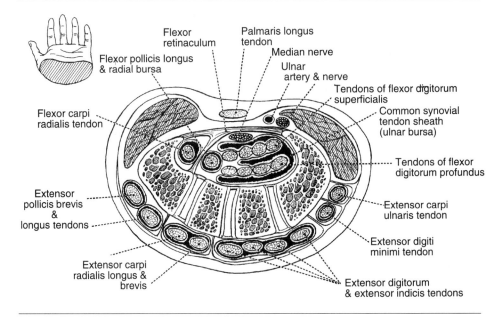

FIGURE 6-4. Transverse section of the wrist across the carpal canal: Synovial membrane is indicated as a *ruffled white line.* Synovial fluid within synovial sheaths is shown in *black;* for purposes of clarity, its quantity is exaggerated. The *inset* shows the level of the section.

---

the thenar muscles as well as the two radial lumbricals. Terminally, the nerve supplies cutaneous innervation to the central area of the palm and the palmar surface of the thumb, index, middle, radial half of the ring fingers, and all of the skin on the distal phalanges and fingernails of these digits. At the wrist, the ulnar nerve divides into a superficial branch that supplies cutaneous innervation to both the palmar and dorsal surfaces of the hand and the small and ring fingers up to a line passing through the midline of the ring finger, and a deep branch that innervates all of the intrinsic muscles of the hand, except those innervated by the median nerve. The deep branch pierces the opponens digiti minimi muscle and passes around the hook of the hamate to cross into the palm. The radial nerve does not innervate any muscles in the hand. Distal to the wrist, it is primarily a sensory nerve supplying cutaneous sensation to the entire dorsum of the hand radial to a line passing through the midline of the ring finger as well as a small area on the palmar surface of the thenar eminence.

History and Physical Examination

Taking a patient's history is somewhat analogous to being a reporter obtaining information for a story, particularly when the patient is a teenager or child. A good reporter asks "who, where, what, when, and how." A good diagnostician needs to know that same information. The who is the patient; where does it hurt—is the pain diffuse or localized, stationary or migratory? What causes the pain and what makes it better? What was the patient doing when the pain started or the injury occurred? When does it hurt? Tumors typically ache at night; arthritis aches more often in the morning. Is the pain related to a particular activity such as pitching, or a particular position, or twisting motion? When did the injury occur—at play, at home, or at work? Finally, how did the injury occur and was the patient involved in an unusual or new activity?

Physical examination includes inspection, palpation, active and passive range of motion, vascular and sensory evaluation, and manual muscle testing.

Inspection

Inspect the skin for bruises, abrasions, lacerations, scars, and swelling. Swelling occurs with inflammation, infection, joint effusions, and after fractures. A comparison to the opposite hand and wrist is useful for subtle cases. An effusion will cause loss of the sharp soft tissue contours. Ecchymosis with swelling is suggestive of fracture or dislocation. Loss of symmetry and soft tissue contours may be secondary to dislocation. This usually presents as deformity with loss of motion.

Deformity of the wrist such as radial deviation of the hand after a fall may be due to Colles' fracture. Ulnar deviation of the fingers may be seen in rheumatoid arthritis. Thenar wasting is suggestive of carpal tunnel syndrome or median nerve injury of any etiology. Dorsal swellings at the wrist are commonly found with ganglions or rheumatoid synovitis. Palmar flexion of the wrist may make a small ganglion more noticeable.

Palpation

Palpate for areas of tenderness or fluctuance. Tenderness in the anatomic snuff box is common with scaphoid fractures but is also seen with wrist sprains and other minor injuries.

Active and Passive Range of Motion

The hand and wrist should be moved actively and passively through a normal and painless range of motion. Observation of active and passive range of motion is a very important part of any examination. Normal wrist motion is 70 degrees dorsiflexion, 75 degrees palmar flexion, 20 degrees radial deviation, and 35 degrees ulnar deviation. Limitations suggest radiocarpal or intercarpal pathology. Pronation of approximately 90 degrees and supination of 90 degrees should be achieved without pain. Although pronation and supination are usually attributed to the forearm and elbow, deformity or pathology at the wrist can also limit forearm rotation. Pain with pronation and supination at the distal radioulnar joint is common with injury to this joint after a Colles' fracture. Limitation suggests a disturbance of the distal radioulnar joint. In the fingers, there should be approximately 0 to 90 degrees active motion at the MCP joints, 0 to 100 degrees of motion at the PIP joints, and 0 to 80 degrees motion of the DIP joints. All of the joints of the fingers are involved in grasping and holding and, therefore, when the patient is asked to make a fist, all of the distal phalanges normally will touch the palm at right angles. A loss of motion at any level will result in an inability to touch the injured finger to the palm. The thumb has a slightly different range from that of the fingers, with approximately 55 degrees of flexion at the MCP joint, and from 20 degrees extension to 80 degrees flexion at the IP joint (100 degrees IP ARC). There should be approximately 60 degrees of abduction of the thumb in a plane at right angles to the palm. Opposition is a composite motion involving abduction of the thumb at right angles to the palm, flexion, and rotation. Normally, the thumb should touch the tip of the small finger. Opposition is achieved by the intrinsic muscles of the thumb; loss of opposition occurs with median nerve pathology as with carpal tunnel syndrome.

Diffuse tenderness is common in all inflammatory conditions, whether or not they are caused by infections. Tenderness and thickening localized to the sheaths of the abductor pollicis longus and extensor pollicis brevis causing pain during thumb abduction are suggestive of de Quervain's tenosynovitis.

Synovitis of the wrist and hand may cause a limitation of normal flexion or extension. Assess the supracondylar area (medial aspect of the arm above the elbow) for an enlarged epitrochlear lymph node that would indicate an infection in the arm or hand. Palpate the bony prominences and check for crepitation. Assess the quality of joint and tendon gliding, feeling for crepitance indicative of intra-articular pathology, adhesions, fractures, or osteoarthritis. Palpate the wrist for tenderness, warmth, or any changes from normal skin tone. Nerves and muscles are then examined.

Sensory Testing and Nerve Function

Paresthesias with percussion of the median or ulnar nerves at the wrist is suggestive of nerve compression. Sensibility evaluation of the thumb, index, and long fingers test the median nerve, whereas sensory testing of the small finger and ulnar half of the ring finger will evaluate the ulnar nerve. The radial nerve provides sensation to the web space on the dorsum of the hand, between the thumb and index finger. Flexor tendon function may be abnormal because of tendon, muscle, or nerve injury (Fig. 6-5).

Median nerve function is checked by testing sensation to the palmar pulp of the thumb, index, and long fingers. Although pinprick testing will give a gross indication of median nerve function, the two-point discrimination test gives a much better evaluation of the status of the nerve at the time of the test. Normal two-point discrimination should be 6 mm or less. The test can easily be performed by bending the prongs of a small paper clip and setting the distance between the prongs to measure 6 mm (Fig. 6-6). The two points of the paper clip are then lightly applied to the volar pulp of the index finger and thumb to test median nerve, and then to the small finger to test the ulnar nerve. The autonomous sensory zone of the radial nerve is on the dorsum of the hand in the web space between the thumb and index fingers (Fig. 6-7). Sensory testing of the radial nerve is more difficult; pinprick and soft touch are usually sufficient.

Muscle function should also be tested: thumb and index finger flexion and thumb opposition tests the median nerve; flexion of the tip (DIP joint) of the small finger and the ability to abduct the small finger away from the ring finger tests ulnar nerve function; and the ability to extend the fingers at the MCP joints and extension of the thumb test the posterior (deep) branch of the radial nerve. The ability to extend

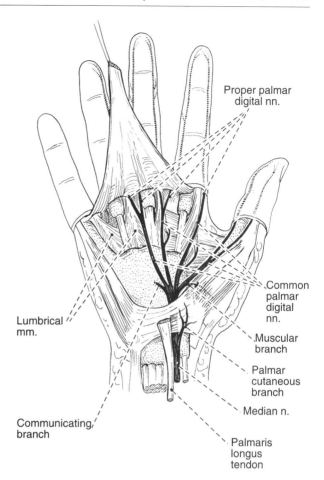

Proper palmar
digital nn.

Common
palmar
digital
nn.

Muscular
branch

Palmar
cutaneous
branch

Median n.

Palmaris
longus
tendon

Lumbrical
mm.

Communicating
branch

FIGURE 6-5. The median nerve in the hand: The palmar aponeurosis has been reflected.

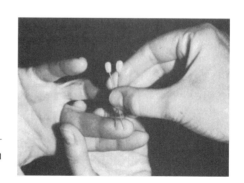

FIGURE 6-6. Two-point discrimination with pins.

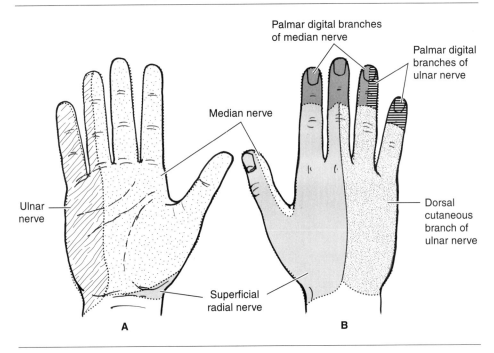

FIGURE 6-7. Normal pattern of sensory distribution on the palmar (**A**) and dorsal (**B**) surfaces of the hand. Note that the palmar nerves provide sensation distal to the midportion of the middle phalanges on the dorsum of the fingers.

the wrist, but not the fingers, points to a lesion of the radial nerve after it has crossed the elbow and become the posterior (deep) interosseous branch of the radial nerve. If the radial nerve is injured above the elbow (as with a displaced humeral shaft fracture), then the patient will also be unable to extend the wrist.

Muscle Testing

Apply resistance to the wrist as the patient flexes and extends the wrist. The wrist is flexed by the flexor carpi radialis and flexor carpi ulnaris. Flexion of the PIP joints of all fingers is done by the flexor digitorum sublimus (median nerve; Fig. 6-8). The DIP joints of the fingers are flexed by the flexor digitorum profundus (FDP). The FDP to the index, long, and part of the ring finger is innervated by the median nerve, and the FDP to the small and part of the ring finger is innervated by the ulnar nerve. The long flexor to the thumb (FPL) flexes the IP joint and is innervated by the median nerve. Extension of the wrist is accomplished by the extensor carpi radialis longus and brevis and extensor carpi ulnaris. Finger extension is done primarily by the extensor digitorum communis, but independent extension of the index and small fingers is performed by the extensor indicis proprius and extensor digiti quinti minimi, respectively. The IP joint of the thumb is extended by the extensor pollicis longus. On the dorsum of the wrist are six compartments for the extensor tendons. The first dorsal compartment contains the EPB and ALP; the second, ECRB and ECRL; the third, EPL; the fourth, EDC and EIP; fifth,

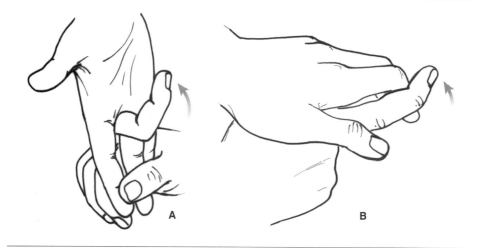

FIGURE 6-8. **(A)** Examination of an intact flexor superficialis tendon using the quadregia effect to eliminate the flexion force of the profundus tendon. **(B)** Examination of an intact flexor profundus tendon.

EDQM; and sixth, ECU. All extensor musculature is innervated by the deep branch of the radial nerve (posterior interosseous nerve).

Special Diagnostic Tests

1. *Allen Test:* Vascular examination to evaluate the distal pulses and capillary refill.

    The circulation of the hand is evaluated by noting the color of the skin and fingernails. The Allen test, which determines the patency of the vessels supplying the hand, is performed as follows:
    a. Compress the radial and ulnar arteries at the wrist.
    b. Have the patient make a tight fist (three or four times to exsanguinate the blood from the hand) and open it into a relaxed position. Avoid forced extension of the fingers; this will maintain blanching.
    c. Release the compression of the ulnar artery while continuing to compress the radial artery. The fingers and palm should fill with blood, and the normal pink color should return.
    d. Repeat steps 1 and 2 and repeat the test for the radial artery. This test can also be carried out on a single finger by expressing the blood from the finger and occluding both digital arteries. The test is performed first for the radial digital artery and then the ulnar digital artery noting the filling of the finger. This helps to evaluate the patency of each digital vessel to the finger.
2. *Tinel Test*

    This test is performed by gently tapping the area over the median nerve at the wrist palmarly. Although this can be done with a reflex hammer, it is better done by using the examiner's long finger bent 90 degrees at the PIP joint, because this joint is more sensitive. The test result is considered positive if this produces tingling or the sensation of electric shocks into the fingers.

3. *Phalen's (Wrist-Flexion) Test*

   The patient actively places the wrist in complete but unforced flexion. If numbness and tingling are produced or exaggerated in the median nerve distribution of the hand within 60 seconds, the test result is considered positive.

Diagnostic Guidelines: Radiographic Examination

Radiographic examination should be performed whenever a fracture, dislocation, or foreign body is suspected. Additionally, radiographs may detect an occult tumor that, although rare, might otherwise be missed.

If a wrist injury is suspected, obtain at least two radiographic views (AP and lateral) of the forearm and wrist. For a suspected scaphoid fracture, a scaphoid series will give AP, lateral, oblique, and longitudinal views of the scaphoid.

For hand and finger fractures and dislocations, it is imperative that in addition to an AP view a "true" lateral is obtained. Fractures of the condylar area of the phalanges will be missed otherwise.

Wrist Injuries: Fractures, Dislocations, and Sprains

Colles' (Distal Radius) Fracture

Distal radius fracture is the most common wrist injury in any age group. Most distal radius fractures are referred to as Colles' fractures whether or not they are true Colles' fractures. The mechanism of injury is a fall on the outstretched arm with the wrist extended. The classic deformity is described as a "silver fork" deformity with dorsal swelling and displacement of the hand and wrist. A splint should be applied from the fingers to above the elbow, and the extremity should be elevated. Many distal radius fractures are intra-articular and require open reduction and internal fixation. Although cast immobilization is often adequate after reduction, newer techniques of internal and external fixation have greatly improved the results of severely comminuted, displaced fractures. After distal radius fractures, patients usually require 6 weeks in a cast, and, after cast removal, many patients require therapy to regain strength and wrist motion. It is important to be sure that active finger flexion and extension exercises are performed while the patient is in the cast. It may require 3 to 6 months after the fracture before the patient is able to return to full activity. Most patients can return to work after 8 to 10 weeks.

Scaphoid Fracture

The scaphoid fracture is one of the most troublesome of the wrist injuries. The scaphoid is one of the eight carpal bones in the wrist and is the one most often fractured. Fracture usually occurs as a result of a fall on the extended wrist with a pronation of the forearm on the fixed hand. Because the scaphoid bone is completely intra-articular in the wrist, it is surrounded by cartilage and has a sparse blood supply. The combination of these factors with the lack of stability of the bone after fracture and the surrounding of the scaphoid by synovial fluid in the wrist joint results in a high rate of nonunion. Patients usually present with complaints of wrist pain and tenderness in the snuff box (Fig. 6-9). Many times, patients (as well as many primary care providers) ascribe the pain to a sprain, and without an x-ray (Fig. 6-10) the fracture will be missed. Radiographs should include AP, lateral, and oblique views of the wrist. For additional definition of the scaphoid, AP radiographs should be taken with the wrist positioned in radial and ulnar deviation. Treatment of nondisplaced fractures differs from fractures with any amount of displacement. If the fracture is nondisplaced, initial treatment is the application of a long arm thumb spica cast and referral to an orthopedist for follow-up. Radiographs should be taken initially at 2- to 3-week intervals to ensure no displacement of the fracture occurs. Displaced fractures should be treated surgically because malunion of the fracture may result and lead to early onset of carpal collapse and degenerative arthritis of the wrist.

If the patient has tenderness of the snuff box at the wrist but no radiographic findings of a fracture, a thumb spica cast should be applied and the patient should be reexamined 2 weeks later. Many times, a fracture may not be "visible" on the initial radiographs but becomes "visible" within 2 weeks after injury. After the fracture heals, it usually takes from 3 to 6 months for wrist motion and grip strength to return to near normal.

Wrist Dislocations

Dislocations of the wrist are usually the result of high-energy trauma such as a motorcycle accident. The dorsal perilunate dislocation is the most frequent (Fig. 6-11). The dislocation is often accompanied by other injuries to the hand and forearm, or it may be only one injury in a multiple-injury patient. This is one of the most commonly missed injuries by those relatively inexperienced at reading wrist radiographs. Radiographs demonstrate a loss of the normal articulation of the lunate and the capitate. On the AP view, the lunate is often triangular and

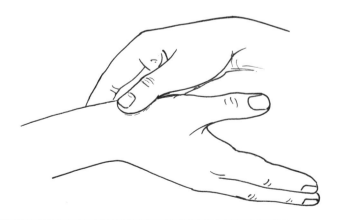

FIGURE 6-9. Palpation of snuff box. Tenderness suggests a navicular fracture.

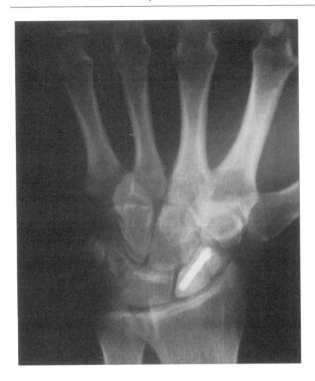

FIGURE 6-10. Scaphoid fracture.

overlaps the capitate by more than one third of its height. On the lateral view, the capitate is seen to be displaced posterior to the lunate; the lunate may be facing palmar. This is commonly referred to as the "spilled teacup" sign. There may also be a fracture of the scaphoid that is best seen on an AP or oblique view.

Physical examination should include documentation of the neurovascular status at the time of initial presentation including ulnar and radial pulses, capillary refill in the fingers, as well as median, ulnar and radial nerve function. If this is not done initially, it will be difficult to tell when a nerve injury occurred should it be noticed after treatment.

Reduction of a dislocated wrist should only be attempted by experienced personnel who have been trained in the evaluation and management of bony injuries, fractures, and dislocations. An attempted reduction of a wrist dislocation by an inexperienced person can result in accidental fracture of the radius or ulna or accidental injury to the radial or ulnar artery or median or ulnar nerves. In most cases, splinting the patient in a comfortable position and immediate referral are all that is necessary.

Radiographs should be taken during the 2 to 3 weeks after reduction to be sure the wrist remains reduced. Patients should be admitted to a hospital overnight to allow monitoring of the neurovascular status of the extremity.

After a wrist dislocation, patients rarely get complete recovery. Wrist range-of-motion exercises (flexion, extension, and radial and ulnar deviation) as well as grip

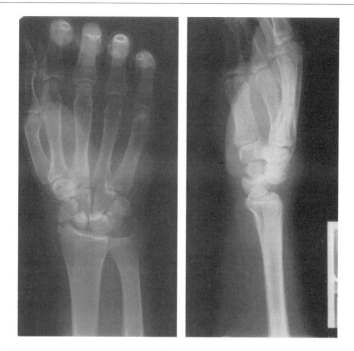

FIGURE 6-11.   Dorsal perilunate dislocation, AP and lateral views.

strengthening will help regain function sooner. It often takes up to 6 months to 1 year for the patient to reach a plateau in wrist motion and grip strength.

Wrist Sprains

After what often seems a relatively trivial injury, many patients will complain of wrist pain with motion of the wrist, especially wrist extension and gripping activities. Most wrist sprains occur as the result of a hyperextension injury to the wrist, either after a fall or catching a heavy object. The diagnosis of wrist sprain should be reserved as one of exclusion when all other possible diagnoses have been ruled out. If one does not look carefully, it is easy to miss a serious ligamentous injury to the radiocarpal or intercarpal ligaments, or a scaphoid fracture. Physical examination may reveal a decreased active and passive range of motion. There may be diffuse tenderness dorsally over the wrist capsule, or an area of point tenderness may be identified. AP, lateral, and oblique radiographs of the wrist should always be obtained. If all studies are negative, it is advisable to place the patient in a short arm cast or a splint for 2 weeks and then examine and x-ray the patient again. Many times, all symptoms will resolve and the patient can return to work, but occasionally an occult fracture or scapholunate dissociation will become obvious at the time of repeat x-rays. If pain is severe, referral to an orthopedic surgeon should be made initially. If there is moderate or mild pain with a negative radiographic examination, it is reasonable to wait until the repeat radiographic examination at

2 weeks. If the patient is symptomatic or a fracture is found, a referral should be made to a hand surgeon.

Triangular Fibrocartilage Complex Injury (TFCC)

The triangular fibrocartilage is a cartilagenous disc found in the wrist similar to the meniscus in the knee. It is located between the lunate and triquetrum and the head of the ulna. Its attachments are the radius and the ulnar styloid. Injury to the TFCC occurs with hyperextension and twisting injuries to the wrist, and presents with ulnar-sided wrist pain. Tears of the TFCC are often confused with wrist sprains. Frequently, diagnosis is delayed until the patient complains that "my wrist sprain seems to be taking an awfully long time to heal." Examination of the patient with a TFCC injury or tear will reveal tenderness in the recess under the ulnar styloid dorsally, volarly, or both. The presence of a "click" or "clunk" with wrist motion should make one suspicious of a ligamentous injury in the wrist. Pain can often be reproduced with forced ulnar deviation of the wrist, and the patient will often complain that there is very little pain at rest but that rotation of the forearm with ulnar deviation is exquisitely painful. Plain radiographs rarely yield any useful information, and an arthrogram or magnetic resonance imaging (MRI) is necessary to make the diagnosis. If diagnosed early, initial treatment is usually cast immobilization in a long arm cast in neutral rotation or supination for 6 weeks. If the wrist is still painful, arthroscopy and debridement or repair of the TFCC will be necessary (Box 6-1).

Box 6-1. Differential Diagnosis of Wrist Pain

Traumatic
  Fractures
  Dislocations
  Ligament injuries (intercarpal ligaments, TFCC)
Degenerative
  Arthrosis (osteoarthritis versus post-traumatic)
Acquired
  Arthritis (rheumatoid)
  Ganglion cysts
  Tumors (bony versus soft tissue)
  Infection (bacterial, tuberculous, fungal)

Diagnostic Studies for Wrist Pain

History and physical examination
Radiographs
Special radiographic studies
  Special radiographic views
  Bone scan
  Arthrogram
  Cineradiography
  CT scan
  MRI
Laboratory studies
  Arthritis screen

Fractures in the Hand

Pain or swelling of the hand or fingers after a twisting or contact injury to the hand should make one suspicious of a fracture in the hand. Physical examination should include palpation along tender areas seeking a point of maximal tenderness. This will usually correspond to the area of the fracture. AP, lateral, and oblique radiographs should be taken. Acute care of most fractures in the hand includes splinting for comfort, elevation of the injured limb, and referral to an orthopedist or hand specialist. Many of these injuries occur in children and adolescents at school. Because most schools do not have access to x-rays or a plaster splint, ice pack and referral to an emergency facility for radiographs should be done initially.

Although most nondisplaced, extra-articular fractures of the phalanges and metacarpals can be treated conservatively by splinting, casting, or "buddy" taping the fingers, it is still necessary to refer these injuries to a qualified orthopedic surgeon for evaluation. Many times, fractures that appear benign will change position, and by the time the patient returns for follow-up the "window" of opportunity for re-reduction and closed treatment will be lost. Intra-articular and displaced fractures should be referred immediately to an appropriate facility where a decision can be made regarding the need for surgical management. Some of the special fractures that usually require surgical treatment include displaced intra-articular fractures at the base of the thumb metacarpal (Bennett's fracture), fracture dislocations of the MCP or PIP joints in the fingers, and fracture dislocations of the base of the fifth metacarpal (Baby Bennett's fracture).

Metacarpal Neck Fractures (Boxer's Fracture)

Fracture of the metacarpal neck of the fifth finger is the most frequent metacarpal fracture and is commonly referred to as a "boxer's fracture" because these often result from a fight. Patients have tenderness and pain just proximal to the MCP joint of the fifth finger over the neck of the fifth metacarpal. Physical examination reveals a loss of the normal prominence of the fifth knuckle. AP and lateral radiographs should be taken. The angulation of the fracture in a palmar direction is best seen on the lateral radiograph. Although this is a displaced fracture, angulation of up to 40 degrees in a volar direction can be accepted. Angulation of index, long, or ring metacarpal neck fractures of greater than 20 degrees is unacceptable and should be treated surgically. If a puncture wound is found over the dorsum of any MCP joint, either alone or in association with a fracture, suspicion should be high that this is due to tooth penetration from a punch to an opponent's mouth. Many of these result in laceration of the extensor tendon over the MCP joint and may communicate with the MCP joint. Infection of the MCP joint can result; prevention consists of treatment with incision and drainage and antibiotics. Joint infection results in cartilage destruction and painful loss of motion. Human bites should be treated with both penicillin (to cover *Eikenella corrodens,* which is an organism specific to the human mouth) and a semisynthetic penicillin or cephalosporin as prophylaxis against *Staphylococcus aureus.* The mouths of cats and dogs carry the organism *Pasteurella multocida,* which is sensitive to penicillin.

Metacarpal Shaft Fractures

Metacarpal shaft fractures usually heal uneventfully in 4 to 6 weeks with splint or cast immobilization. Simple, nondisplaced fractures should not need surgery, but displaced or shortened transverse, or oblique fractures are unstable and may need open reduction and internal fixation.

Phalanx Fractures

Phalanx fractures usually heal in 4 to 5 weeks. The greatest pitfall in the management of phalanx fractures is missing a rotatory deformity of the bone. This is easy to do because during the acute fracture period swelling of the hand and fingers will make flexion difficult. Once the swelling has resolved and flexion of the finger becomes possible, rotational abnormalities become evident.

Dislocations in the Hand

Metacarpophalangeal Joint

Dislocation of the MCP joint of the fingers and thumb usually results from a hyperextension injury. The index finger is the most commonly involved, followed by the thumb and small fingers. On physical examination, the proximal phalanx is held in extension or hyperextension and there may be dimpling of the palmar skin over the protruding metacarpal head. A lateral radiograph will show the base of the proximal phalanx dorsal to the metacarpal head. On the AP view, there is obliteration of the normal joint space because of the overlap of the bones. Reduction can be attempted by hyperextending the finger at the MCP joint followed by traction, distraction, and flexion of the finger. Reduction is frequently unsuccessful because the volar plate may become trapped in the joint and often can only be extricated surgically. In the thumb and index finger, there is a sesamoid bone in the volar plate that acts as a further block to reduction. If reduction is accomplished, a posterior splint should be applied as a block to extension with the MCP flexed 70 degrees. Motion (flexion and extension of the MCP joint) should be started in the splint at about 1 week, and the splint can be discontinued after 3 to 4 weeks. It is important to check the range of flexion and extension of the MCP joint after reduction and before applying the splint to be certain there is no obstruction to motion (particularly extension). As always, postreduction radiographs should be taken (AP, lateral, and oblique views of the MCP joint). Occasionally, a fracture will become obvious that could not be well visualized previously.

Proximal Interphalangeal Joint

This is probably the most common dislocation. Dorsal dislocation of the middle phalanx on the proximal phalanx is the most commonly seen type. These occur by hyperextension or a "jamming" injury, often while playing basketball or baseball. The finger appears swollen and malformed with limitation of flexion. There is obliteration of the joint space on AP radiographs and dorsal dislocation of the middle phalanx on the lateral view. Occasionally, a fracture will be seen from the volar margin of the middle phalanx. If there is a fracture of the joint associated with the dislocation, surgical reattachment of the fragment may be necessary. Reduction is usually easily accomplished by direct longitudinal traction. Anesthesia should be administered, blocking the digital nerves in the palm at the level of the metacarpal neck rather than in the finger. Instillation of anesthesia into the base of the finger can cause compression of the digital arteries and ischemia to an already injured digit. Lidocaine (0.5% or 1%) *without epinephrine* should be used. After reduction, a dorsal extension block splint should be applied, blocking the last 15 degrees of extension. Motion can be started in the splint after the first week, and the splint can be removed at 3 weeks. "Buddy" taping the fingers after splint removal will help regain motion and overcome stiffness. Stiffness of the PIP joint (usually loss of range of flexion and extension) may be present for 3 to 6 months. Patients often require treatment by a therapist with specialized flexion and extension splints to regain motion.

Volar dislocation of the finger PIP joint occurs by a hyperextension injury at the PIP joint in the extended finger. AP and lateral radiographs should be taken of the finger. Lateral x-rays will show that the base of the middle phalanx is palmar to the head of the proximal phalanx. Volar dislocation of the middle phalanx is much less common and after reduction should be splinted in full extension of the PIP joint. A splint should be applied on the volar side of the finger and left in place for 4 to 6 weeks. Volar dislocations often cause traumatic rupture of the central extensor tendon insertion into the base of the middle phalanx. If these are not recognized and treated appropriately, a traumatic boutonnière will result and the patient will be unable to extend the PIP joint. AP and lateral radiographs should be checked postreduction to look for any fractures that may have been missed. Flexion and extension of the PIP joint should be started at 4 to 6 weeks postinjury.

Sprains

Collateral Ligaments at the MCP Joints of the Fingers

Twisting or lateral stress injuries of the fingers can result in traction on the collateral ligaments at the MCP joints. Patients with sprains of the collateral ligaments will usually present with complaints of a dull, aching pain in the hand between the metacarpal heads, particularly while gripping or shaking hands.

These injuries usually do not require surgery and can be treated by simple buddy taping of the injured finger to the adjacent finger. Healing is usually slow, however, and it is not uncommon for the tenderness to persist for 12 weeks or longer. It is important to stress to the patient that buddy taping should be continued until all pain has subsided or the injury may recur.

Gamekeeper's Thumb

This term is commonly used to describe a sprain or tear of the ulnar collateral ligament of the thumb. Disruption occurs after acute radial deviation of the thumb at the MCP joint (Fig. 6-12). Although this is often called "gamekeeper's thumb," it is commonly caused when the thumb is forcefully radially deviated by a ski pole

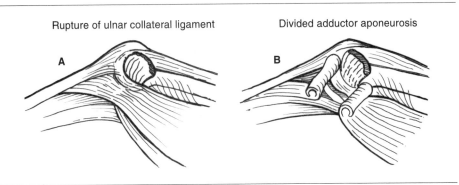

Rupture of ulnar collateral ligament   Divided adductor aponeurosis

FIGURE 6-12. The ulnar and colateral ligament of the thumb when ruptured (**A**) can only be identified and sutured after division of the adductor aponeurosis (**B**).

or strap when the hand hits the ground after a fall while skiing. Physical examination usually reveals tenderness over the ulnar side of the thumb MCP joint or at the head of the thumb metacarpal. Swelling or ecchymosis is also frequently seen along the ulnar side of the thumb MCP joint. It is important to compare the joint stability of the injured thumb with the patient's uninjured thumb. If there is radial deviation of the injured thumb of 15 degrees greater than the uninjured thumb, or 45 degrees radial deviation is possible, then the collateral ligament is probably disrupted (Fig. 6-13). AP and lateral radiographs should be taken. Although radiographs are usually negative, occasionally a bony avulsion will be seen where the collateral ligament inserts into the base of the proximal phalanx. For acute injuries with bony avulsion on the AP radiograph, a short arm thumb spica cast is applied and the x-rays are repeated. If the bone fragment is reduced into anatomic or near anatomic position,

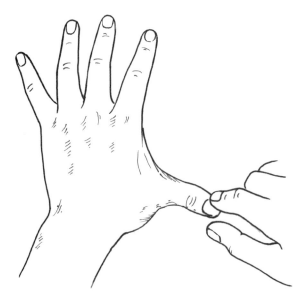

FIGURE 6-13. Complete instability to radial stress of the MP joint of the thumb.

immobilization for 4 to 6 weeks in a cast should be adequate. If no fracture or avulsion is seen on the x-ray, the optimum treatment is either primary surgical exploration and repair or immobilization in a thumb spica cast for 4 to 6 weeks (author's preference is surgical repair).

Tendon and Tendon Sheath Injuries

Mallet Finger

In a mallet finger injury, the DIP joint is held in a permanent position of flexion and the patient is unable to extend the distal joint of the finger. The etiology is either a tear of the terminal extensor tendon close to its insertion into the distal phalanx or a fracture of the dorsal base of the distal phalanx as the result of trauma. Many occur after a "jamming" injury to the extended distal phalanx causing a forced flexion injury. This is why the common name for a mallet finger is a "baseball" finger. Treatment is with a metal or prefabricated splint holding the DIP joint in full extension for 6 weeks. It is important to emphasize to the patient that the splint should not be removed at any time during the healing period (6 weeks) because this will allow the terminal phalanx to drop down into flexion and pull apart the healing tendon. Untreated mallet fingers may be complicated by a swan neck deformity with hyperextension of the PIP joint. This is usually not problematic and, if it occurs, does not usually require treatment.

Mallet Thumb

This is usually due to rupture of the extensor pollicis longus (EPL) tendon. Although delayed rupture of the EPL tendon may occur after Colles' fracture, it is more commonly seen in patients with rheumatoid arthritis. Direct repair is usually not possible because these are mostly attritional ruptures and transfer of the extensor indicis proprius tendon is usually necessary.

Boutonnière Deformity

Traumatic injuries to the PIP joint of the finger may result in detachment of the central slip of the extensor tendon from its attachment at the base of the middle phalanx. This can be secondary to a "jammed" or dislocated finger that occurred during sports activity or attrition of the joint capsule in rheumatoid arthritis. The characteristic deformity is flexion of the PIP joint with hyperextension at the DIP joint. Physical examination after a traumatic injury will usually elicit tenderness dorsally over the base of the proximal phalanx where the central slip of the extensor tendon inserts. In the rheumatoid patient, the deformity usually develops progressively and is not usually tender. Early traumatic lesions can usually be successfully treated by splinting the PIP joint in extension while leaving the DIP joint free for 6 weeks. Late deformity with fixed flexion contracture often requires fusion of the PIP joint in a functional position (they rarely respond to splinting).

Extensor Tendon Lacerations

Extensor tendon lacerations on the back of the hand are best treated by primary repair and splinting for approximately 4 weeks. These injuries have an excellent prognosis.

Flexor Tendon Injuries

In the fingers, laceration of either the FDP or flexor digitorum sublimus (FDS) can be easily diagnosed by physical examination and history. With isolated laceration of an FDP, patients are unable to flex the distal IP joint. With laceration of both FDS and FDP, neither the proximal IP nor the distal IP joint can be actively flexed. Isolated injury to the FDS occurs with lacerations proximal to the wrist flexion crease or in the forearm. Flexor tendon injuries in the fingers are often accompanied by digital nerve or nerve and artery laceration. Patients should be examined closely to determine the circulatory status. These injuries all require rapid surgical repair and should be referred to a hand surgeon for care.

Nontraumatic Conditions

Ganglions

Ganglions are extremely common about the wrist and hands and often present as painless swellings (Fig. 6-14). They vary in size between the tiny ganglions found in the fingers to the often large, fluctuant ganglions found on the dorsum of the wrist. In most cases, dorsal wrist ganglions communicate with the radiocarpal joint, and ganglions in the fingers communicate with the flexor tendon sheath. Diagnosis is not usually difficult unless the swelling is slight. AP and lateral radiographs of the hand and wrist are usually negative but should be taken in an attempt to rule out any other cause of pain or wrist swelling. Dorsal swelling and tenderness may only be obvious when the wrist is palmar flexed. This type of ganglion is often the cause of persistent wrist pain in young women. Their symptoms are often labeled as functional when the difficulty in examination has not been appreciated. Dorsal ganglions can be aspirated with a large-bore needle (16 or 18 gauge) and splinted

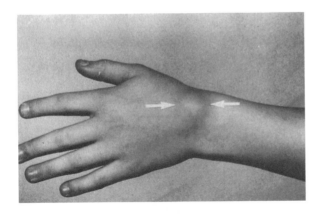

FIGURE 6-14. The most common location of a ganglion is on the dorsal wrist over the scapholunate joint.

for 2 to 3 weeks. Up to 50% will respond to this form of treatment. Volar wrist ganglions are usually deep to the radial artery, arising from the volar wrist capsule. Aspiration of these is more difficult because the radial artery is often compressed over the top of the ganglion and aspiration may result in accidental puncture of the artery. Excision is recommended for volar ganglions and those ganglions resistant to conservative treatment.

Trigger Finger and Thumb

This condition results from a thickening of either the fibrous tendon sheath or nodular thickening in a flexor tendon. In young children, the thumb is held flexed at the MCP joint, and a nodular thickening in front of the MCP joint is palpable. Frequently, the deformity is incorrectly considered untreatable. In adults, the middle or ring finger is most frequently involved. When the fingers are extended, the affected finger lags behind and then suddenly straightens with a painful snap. There is usually a palpable nodular thickening at the level of the MCP joint. Treatment with steroid injection into the flexor tendon sheath and splinting of the thumb for 3 weeks is usually successful. For unresponsive or recurrent cases, division of the tendon sheath at the level of the MCP joint (A1 pulley) gives an immediate and gratifying cure.

De Quervain's Syndrome

Tenosynovitis involving the abductor pollicis longus and extensor pollicis brevis is known as de Quervain's disease. It occurs most often in middle-aged women. The walls of the fibrous tendon sheaths on the lateral aspect of the radius are greatly thickened, and there is often marked underlying swelling. The patients often complain of pain with thumb flexion and extension, as well as grip. This is a very common occupational injury as a complication of repetitive movement of the thumb. Treatment is injection of a combination of 1% lidocaine and 40 mg methylprednisolone (Depo-Medrol) into the inflamed tendon sheath, followed by splinting in a radial gutter splint with the thumb immobilized for 3 weeks. For cases resistant to immobilization, surgical release of the lateral wall of the tendon sheath is necessary.

Extensor Tenosynovitis

Acute frictional tenosynovitis occurs most frequently in those 20 to 40 years of age, generally after a period of excess activity. Any or all of the extensor tendons may be involved. The condition has a benign course and is usually resolved if the wrist is immobilized in neutral to 20 extension for 3 weeks. If the pain has resolved after this period of immobilization, the patient can return to the previous level of activity at work or sports.

Carpal Tunnel Syndrome

This condition occurs most commonly in women, 30 to 60 years of age. Compression of the median nerve as it passes through the carpal tunnel under the transverse carpal ligament leads to signs and symptoms in the distribution of the median nerve.

In some cases, premenstrual fluid retention, early rheumatoid arthritis with synovial tendon sheath thickening, and old carpal fractures may be responsible because they restrict the space left for the nerve in the carpal tunnel. The condition is sometimes seen in association with myxedema, acromegaly, and pregnancy. Often, however, no obvious cause can be found.

People in occupations that require chronic repetitive wrist motion in flexion, extension, and gripping are prone to develop carpal tunnel syndrome. Another factor in the development of carpal tunnel syndrome is any activity, such as that of a jackhammer operator, that results in chronic trauma to the volar side of the wrist. More common occupations that are prone to develop carpal tunnel syndromes are assembly line workers, construction work involving repetitive hammering, carpentry, and electrical. Many times, it is helpful if patients can perform different types of activities during an 8-hour shift (part-time on the assembly line, part-time doing another job within same factory).

Patients typically complain of paresthesias in the hand. Often, they claim that all the fingers are involved and, although theoretically sensation of the little finger should be spared, approximately 30% of patients will also have paresthesias in the ulnar nerve distribution. Pain may radiate proximally to the elbow or shoulder, and weakness of grip is common. Symptoms may become most marked at night, often awakening the patient (nocturnal paresthesias) and causing the patient to shake the hand or hang it over the side of the bed. In many cases, the history and clinical examination are unequivocal. In others, it may be difficult to differentiate the patient's symptoms from those produced by cervical spondylosis or diabetic peripheral neuropathy; indeed, both conditions may be present at the same time as carpal tunnel syndrome.

Two-point discrimination testing is useful when screening for any of the compression neuropathies such as carpal tunnel syndrome. The test is performed by either bending the prongs of a small paper clip so there is a 6-mm distance between the tips or by using one of the commercially available two-point discrimination calipers. The tips are placed against the volar pulp of the index finger, long finger, and thumb (all fingers should be tested, but these three are innervated by the median nerve) until there is a slight blanching of the skin under the prongs. The patient is then asked if he or she feels (is able to discriminate between) one or two points. Normal two-point discrimination is 6 mm or less. On physical examination, two-point discrimination may be abnormal (greater than 6 mm), grip strength may be diminished, and thenar atrophy may be present. Flexion of the involved wrist for 60 seconds (Phalen's test) may reproduce the symptoms, or gentle percussion of the median nerve at the wrist may produce paresthesias radiating into the fingers (Tinel's sign). For patients seen early, before the development of abnormal two-point discrimination or thenar atrophy, splinting of the wrist with or without injection of steroids into the carpal canal may prove successful. If conservative treatment does not relieve the symptoms electrodiagnostic testing (EMG, NCV) may prove useful when contemplating surgery or trying to rule out another etiology. If, at the time of presentation, there is either thenar atrophy or abnormal two-point discrimination in the distribution of the median nerve then surgical release of the transverse carpal ligament is the best treatment.

Postoperatively, patients should be protected in a removable volar wrist extension splint for 2 to 3 weeks. During this time, finger motion is encouraged. After the splint is removed, wrist range-of-motion exercises and grip strengthening are started. Most patients will return to their preoperative level of grip strength and wrist motion by 3 months. Not all patients require therapy after surgery, but if progress appears slow, referral to an occupational or hand therapist should be made. Patients are usually ready to return to work between 6 and 12 weeks postoperatively.

Ulnar (Guyon's) Tunnel Syndrome

Ulnar nerve compression at the wrist may be confused with carpal tunnel syndrome. The most frequent presenting symptoms are paresthesias in the hand, tenderness of the nerve at the wrist, a positive Tinel sign on percussion of the nerve as it passes across the wrist and through Guyon's canal, and wasting of the small muscles of the hand. Differential diagnosis of ulnar nerve symptoms at the wrist should include metabolic abnormalities such as diabetes or rheumatoid arthritis and infectious diseases such as lepromatous leprosy, which often presents with ulnar nerve palsy.

The ulnar nerve may be compressed as it passes through the ulnar carpal canal (Guyon's canal) between the pisiform and the hook of the hamate. Although isolated ulnar nerve compression at the wrist is much less common than compression of the median nerve, 30% of patients with median nerve compression have concomitant compression of the ulnar nerve. Both the sensory and motor divisions of the nerve may be affected, but often only one division is involved.

Symptoms may include weakness or wasting of the small muscles in the hand, or diminished sensibility on the volar aspect of the ring or small finger. Pain is rarely seen with ulnar nerve compression at the wrist. Because the ulnar sensory branch to the dorsum of the hand branches 5 cm proximal to the wrist in the forearm, sensory disturbance on the dorsum of the hand and little finger usually excludes a lesion of the ulnar nerve at the wrist level, and points toward a more proximal lesion.

Physical examination includes grip strength, sensory testing of the small and ring fingers, motor examination of the ulnar innervated flexors, examination of the small muscles of the hand for wasting, and palpation of the ulnar nerve at the elbow. If on initial presentation there is no evidence of muscle wasting in the hand (compare the involved and uninvolved hands), and the sensory examination of the palmar pulp of the small finger is normal (two-point discrimination is less than or equal to 6 mm), then initial treatment is conservative with splinting of the wrist in extension for 3 to 6 weeks to rest the nerve as well as the use of nonsteroidal anti-inflammatory drugs (NSAIDs). For patients who are unable to take NSAIDs because of gastric intolerance, sensitivity, or allergy, many homeopathic anti-inflammatories such as Traumeel (Heel/BHI, Albuquerque, NM) are sold in health food stores. These can be very effective and better tolerated by patients. Homeopathic preparations rarely have any reported side effects.

An effort should always be made to exclude a more proximal cause for the patient's symptoms such as ulnar neuritis at the elbow or cervical spondylosis. Nerve conduction studies are often useful. The most common causes of ulnar nerve involvement at the wrist are compression by a ganglion or thrombosed ulnar artery, occupational trauma, and old carpal or metacarpal fractures. After establishing a diagnosis of a lesion localized to the ulnar tunnel (Guyon's canal) at the wrist, surgical exploration of the nerve and decompression may be necessary.

Dupuytren's Contracture

In this condition, there is nodular thickening and contracture of the palmar fascia. The palm of the hand is most often affected first, with the fingers becoming involved at a later stage (Fig. 6-15). The ring finger is most frequently affected, followed by the little and middle fingers. The index and even the thumb may be involved. Progression of flexion of the affected fingers into the palm interferes with hand function. Flexion may be so severe that the fingernails dig into the palm making hygiene difficult or impossible. The condition predominately affects men over age 40. In some cases, there may be a hereditary tendency, and an association with epilepsy or alcoholism has been reported. The condition may occur in either gender at an earlier age and may be precipitated by trauma. Indications for surgical treatment are flexion of the MCP joint greater than 30 degrees or any flexion contracture of the PIP joint. Splinting in an extended position at the MCP joint is rarely successful in either correcting or halting the progression of deformity.

When the flexion contracture of the MCP joint is less than 30 degrees and full extension of the PIP joint is possible, patients should be told that surgery will not be necessary unless the contracture progresses further. Many patients are concerned with how rapidly deformity will progress. Unfortunately, there is no way of predicting this other than by observation and regular follow-up. At surgery, the contracted palmar fascia and fibrous bands are released and excised, which allows improved extension. Postoperatively, a splint should be worn on the palmar side of the hand and forearm; the splint holds the MCP and PIP joints in extension. The splint is worn for 6 weeks (day and night) and then for an additional 3 months (night only). Most patients need hand therapy after surgery to regain motion and will not be able to return to work for approximately 3 months.

Arthritis

Rheumatoid Arthritis of the Wrist

Involvement of the wrist is common in rheumatoid arthritis, and extensive synovial thickening of the joint and related tendon sheaths leads to gross swelling, increased local heat, pain, and stiffness. Rarely, tuberculosis of the wrist may produce a similar

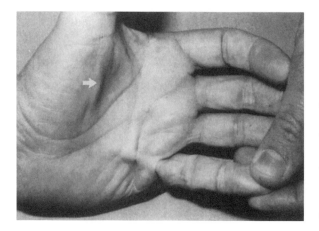

FIGURE 6-15. Photograph of the palm of a hand with Dupuytren's disease. A thick fibrous band (*arrow*) can be seen extending from the mid-palm up across the base of the thumb to the left of the picture.

clinical picture, but the multifocal nature of rheumatoid arthritis usually makes differentiation easy. Anti-inflammatories, intra-articular cortisone injections, and wrist splinting may provide relief during painful periods, but arthrodesis or arthroplasty is often necessary for lasting pain relief.

Rheumatoid Arthritis of the Hand

Patients with rheumatoid arthritis commonly have hand and wrist involvement. As the disease progresses, joints, tendons, muscles, and nerves are affected, resulting in severe deformities and crippling effects on hand function. In the earliest phases, the hands are warm and erythematous; later, the joints become swollen and tender. Synovial tendon sheath and joint thickening with effusion, muscle wasting, and deformity then become apparent. Tendon rupture and joint subluxation are the main factors leading to more severe deformities. Surgery of the rheumatoid hand is highly specialized and requires particular skills and experience in judgment, timing, and technique. In the earliest stages of the disease, analgesic and anti-inflammatory drugs are used, along with physiotherapy and splinting to alleviate pain, preserve motion, and minimize deformity. When synovial thickening is present without joint destruction, and is unresponsive to medical management or steroid injections, synovectomy is often useful in alleviating pain and delaying the progression of deformity. As joint destruction and deformity progress, reconstructive surgery often becomes necessary. It is important to watch for tendon rupture (particularly the common extensors to the ring and small fingers) because immediate exploration, synovectomy, and repair are recommended. Once tendon rupture occurs, it is usually a sign of impending rupture of additional tendons.

Osteoarthritis of the Wrist

Osteoarthritis of the wrist is surprisingly rare considering the frequency with which the wrist joint is involved in fractures. Osteoarthritis may be seen after comminuted fractures involving the articular surface of the radius, nonunion of fractures of the scaphoid, and avascular necrosis of the scaphoid or lunate. Patients commonly present with symptoms of increasing pain with gradual loss of motion, principally in extension. Initial treatment is with anti-inflammatory medications and splinting with a volar wrist splint during particularly painful periods. When symptoms are severe, fusion of the wrist (radiocarpal joint) may be necessary.

Osteoarthritis of the Hands

Nodular swellings over the dorsum and sides of the DIP joints (Heberden's nodes) and PIP joints are the most common findings of osteoarthritis of the finger joints. These occur frequently in women after menopause and are often familial. Early in the disease, they are usually symptom free, but, as the joint deformity progresses, pain becomes more frequent. Analgesics and anti-inflammatory drugs can usually control the pain. If not, joint arthrodesis will be necessary to alleviate the pain.

Carpometacarpal (Basal) Joint of the Thumb

The carpometacarpal joint lies between the thumb metacarpal and the trapezium and is the most commonly involved with osteoarthritis in the hand (Fig. 6-16). Pain is often disabling, leading to impaired hand function, particularly pinch and grip. There may be a history of a previous Bennett's fracture or of occupational overuse, particularly if the job requires repetitive pinching or picking up of small objects. Initial treatment with anti-inflammatory drugs, splinting, and intra-articular steroid injections may provide temporary relief. Once symptoms become severe, however, surgical intervention provides pain relief with minimal loss of function.

Tumors in the Hand

Tumors in the hand are not uncommon. Most involve the soft tissues and are benign, but it must be stressed that whenever the diagnosis is in question, malignant potential must be fully investigated. The most common are *ganglions* that occur in the fingers, most commonly along the volar aspects of the flexor tendon sheath between the A1 and A2 pulleys. They are small, spherical masses, usually tender to the touch and may be particularly painful during gripping activities. They are often unresponsive to conservative management and usually need to be surgically removed. Differential diagnosis should include *inclusion cyst* and foreign body granulomas that can also occur along the volar surfaces of the fingers and palms.

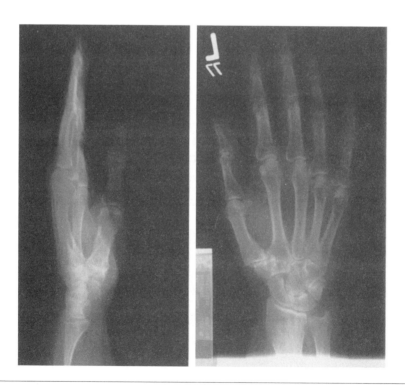

FIGURE 6-16.   Basal joint degenerative joint disease.

Hemangiomas are small, tender, bluish swellings also found in fingers. *Glomus tumors* are less common. They are small vascular tumors, presenting with exquisite tenderness under the nail bed. They are benign but respond only to surgical removal. *Enchondromas* are most common in the hands, may be multiple, and are often a cause of pathologic fracture. They are benign but may be expansile. Their presence may not be noted until a radiograph of the hand is taken after injury or fracture, but, in other cases, there may be gross swelling and deformity. There is rarely any evidence of an enchondroma on physical examination. These are usually best treated by curettage and bone grafting. If a fracture is present, allow it to heal before curettage of the lesion.

Infections

Wrist: Septic Arthritis

Although idiopathic septic arthritis of joints is more common in children, it can also occur in adults. Complaints of a hot, painful, swollen wrist, particularly with normal radiographs, should raise a high index of suspicion of septic arthritis of the wrist joint. Routine evaluation includes a complete blood count, sedimentation rate, and aspiration of the joint with a large-bore needle (pus is thicker than normal joint fluid). Any aspirate should be sent first for culture and Gram's stain, and second for cell count if any fluid is left. If there is a cloudy or purulent aspirate, an open lavage of the joint should be done. The only organism that may be treated without joint incision and drainage is gonnococcus.

Tuberculosis of the Wrist

Although tuberculosis of the wrist is rare, the diagnosis should be considered when a low-grade chronic infection is present. Marked swelling of the joint is followed by muscle wasting in the forearm, erosion, destruction, and anterior subluxation of the carpus. Radiographs show marked osteopenia on both sides of the joint with loss of the normal articular joint space. Diagnosis is confirmed by synovial biopsy and culture for mycobacterium tuberculosis. Differential diagnosis includes monoarticular rheumatoid arthritis.

The AP chest x-ray may be typical for tuberculosis, or the diagnosis may not be obvious. If tuberculosis is suspected, consultation should be made to an infectious disease specialist. Treatment should include antituberculosis drugs combined with synovectomy and drainage of the wrist joint. Late presenting cases often need wrist fusion as a result of the longstanding joint destruction and cartilage loss.

Infections in the Hand

1. *Paronychia* is the most common of all infections in the hand, occurring between the base of the nail and the cuticle. Infection usually results from introduction of *Staphylococcus aureus* into the paronychial tissue by a sliver of a nail or a hangnail, a manicure instrument, or a tooth. Continuity of the nail fold around the base of the nail may cause infection to extend from one side of the finger to the other. In the very early stages, this pro-

cess can be aborted by soaks in warm saline solution, systemic oral antibiotics, and rest of the affected part. If there is no response to soaks and oral antibiotics after 24 to 48 hours, treatment by removing a portion of the nail, drainage of the abscess, and oral antibiotics usually results in cure.

2. A *felon* is a pulp space infection occurring in the fibrofatty tissue of the fingertips and is extremely painful. There is often, but not always, an injury preceding the development of a felon. Pain and swelling usually develop rapidly. If untreated, infection frequently leads to osteomyelitis of the distal phalanx. Treatment should be by surgical drainage and oral antibiotics.

3. *Tendon sheath infections (flexor tenosynovitis)* lead to rapid swelling of the finger and pressure buildup within the tendon sheath. There is always a serious risk of tendon sloughing or disabling adhesion formation.

    On physical examination, patients will usually demonstrate Knavel's four classic signs: swollen digit, tenderness along flexor tendon sheath, flexed posture of digit, and pain with passive extension of digit. The finger may also have a palpable area of fluctuance with erythema and increased warmth. These infections are often secondary to a puncture wound but may also occur with no identifiable etiology. Infection and swelling spread rapidly. Before the common use of antibiotics, these infections were associated with a mortality rate as high as 50%. Rapid treatment will decrease the incidence of adhesions and loss of finger function. In the case of the fifth finger, there may be retrograde spread to involve the ulnar bursa, and in the thumb, retrograde spread proximally involves the radial bursa. These two bursae communicate proximal to the wrist at Parona's space, and infection may develop in the wrist proximal to the flexor retinaculum, or infection may spread between the thumb and the small finger. Flexor sheath infections should all be treated surgically by incision, drainage, and parenteral antibiotics. Postoperatively, patients are usually hospitalized for 3 to 7 days and the wound may take up to 3 weeks to heal. Most patients require therapy after surgery, and 3 months may pass before finger motion returns to near normal.

4. *Web space infections* are usually accompanied by pain as well as swelling and redness in the palm and affected web space. Physical examination reveals erythema with exquisite tenderness in the web space. Infection may follow a puncture wound or rupture of a blister in the web. Infection may spread along the volar aspects of the related fingers or to adjacent web spaces across the anterior aspect of the palm. If seen early, most web space infections respond to antibiotics, splinting, and elevation. After abscess formation, however, surgical drainage is usually necessary. Postoperatively, most patients do not need therapy and are able to return to work in approximately 4 weeks.

5. *Mid palmar and thenar space infections* usually occur in these two compartments of the hand that lie between the flexor tendons and the metacarpals. Infection may spread to these areas from web space or tendon sheath infections, and dissemination through the hand is then rapid. In either case, there is usually gross swelling and tenderness of the hand. Un-

less there is a rapid response (24 hours) to antibiotics, elevation, and splinting, early drainage should be performed.

6. *Human bites* should be suspected when a patient presents with puncture wounds over the MCP joints. These probably originated from a human tooth during a fight. Some patients will, however, admit that they were bitten. The flora of the human mouth include *Eikenella corrodens,* a facultative anaerobe that is sensitive to penicillin, as well as *Staphylococcus aureus* and other oral flora. Patients should be treated with incision and drainage and high-dose penicillin as well as a cephalosporin or other antibiotic effective against *Staphylococcus aureus.*

Recommended Readings

Gellman, H., & Campion, D. (1996). In-situ decompression of the ulnar nerve. *Hand Clinics, 12*(2), 405.

Gellman, H., Caputo, R., Carter, V., Aboulofia, A., & McKay, M. (1989, March). Comparison of short and long thumb-spica casts for non-displaced fractures of the carpal scaphoid. *Journal of Bone and Joint Surgery, 71A,* 354.

Gellman, H., Gelberman, R. H., Tan, A. M., & Botte, M. J. (1986). Carpal tunnel syndrome. An evaluation of the provocative diagnostic tests. *Journal of Bone and Joint Surgery, 68A,* 735.

Grover, R. (1996). Clinical assessment of scaphoid injuries and the detection of fractures. *Journal of Hand Surgery, 21*(3), 341.

Kuklick, R. G. (1996). Carpal tunnel syndrome. *Orthopaedic Clinics of North America, 27*(2), 345.

Kuschner, S. H., Brien, W., Johnson, D., & Gellman, H. (1991, April). Complications associated with carpal tunnel release. *Orthopaedic Review, 20*(4), 346.

Kuschner, S. H., Lane, C. S., Brien, W. W., & Gellman, H. (1994). Scaphoid fractures and scaphoid nonunion: diagnosis and treatment. *Orthopaedic Review, 23*(11), 861.

Pomerance, J. F. (1995). Painful basal joint arthritis of the thumb. Part I: anatomy, pathophysiology and diagnosis. *American Journal of Orthopaedics, 24*(5), 401.

Pomerance, J. F. (1995). Painful basal joint arthritis of the thumb. Part II: treatment. *American Journal of Orthopaedics, 24*(6), 466.

Rettig, A. C., & Patel, D. V. (1995). Epidemiology of the elbow, forearm and wrist injuries in the athlete. *Clinical Sports Medicine, 14*(2), 289.

Chapter 7

The Hip and Pelvis

Pekka A. Mooar, MD

Anatomy and Function

The pelvis (Fig. 7-1) consists of a complex of bone and ligamentous structures that connects the spine to the hip joint and provides a broad surface for the articulation of the powerful muscles of the lower extremity that are needed for ambulation and to provide a stable attachment of the spine to the lower extremities. The pelvis also protects the abdominal viscera.

The spine is attached to the pelvis through the sacrum. It is secured in all planes by a complex of ligamentous supports and secondary muscle stabilizers. The pelvis is made up of two paired innominate bones that articulate at the symphysis pubis and the sacroiliac (SI) joints. Each innominate has three separate bones: the ilium, ischium, and pubis. The confluence of these three bones is in the acetabulum. In the young, this confluence provides for acetabular growth. This growth area fuses around 16 years of age.

The ilium is the most prominent of the pelvic bones and forms the superior and lateral borders of the pelvis. It also provides for protection of the abdominal viscera and for the broad insertion of the gluteal muscles. It also provides stress transference during standing.

The ischium (Fig. 7-2) is posterior and provides for stress transference during sitting. The pubis is the most anterior structure and performs a tie rod mechanism to prevent lateral displacement of the two innominate bones during weight bearing.

The hip joint is a ball-and-socket joint composed of the acetabulum (socket) and femoral head (ball). Stability of this joint is produced by capsular ligaments, acetabular labrum, and secondary muscles stabilizers. The forces acting across the hip joint are three times body weight during walking and four times body weight during running. Blood is supplied to the hip through the fovial artery in the acetabulum and by the medial and lateral circumflex arteries. Dislocations and fractures may disrupt the blood supply to the femoral head resulting in avascular necrosis.

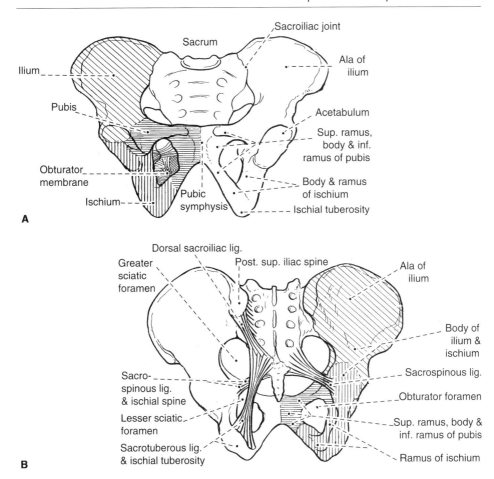

FIGURE 7-1. The bony pelvis, tilted slightly backwards and seen from (**A**) an anterior and (**B**) a posterior view. The three component bones of the pelvic girdle are shaded differently. The posterior view shows the chief bracing ligaments between the sacrum and the coxal bone.

The hip moves in four planes and two rotations; flexion, extension, abduction, adduction, and internal and external rotation (Table 7-1).

Physical Examination of the Hip and Pelvis

The hip and pelvis are examined in a sequential fashion: inspection and palpation of the bone and soft tissues, evaluation of active and passive range of motion, and assessment of motor strength.

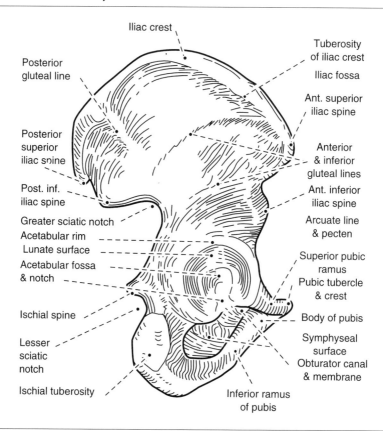

FIGURE 7-2.   Lateral view of the right coxal bone.

Inspection

Inspection is first performed when the patient enters the examining room. Observe for antalgic gait or Trendelenburg gait (lurching gait). Examine the ease with which the patient stands, walks, sits, and arises from sitting. While the patient is standing, observe for equal weight distribution, symmetry of the pelvis, and height of the pelvis. Look for a tilt of the pelvis that may indicate a leg length discrepancy. Examine the lumbosacral spine for normal contours. Increased lordosis is seen with weak abdominal muscles and with hip flexion contractures. Absence of lordosis may be secondary to muscle spasm. The buttocks should be symmetric, and the gluteal fold should be at the same level. Observe for ecchymosis, abrasions, draining sinuses, and erythema.

Palpation

Palpation is performed to gauge skin temperature and areas of tenderness. The patient should be in undergarments and may be standing or supine.

Beginning anterior with the patient directly in front of the examiner, place the examining hands on the patient's waist and slide them down toward the thigh to

TABLE 7-1
Muscles of the Hip and Pelvis

	Primary	Secondary
Hip extensors	Gluteus maximus ischial portion of adductor magnus	Hamstrings Gluteus medius Piriformis
Hip flexors	Iliopsoas Rectus femoris	Adductors Tensor fasciae lata
Hip abductors	Gluteus medius Gluteus minimus	Tensor fasciae lata
Hip adductors	Adductor magnus Adductor longus Adductor brevis	Gracilis Obturator externus Hamstrings Gluteus maximus
External rotators	Gluteus maximus Piriformis Obturator internus Gemelli Obturator externus Quadratus femoris	Iliopsoas
Hip internal rotators	Tensor fasciae latae Gluteus medius Gluteus minimus	

the bony prominences. This is the iliac crest. With the thumbs, palpate inferiorly to locate the most anterior bony prominence. This is the anterior superior iliac spine and the origin of the sartorius. By sliding the thumbs inferiorly, the examiner will come upon the pubic ramus (usually just at the line of pubic hair and the prepubic fat). The pubic symphysis is at the level of the greater trochanters laterally. Palpate the trochanters laterally for tenderness of the bursa and tenderness of the iliotibial band. The posterior aspect of the pelvis is palpated directly over the posterior brim of the iliac crest (the origin of the gluteus medius).

Palpate the iliac crest posteriorly to the iliac tubercle posteriorly. Deep in this most posterior portion of the iliac crest is the SI joint, which is not directly palpable. Next, palpate the ischial tuberosity, the origin of the hamstrings. This is located in the middle of the buttock usually in the gluteal fold. Flexion of the hip to move the gluteus maximus upward allows for easier palpation of the ischial tuberosity. Perform soft tissue palpation on all muscles to examine for masses, tenderness and defects. Palpation of the adductors is facilitated by placing the lower extremity in the figure-four position with the hip flexed and externally rotated, and the foot resting on the contralateral knee. Adductors are now easily palpated at their origin in the groin. Evaluate for range of motion. Range of motion is tested actively and passively and includes flexion, extension, abduction, adduction, and internal and external rotation.

Normal hip range of motion (Fig. 7-3) is: flexion, 120 degrees; extension, 30 degrees; internal rotation, 35 degrees; external rotation, 45 degrees; abduction, 45 degrees; and adduction, 25 degrees. Test muscle strength providing resistance in

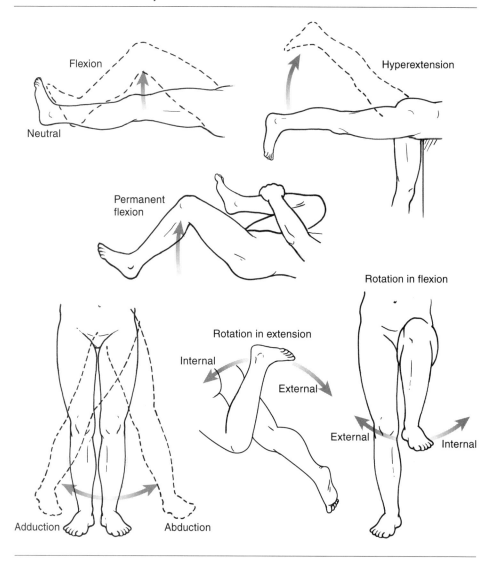

FIGURE 7-3. Normal range of motion of the hip.

all planes against motion and grade using a scale of 0 to 5 (see Fig. 2-2 for motor grading scale).

Special Tests

Trendelenburg Test

The Trendelenburg test (Fig. 7-4) is used to evaluate gluteus medius strength. The patient is observed from behind and asked to stand on one leg. The pelvis should remain level or slightly elevated (this assesses the gluteus medius of the weight-bearing leg). If the pelvis drops, the gluteus medius is weak.

A.
Negative (Normal) Trendelenburg Test

B.
Positive (Abnormal) Trendelenburg Test

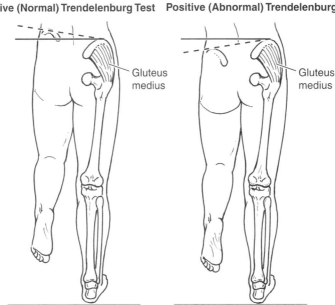

FIGURE 7-4. (**A**) The Trendelenburg test as performed while standing on the left lower extremity. This person has a negative Trendelenburg test. Note that the right side of the pelvis does rise slightly because the gluteus medius and minimus of the right side act by origin-insertion inversion to straighten the pelvis. (**B**) This person is also performing the Trendelenburg test while standing on the left lower extremity. This is a positive Trendelenburg test in that the pelvis tilts to the right side and cannot be recovered to a straight position. This person is suffering from either (**a**) paralysis of the gluteus medius and minimus muscles; (**b**) dislocation of the hip joint, or (**c**) an abnormal angle of femoral inclination.

Gaenslen's Sign

To be examined for Gaenslen's sign (Fig. 7-5), the patient is supine with both legs drawn to the chest, and with one buttock extended over the edge of examining table. The unsupported leg is dropped over the edge of the table. This will provoke pain in the SI joint in the presence of SI disease. The affected hip is hyperextended against a stabilized pelvis. With the patient's unaffected leg flexed to the chest, place one hand on the iliac crest of the affected hip. With the other hand on the knee, move the affected hip into hyperextension. Reproduction of SI pain indicates a positive test.

Thomas Test

The Thomas test (Fig. 7-6) demonstrates a hip flexion contracture. The patient is placed supine and both hips are flexed maximally, reversing the normal lumbar lordosis of the spine. While holding one hip maximally flexed, the opposite hip

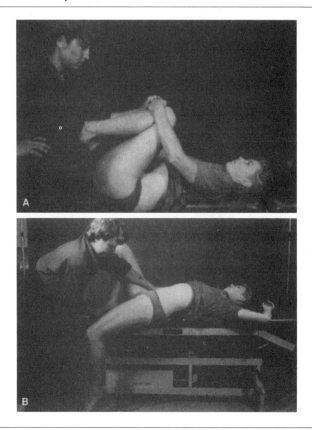

FIGURE 7-5. (**A**) Gaenslen's sign. (**B**) Lower limb of unsupported side is lowered over the side of the table.

is extended. Lack of complete extension is indicative of a hip flexion contracture.

The Painful Hip and Pelvis

Pain in the pelvis and hip region is a common complaint and may be due to traumatic or nontraumatic causes (Fig. 7-7). Referred pain from the spine or viscera must always be included in the differential diagnosis. Trauma is either repetitive, persistent microtrauma leading to overuse or "stress" syndromes, or macrooverload resulting in the failure of muscle and bone units (ie, as in a muscle pull or fracture).

Nontraumatic causes of hip and pelvic pain include inflammatory conditions, infections, tumors, referred pain, metabolic bone disease, and degenerative arthritis. Inflammatory conditions of the pelvis and hip will usually present in the hip joint or SI joint. They include rheumatoid arthritis, ankylosing spondylitis, and Reiter's syndrome.

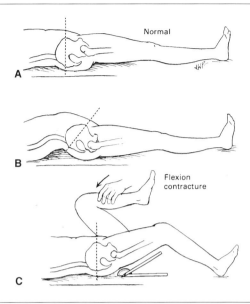

FIGURE 7-6. The Thomas test for the detection of hip flexion contracture. The subject is lying supine on a hard surface with hips and knees extended. (**A**) If there is no contracture, the pelvis remains neutral with the anterior superior iliac spine lying vertically above the posterior superior iliac spine. (**B**) If a flexion contracture is present, to keep the legs on the table, the subject arches his or her back, compensating for the forward tilt of the pelvis. (**C**) To test the right hip, the left thigh is flexed passively until the anterior superior iliac spine directly overlies the posterior superior iliac spine. This places the pelvis in the neutral position and brings the lumbar spine down flat on the table. If there is a flexion contracture, the right thigh cannot remain on the table and will make an angle with it that equals the angle of the deformity.

Nontraumatic Conditions of the Pelvis and Hip

Ankylosing Spondylitis

SYMPTOMS. Ankylosing spondylitis presents as low back pain in the buttocks or thighs with protracted morning stiffness that is relieved with activity.

SIGNS. Localized pain over the SI joint, and decreased spine motion and chest expansion are two important signs.

LABORATORY EVALUATION. Collagen vascular screen (RF, ANA, erythrocyte sedimentation rate [ESR], HLA B-27) is usually negative in these seronegative spondyloarthropathies.

RADIOGRAPHIC EVALUATION. Sclerosis in the SI joints is seen on x-rays. Computed tomography (CT) scan may diagnose sclerosis earlier. Bone scan is useful when x-rays are negative, showing increased activity in the SI joint.

TREATMENT. Indomethacin usually provides prompt relief. Thoracic extension flexibility exercises at least twice each day help to maintain normal spinal curves.

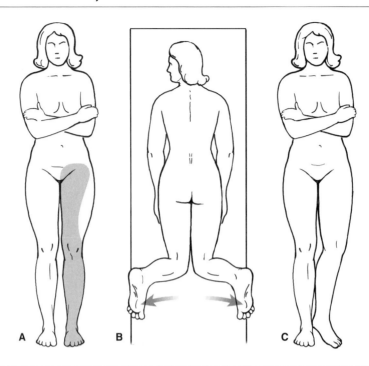

FIGURE 7-7. Characteristics of hip joint pain. (**A**) Location of the pain: Initial location over the groin and/or anterior aspect of the knee; referral of pain along the anterior aspect of the thigh, and eventually into the leg as well. (**B**) Painful manipulation. (**C**) Posture of the joint.

REFERRAL. The patient should be referred to an orthopedic surgeon or rheumatologist.

OUTCOME. The outcome can be variable.

Paget's Disease

SYMPTOMS. Paget's disease presents in the adult as pelvic or hip pain. Pain is increased with weight bearing with acetabular involvement, often resulting in degenerative arthritis. Significant acetabular protrusion may be present.

SIGNS. The signs for Paget's disease are the same as the symptoms.

LABORATORY EVALUATION. The laboratory evaluation includes increased serum alkaline phosphatase.

RADIOGRAPHIC EVALUATION. Mixed areas of sclerosis and osteolysis are the hallmarks of Paget's disease.

TREATMENT. See Chapter 10.

Inflammatory Arthritis

The hip joint may also be involved in any inflammatory collagen vascular disease.

SYMPTOMS. These diseases present with morning stiffness and painful motion. The stiffness usually decreases with activity. With longstanding inflammation, joint motion may be lost.

SIGNS. The signs for inflammatory arthritis are the same as the symptoms.

LABORATORY EVALUATION. A collagen vascular screen should be performed (RF, ANA, ESR).

RADIOGRAPHIC EVALUATION. The radiographic evaluation consists of a standing anteroposterior (AP) with lateral (LAT) views. These may show joint space narrowing, subchondral cyst formation, and peripheral osteophytes. A bone scan may be useful to demonstrate synovitis. Early disease may be represented with widening of the joint space. This is indicative of a joint effusion.

TREATMENT. See Chapter 10.

Crystalline Arthritis

SYMPTOMS. Gout and pseudogout can present with an acutely painful hip. Pain is exacerbated by motion and weight bearing.

SIGNS. The hip is held in flexion and external rotation. Movement in any plane increases the discomfort. A low-grade fever may be present. Pain is increased with weight bearing.

LABORATORY EVALUATION. Joint aspiration and synovial fluid analysis must be performed to confirm the diagnosis. Crystals will be seen on polarized microscopy. Serum uric acid may be elevated in gout. ESR may be elevated. Cultures should be obtained to exclude infection.

RADIOGRAPHIC EVALUATION. In an acute attack, the routine radiographs may be normal or show joint space widening consistent with an effusion. With longstanding disease, joint space narrowing with cyst formation on both sides of the joint may be seen. Calcification in the cartilage (chondrocalcinosis) may be seen in pseudogout. A bone scan will show synovitis in the acute attack.

TREATMENT. See Chapter 10.

Osteoarthritis

Arthritis is a common finding in the aging patient. It is a result of the gradual loss of articular cartilage secondary to increased stresses (overload), abnormal cartilage metabolism (chondrocalcinosis), or persistent inflammation (crystal-induced arthritis).

SYMPTOMS. Pain is increased with activity. As the disease progresses, there is loss of hip rotation and abduction. The end stage hip is an uniaxial hip allowing only for flexion and extension.

SIGNS. These include pain with weight bearing and limited hip motion with an antalgic gait.

DIAGNOSTIC STUDIES. AP and LAT radiographs of the pelvis and hip in weight bearing are necessary. These will demonstrate joint space, narrowing, cyst formation, sclerosis, and osteophyte formation.

TREATMENT. Consists of muscle strengthening, nonsteroidal anti-inflammatories, and use of ambulatory aides, such as a cane in the opposite hand (see Appendix D). Surgery is recommended in those patients who have pain that is unrelieved with conservative measures and in those whose pain interferes with their activities of daily living.

REFERRAL. Referral to an orthopedic surgeon or rheumatologist is recommended.

Avascular Necrosis

Avascular necrosis is the loss of blood supply to the femoral head and the resultant death to all or part of the femoral head. It may occur in any age group.

ETIOLOGY. The etiology may be posttraumatic after hip dislocation or fractures or may be secondary to steroid use or alcohol abuse. The vast majority, however, is idiopathic.

SYMPTOMS. Hip pain occurs with weight bearing. Pain is localized to the groin.

SIGNS. Signs include pain on weight bearing and with activity that is relieved with rest, and progressive loss of joint motion as the disease progresses. Loss of rotation occurs first.

DIAGNOSTIC EVALUATION. Radiographs are initially within normal limits with progression seen over time. The weight-bearing surfaces of the femoral head collapse with loss of sphericity of the femoral head. Crescent sign formation on the LAT x-ray is diagnostic for avascular necrosis and indicates separation of the articular surface from the underlying bone. Earliest diagnostic imaging is with magnetic resonance imaging (MRI). Three-phase bone scanning is also a diagnostic tool.

TREATMENT. Treatment, in the early stages of the disease before collapse, is with protected weight bearing. Conflict exists as to whether core decompression of the femoral head is useful in the treatment of this disease. Joint reconstruction for the elderly and hip fusion for the younger patient are the treatments for late disease. For bilateral involvement, hip replacement is indicated even in younger patients.

OUTCOME. This depends on the stage of the disease when first diagnosed and patient compliance with protected weight bearing.

REFERRAL. An orthopedic surgeon is recommended for treatment.

Infection

ETIOLOGY. The etiology can be drug use, sexually transmitted diseases, immunosuppression, and dissemination from other sources.

SYMPTOMS. Severe pain that is increased with any motion, and pain that is localized to the groin but may radiate to the thigh or knee are important symptoms. There is also a loss of joint motion, and fever and night sweats are usually present.

SIGNS. The patient presents with a flexed, abducted, and externally rotated hip, as position of comfort. Fever is usually present. The patient resists any motion because it increases pain. Inguinal lymphadenopathy may be present.

LABORATORY EVALUATION. The laboratory evaluation will show an elevated white cell count, often with an elevated ESR. Blood cultures may be useful but are often negative. An aspiration of the hip joint is mandatory and is diagnostic. It will show an elevated white cell count with a predominance of polys. Routine Gram's stain and cultures of the synovial fluid are mandatory. Cultures for gonorrhea should also be obtained. Tuberculosis cultures should also be considered.

RADIOGRAPHIC EVALUATION. Radiographs may show joint space widening. A bone scan is performed to rule out osteomyelitis. MRI is useful to exclude bone involvement.

TREATMENT. Aspiration for culture followed by surgical drainage for all infections other than gonococcal arthritis is recommended.

REFERRAL. Immediate referral to an orthopedic surgeon is mandatory if infection is suspected.

OUTCOME. If treated early, the outcome should be good. If treated late, chondrolysis from lysosomal enzymes leads to rapid joint degeneration.

Infection After Total Hip Arthroplasty

ETIOLOGY. This infection may be either primary or secondary after a total hip arthroplasty. Primary infections result from infections from innoculum at the time of surgery and occur immediately in the perioperative period. Secondary infections usually are due to a secondary transient bacteriemia from dental work, gastrointestinal or genitourinary instrumentation, or urinary tract infection and are primarily gram negative. It is recommended that antibiotic prophylaxis be performed in patients undergoing these procedures.

SYMPTOMS. The patient presents with painful antalgic gait and may present with an acute dislocation.

SIGNS. Pain with loss of ambulatory range is the primary sign. CBC may show an elevated white count, and the ESR may be elevated.

RADIOGRAPHIC EVALUATION. Radiolucent lines about the prosthesis indicate loosening. Sequential bone scan/gallium scan may be useful in determining septic versus aseptic loosening. Indium white cell scanning is useful. Aspiration is diagnostic only if positive.

TREATMENT. Treatment includes débridement, irrigation, and antibiotics with immediate or delayed exchange of the prosthesis, depending on the organism. For a highly virulent, drug-resistant organism, resection arthroplasty (Girdlestone procedure) or fusion is the treatment of choice.

REFERRAL. Refer the patient to an orthopedic surgeon experienced in revision arthroplasty.

OUTCOME. The outcome is highly variable and depends on the organism infecting the joint and underlying bone stock.

Gram-positive infections have better outcomes than gram-negative infections.

Tumors

Tumors may be either benign or malignant and either primary or metastatic. Primary bone tumors are primarily a disease of the adolescent. Metastatic disease and multiple myeloma are primarily diseases of the mature adult and the elderly. Tumors should always be suspected when pain is disproportionate to the physical findings and with the presence of night pain. Visceral tumors should also be considered as sources of pelvic and hip pain.

ETIOLOGY. The etiology of musculoskeletal tumors is unknown.

SYMPTOMS. Tumors should always be suspected when pain is disproportionate to the physical findings. Tumors characteristically present as night pain. They are often discovered after minor trauma and often present as persistent discomfort after relatively minor injury exacerbated by activity.

SIGNS. Physical examination may reveal localized tenderness, swelling, and loss of normal motion. There may be localized erythema and rubor.

EVALUATION. Evaluation should include complete history and physical with abdominal, vaginal, and rectal examination. Laboratory evaluation includes alkaline phosphatase (elevated), serum calcium (elevated), CBC (hemoglobin is decreased, white count ±), SPEP (monoclonal spike), UA (proteinuria), and PSA.

RADIOGRAPHIC IMAGING. Plain films in early lesions are often negative, especially in osteoid osteomas. They may show early areas of sclerosis or periosteal elevation. Tomography and CT scanning are useful to show the nidus of the osteoid osteoma. Bone scanning with tomography is usually diagnostic for malignancies and will localize a tumor except for myeloma. An MRI with and without gadolinium is highly diagnostic.

DIFFERENTIAL DIAGNOSIS OF TUMORS. Adolescent tumors may be either benign or malignant. Benign tumors include osteoid osteoma, osteoblastoma, bone cyst, benign chondroblastoma, and chondromyxoid fibroma. Malignant tumors of the pelvis and hip include periosteal osteosarcoma and chondrosarcoma. Multiple myeloma is the most common primary malignancy of bone and should always be considered in the differential diagnosis in all patients over the age of 60 with pelvic and hip pain. Metastatic tumors are the second most common.

OUTCOME. Outcome is highly variable depending on the malignancy tissue type and degree of local and distant spread. Excision of benign tumors with curettage and bone grafting is usually curative. Sarcomas may require amputation, although limb salvaging surgery is available for early lesions.

REFERRAL. Referral should be immediate after suspicion of any malignancy. The long-term outcome depends on staging. In metastatic disease, early intervention may prevent development of pathologic fractures. This includes localized radiation, surgical stabilization, and chemotherapy. Referrals to multiple disciplines may be required, such as oncology, radiation oncology, and orthopedic oncology.

Traumatic Conditions of the Pelvis and Hip

Contusions (Table 7-2)

ETIOLOGY. Contusions result from a direct blow to a soft tissue area that has little soft tissue padding; the iliac crest, greater trochanter, and ischial tuberosity are at greater risk for a more painful contusion.

SYMPTOMS. Symptoms include pain, localized tenderness, ecchymosis, and swelling.

SIGNS. Signs are the same as the symptoms.

TREATMENT. Ice, compression, and rest will control local bleeding. When pain decreases, therapy is necessary to restore normal flexibility and strength before returning to activity. Heat should not be used acutely because it is associated with the development of myositis ossificans.

Bursitis (Table 7-3)

ETIOLOGY. Bursitis usually results from repetitive stress or direct trauma.

SYMPTOMS. Symptoms are characterized by pain that may be aggravated with motion.

SIGNS. Pain on palpation of the bursa is one sign of bursitis. Erythema and rubor also may be present.

TREATMENT. Treatment consists of rest and ice with adjunctive use of nonsteroidal anti-inflammatory medication, and the identification of the etiology and correction of the underlying causes. Therapy to restore normal flexibility, range of motion, and strength completes the treatment. Bursal injections with a steroid preparation may be useful in an acutely painful bursitis.

TABLE 7-2
Common Contusions

Location	Etiology	Signs
Greater trochanter	Direct blow or fall onto trochanter	Pain with hip abduction, external rotation
Ischial tuberosity	Fall onto buttocks	Pain with straight leg raising Active resisted contraction of hamstring
Pubic ramus	Fall across bar, as in gymnastics	Pain on palpation of pubis
Iliac crest	Direct fall on crest	Difficulty walking, standing upright, pain along the iliac crest

TABLE 7-3
Bursitis

Location	Etiology	Signs
Trochanteric bursitis	Leg length discrepancy Board pelvis in females Tight tensor fascialata Poor running mechanics Running on banked surfaces	Pain localized to trochanter Increased with abduction, external rotation Positive Ober test
Ischial bursitis	Direct blood Saddle irritation	Pain with sitting, especially increased with legs crossed Direct tenderness on palpation
Iliopectoneal bursitis	Microtrauma	Anterior hip pain and antalgic gait Hip flexion, externally rotated for comfort

Muscle Strains

These are the most common injuries encountered in athletes and are a result of stretching the muscle and tendon beyond their normal length. Injury may occur anywhere along the muscle but usually occurs in the muscle tendon junctions. Lack of warm-up or preparation for activity is the common etiology. All muscle groups crossing the hip are at risk for muscle strain (Table 7-4).

TABLE 7-4
Muscle Strains

Location	Etiology	Signs/Symptoms
Adductors	Most common in the older athlete Forced external rotation of the adducted leg and forced abduction Additional adductor imbalance	Localized tenderness Pain with passive abduction and forced adduction
Hamstrings	Forced flexion of hip with the knee extended	Localized tenderness Pain over muscle and ischial tuberosity with straight leg raising Pain increased with active/resisted hip extension
Iliopsoas	Kicking injury Blocked kick resulting in muscle overload; the thigh fixed or pushed into extension	Deep groin pain May extend into abdomen External rotation of hip in extension increases pain
Rectus femoris	Jumping activities requiring hip flexion and knee extension (ie, long jump)	Groin pain increased with knee extension while prone; pain increased with passive hip extension and rotation
Gluteus medius	Usually chronic overuse Ice hockey	Pain and attachment to greater trochanter

TREATMENT. Treatment consists of rest, ice compression, elevation, and a gradual restoration of activity as symptoms subside and normal, painless range of motion and flexibility, endurance, and strength are established.

Before returning to sports, individuals must have:

1. Full, painless range of motion
2. Normal flexibility
3. Normal strength
4. Endurance strength
5. Ability to perform the sport without pain

Sacroiliac Strains

ETIOLOGY. Sudden twisting motions of the trunk, pulling while bending forward (eg, weed pulling), or falling on unilateral buttocks can cause SI strains.

SYMPTOMS. Pain that usually presents a day after injury, with ache and stiffness over the SI joint posteriorly with difficulty bending forward are frequent symptoms.

SIGNS. Limited lumbosacral motion and forward flexion as well as pain over the SI joint, a positive Gaenslen's sign, and a positive Lasègue's sign.

DIAGNOSTIC IMAGING. This is not needed in SI strains.

TREATMENT. Treatment includes rest, ice, and analgesics followed by postural education and back rehabilitation programs for both flexion and extension exercise (see Appendix E for back exercises).

Fractures of the Hip and Pelvis

Apophyseal Avulsion Injuries

ETIOLOGY. Apophyseal avulsion injuries usually occur in the adolescent before cessation of growth. These injuries are associated with avulsion of the secondary growth centers or apophysis. Injury may occur before the appearance of the secondary ossification centers that develop late in adolescence. A high index of suspicion is needed to diagnose these cases. Diagnosis is confirmed with the development of callus several weeks after injury; this callous formation may be mistaken for tumor (Table 7-5).

TREATMENT. Treatment is usually conservative and consists of rest, ice, and resolution in 4 to 6 weeks.

STRESS FRACTURES

Stress fractures are usually the result of overuse and are generally seen several weeks after a sudden increase in activity levels. They present as pain with weight bearing and increase with activity. Pain is increased with extremes of hip rotation. Diagnosis is made with imaging studies. Plain x-rays may show fractures with periosteal reaction. A bone scan provides diagnosis before radiographs. MRI will demonstrate bone marrow edema. Pain in the groin is the hallmark of a proximal femoral stress fracture and requires prompt intervention to prevent subsequent fracture displacement. If the fracture line progresses across the neck, percutaneous

TABLE 7-5
Apophyseal Injuries

Location	Etiology	Signs/Symptoms
Iliac crest	Sudden twisting motions Direct trauma	Pain and discomfort over crest Pain with resisted abduction of hip
Anterior superior iliac spine	Forceful contraction of sartorius with running or jumping	Pain over the anterior thigh Pain increased with active hip flexion and passive hip extension
Anterior inferior iliac spine	Kicking activity	Pain and weakness with hip flexion and an antalgic gait
Ischial apophysis	Sudden hamstring contraction with the hip and pelvis flexed and the knee extended. Results in a hamstring avulsion (hurdler's position) Splits during dancing Avulsion—adductor magnus	Pain with antalgic gait Pain with sitting Pain increased with hip flexion when the knee is extended
Lesser trochanter	Rare—sudden contraction of iliopsoas with the thigh flexed and hip extended (eg, a blocked kick at the point of contact with the ball)	Antalgic gait Pain over trochanter Pain with hip flexion with leg extended Position of comfort, flexed and abducted hip

pinning should be performed (Table 7-6). Activity modification is required to prevent displacement. Activity modification may be required for 12 to 26 weeks to allow healing.

Pelvic Fractures

ETIOLOGY. Pelvic fractures are usually associated with high-energy accidents such as a motor vehicle accident or a fall from a significant height. Injury may occur to a pedestrian struck by a car or to a person who falls from a horse or scaffolding.

TABLE 7-6
Stress Fractures

Location	Etiology	Signs/Symptoms
Pelvic stress fractures	Usually female runners Ischial ramus most common Overuse	Pain over ischial ramus
Pubic ramus	Repetitive trauma Gymnastics	Pain over pubic ramus
Femoral neck	Repetitive jumping activities or running	Pain, antalgic gait Pain with flexion and internal rotation May also present as thigh pain

These injuries carry associated high morbidity and mortality secondary to associated other injuries. The geometry of injury depends on the direction of the injury and the force that is applied.

SYMPTOMS. Pain, swelling, visible ecchymosis, hematoma, and inability to bear weight are several symptoms. There may be a shift of the iliac crest with vertical or horizontal instability appreciated on palpation. General pressure applied to the iliac wings in compression and distraction may demonstrate this instability.

SIGNS. The signs are the same as the symptoms. Significant hypotension may be present.

TREATMENT. The patient must be referred immediately to a trauma center. Vascular support is necessary because bleeding may be life threatening. The use of military anti-shock trousers (MAST) in the acute setting with a comminuted fracture may be beneficial in maintaining vascular volume and controlling pelvic bleeding.

RADIOGRAPHIC IMAGING. Imaging consists of AP/LAT, both obliques, and inlet and outlet views to define the planes of displacement. CT scanning is used to define the fracture geometry before surgical stabilization.

DEFINITIVE TREATMENT. Stable injuries are treated with protected weight bearing. Unstable injuries require stabilization with either internal or external fixation.

OUTCOME. The long-term results depend on the severity of the injury. Pelvic fractures associated with SI joint dislocation and fracture comminution are associated with chronic pain. Fractures involving the acetabulum are associated with late degenerative arthritis.

Hip Dislocation

ETIOLOGY. Hip dislocation is usually the result of a motor vehicle accident with direct axial loading of the hip in a flexed position. Posterior dislocations are a result of this position, with the hip in an adducted position. Anterior dislocations are the result of abduction, external rotation and forced extension of the hip.

SYMPTOMS. Severe pain and inability to walk or stand are two symptoms. Any motion is painful. For *anterior dislocation,* the hip is held *abducted, externally rotated,* and slightly flexed. For *posterior dislocation,* the hip is held *adducted, internally rotated,* and flexed (Fig. 7-8).

SIGNS. The signs are the same as the symptoms.

TREATMENT. This is an orthopedic emergency requiring immediate referral for closed, possible open reduction of the hip dislocation. Delays in relocation result in higher incidence of avascular necrosis. Dislocations may occur in conjunction with acetabular or femoral head fractures. Treatment is based on the position of the fragments and the degree of displacement. For displaced fractures, ORIF is the preferred treatment with removal of acetabular loose bodies.

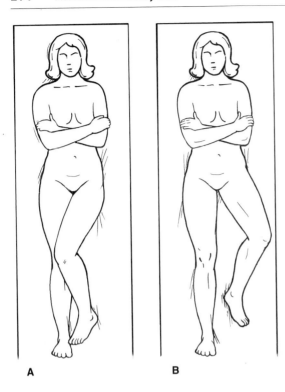

FIGURE 7-8. Postures of hip disloca-
tion. (**A**) Posterior dislocation. (**B**) Anterior dislocation.

FEMORAL NECK FRACTURES

In the adolescent and early adult, femoral neck fractures occur as a result of high-energy accidents. In the elderly, they may occur with relatively minor trauma secondary to osteoporosis. Fractures may result from a direct fall on the greater trochanter or from a rotational force along the shaft of the femur.

SYMPTOMS. Symptoms include excruciating groin pain, inability to bear weight, and the extremity held in *external rotation* and *mild adduction.* The pain is exacerbated by motion, particularly internal rotation. In the elderly person with an impacted fracture, symptoms may consist of pain with ambulation in the groin, thigh, or knee.

SIGNS. The impacted fracture presents with an antalgic gait. The fracture may be associated with an inability to bear weight, and it may have associated swelling and ecchymosis in the thigh.

DIAGNOSTIC IMAGING. AP and LAT radiographs usually confirm the diagnosis. In the elderly with groin pain and osteopenia, tomograms and a bone scan may be necessary to confirm the diagnosis. MRI is also useful to confirm a diagnosis of hip fracture.

TREATMENT. In children and young adults, all fractures should be reduced and internally fixed. A high percentage of displaced fractures will undergo avascular necrosis secondary to disruption of the blood supply along the femoral neck. In the elderly, displaced fractures should be treated with hemiarthroplasty or total hip arthroplasty in the presence of acetabular disease. Nondisplaced fractures should be treated with in situ pinning. Failure of fixation may occur secondary to osteopenia. Avascular necrosis is a late sequela in both displaced and nondisplaced fractures.

Adolescent Slipped Capital Femoral Epiphysis

ETIOLOGY. The etiology of adolescent slipped capital femoral epiphysis is uncertain, but occurs in adolescents who are short and obese or tall and thin. Displacement occurs at the junction of the proliferative cartilage and the provisional zone of calcification. This should be suspected in any adolescent complaining of groin, thigh, or knee pain.

SYMPTOMS. Groin pain often referred to the anterior medial thigh is one symptom. Antalgic gait with external rotation position of the hip and loss of internal rotation are also symptoms. For an acute slip, there is usually a history of a fall or direct trauma associated with sudden pain, spasm, or inability to fully bear weight. Chronic slips have a history of mild, aching pain in the groin and a limp. An acute slip may occur in the presence of chronic slippage.

SIGNS. The signs are the same as the symptoms.

TREATMENT. Early diagnosis before a significant slip occurs is important. Surgical in situ pinning is the treatment of choice.

DIAGNOSTIC IMAGING. AP and LAT radiographs are the appropriate studies.

Intertrochanteric Hip Fractures

ETIOLOGY. In the young, an intertrochanteric hip fracture is a result of violent trauma. In the elderly, it is usually the result of a fall from a standing position, and a result of secondary underlying osteopenia.

SYMPTOMS. Pain and an inability to bear weight with ecchymosis are symptoms.

SIGNS. A flexed, shortened, externally rotated hip, thigh swelling, and ecchymosis are several signs.

TREATMENT. Immediate referral for surgery with open reduction, and internal fixation are necessary.

DIAGNOSTIC IMAGING. AP and LAT hip radiographs are required.

OUTCOME. The outcome depends on the premorbid state of the patient. In a compromised patient, the outcome may result in the loss of one level of activity. In an active, healthy patient, resumption of normal lifestyle after healing usually occurs.

Recommended Readings

American Academy of Orthopedic Surgeons. (1991). *Athletic training and sports medicine.*

Bonjour, S. P., Schurch, M. A., & Rizzoli, R. (1996). Nutritional aspects of hip fractures. *Bone, 18*(3S), 139S.

Dandy, D. (1993). *Essential orthopedics and trauma.* New York: Churchill-Livingstone.

Fullerton, L. R. Jr. (1990). Femoral neck stress fractures. *Sports Medicine, 9*(3), 192.

Gross, J., Fetto, J., & Rosen, E. (1996). *Musculoskeletal examination.* Oxford: Blackwell.

Hoppenfeld, S. (1976). *Physical examination of the spine and extremities.* East Norwalk, CT: Appleton-Century-Croft.

Johansson, C., Ekenman, I., Tornkvist, H., & Eriksson, E. (1990). Stress fractures in the femoral neck in athletes: the consequence of a delay in diagnosis. *American Journal of Sports Medicine, 18*(5), 524.

Kanis, J. A., & McClosky, E. V. (1996). Evaluation of the risk of hip fracture. *Bone, 18*(3S), 127S.

Karagas, M. R., LuYao, G. L., Barrett, J. A., Beach, M. L., & Baron, J. A. (1996). Heterogeneity of hip fracture, age, race, sex and demographic patterns of femoral neck and trochanteric fractures among the US elderly. *American Journal of Epidemiology 143*(7), 677–682.

McLatchie, G. R., & Lennox, C. M. E. (1996). *The soft tissues: trauma and sports injuries.* London: Butterworth-Heinemann.

Mellion, M. B. (1994). *Sports medicine secrets.* Philadelphia: Hanley & Belfus/Mosby.

Norden, M., Gunnar, A., Pope, M. (1997). *Musculoskeletal disorders in the work place: principles and practices.* St. Louis: Mosby.

Norris, C. M. (1993). *Sports injuries: diagnosis and management for physiotherapists.* London: Butterworth-Heinemann.

Obrant, K. (1996). Orthopaedic treatment of hip fracture. *Bone, 18*(3S), 145S.

Raheb, J. (1995). Water fluoridation, bone density and hip fractures, a review of recent literature. *Community Dentistry and Oral Epidemiology, 23*(5), 309.

Reid, D. C. (1992). *Sports injury assessment and rehabilitation.* New York: Churchill-Livingstone.

Rosemartz, IL. *American Journal of Epidemiology, 143*(7), 677–682.

Snider, R. (1997). *Essentials of musculoskeletal care.* Rosemont, IL: American Academy of Orthopedic Surgeons. American Academy of Pediatrics.

Chapter 8

The Thigh, Knee, and Patella

Pekka A. Mooar, MD

The Knee

Anatomy and Function

The knee joint consists of two joints: the tibiofemoral joint and the patellofemoral joint. The motion at the knee joint is a complex interaction of flexion, extension, rotation, gliding, and rolling. These complex movements are allowed by the controlled instability of the knee joint. When motions outside of the range of this controlled instability take place, injury occurs. The injury is to the structure or structures that resist the applied force. Knowledge of the anatomy of the stabilizing knee structures is necessary to understand the patterns of injury.

The knee provides motion and stability, allows forces to propel the body forward, and absorbs high loads. Figure 8-1 depicts the structures of the knee. The femur, tibia, and patella are covered on their articulating surfaces with a layer of cartilage. This cartilage derives its nutrition from the synovial fluid and is subjected to the stresses imposed on it by both normal and abnormal knee motions.

The Meniscus

The menisci (medial and lateral) are crescent-shaped pieces of cartilage interposed between the femur and tibia; they absorb energy and distribute the load across the knee joint. They also provide secondary stability by deepening the tibial plateau. The ligaments of the knee are the medial and lateral collateral ligaments, and the anterior and posterior cruciate ligaments. They function in conjunction with the joint capsule to limit varus (medial), valgus (lateral), and anterioposterior translations of the knee.

The medial stabilizers of the knee are the joint capsule and the medial collateral ligament. These structures resist valgus laxity and external rotatory instabilities.

217

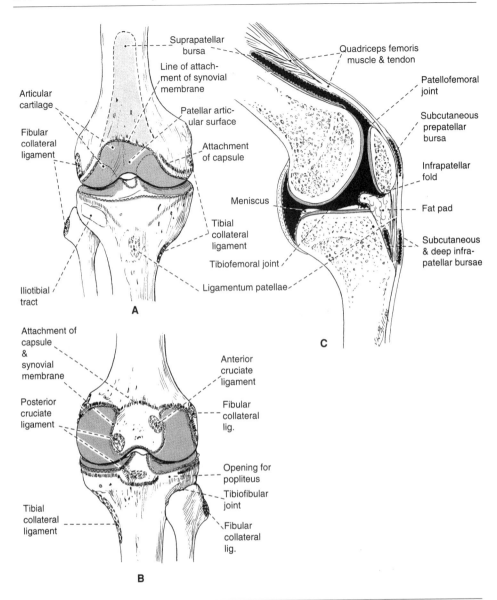

FIGURE 8-1. The anatomy of the knee joint, showing the attachments of the capsule, synovial membrane, ligaments, and menisci: (**A**) anterior view; (**B**) posterior view; (**C**) sagittal section cut to one side of the midline. The attachment of the capsule is indicated with a *dashed black line;* that of the synovial membrane with a *red line.* Cavities filled with synovial fluid are shown in *black* in C.

They have a firm attachment to the medial meniscus that make it less mobile and therefore at risk for injury during flexion and rotation of the knee. The pes anserine group (sartorius, gracilis, semitendinosus muscles) dynamically protects the knee against valgus and rotatory stresses.

The lateral stabilizers of the knee are the lateral collateral ligament and the lateral joint capsule (Fig. 8-2). These structures resist varus laxity and internal rotatory instability. Secondary contributions to lateral stability are supplied by the iliotibial band, biceps tendon, and the popliteal arcuate complex in the posterolateral corner of the knee.

The cruciate ligaments are the primary stabilizers for anterior and posterior displacement of the tibia on the femur (Fig. 8-3). The anterior cruciate runs from anterior on the tibia just medial to the anterior tibial spine to the posterior aspect of the lateral femoral condyle in the intercondylar notch. This ligament prevents anterior displacement of the tibia and helps control rotation and hyperextension of the knee during cutting, twisting, and turning activities.

The posterior cruciate runs from the posterior aspect of the tibial plateau to the anterior aspect of the medial femoral condyle in the intercondylar notch. This ligament prevents posterior displacement of the tibia on the femur, especially during flexion.

The posterior aspect of the knee contains a hollow space (popliteal fossa) bounded by the biceps femoris laterally and the semimembranosus and semitendinosus medially. Inferiorly, it is bounded by the two limbs of the gastrocnemius muscle. Found within the popliteal space are the popliteal artery and vein, and the peroneal and tibial nerves.

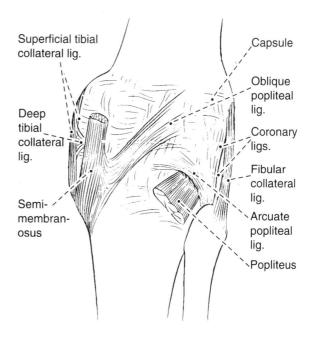

FIGURE 8-2. Posterior view of the capsule of the knee joint.

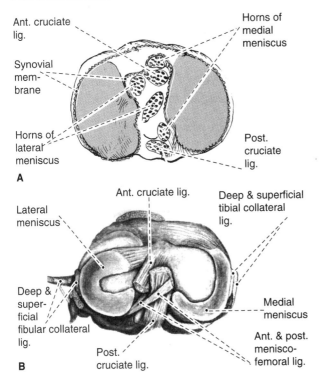

Ant. cruciate lig.

Synovial membrane

Horns of lateral meniscus

A

Horns of medial meniscus

Post. cruciate lig.

Ant. cruciate lig.

Lateral meniscus

Deep & superficial tibial collateral lig.

Deep & superficial fibular collateral lig.

Post. cruciate lig.

Medial meniscus

Ant. & post. menisco-femoral lig.

B

FIGURE 8-3. The menisci: (**A**) bony attachments of structures on the tibial plateau; (**B**) the menisci and associated ligaments, drawn from a specimen in the Anatomy Museum of the Royal College of Surgeons of England. (**B** adapted from McMinn, R.M.H. [ed.] *Last's anatomy, regional and applied* [8th ed.]. New York: Churchill Livingstone, 1990.)

The Muscles

The muscles about the knee are important to:

1. Provide locomotion
2. Absorb energy
3. Provide dynamic stability

The quadriceps are the anterior thigh muscles and consist of four muscles. These muscles function to extend the knee (Fig. 8-4).

They converge to form the quadriceps tendon that inserts on the patella. The patella acts as a pulley across the knee joint and increases the biomechanic advantage of the quadriceps. The patellar tendon originates at the inferior pole of the patella and inserts into the tibial tubercle.

The vastus medialis has a secondary function as a dynamic stabilizer of the patellofemoral joint. It is also a sensitive indicator of muscle weakness because it is the first of the quadriceps muscles to atrophy after injury.

The sartorius, gracilis, and semitendinosus form the pes anserine group, which originates from the pelvis and inserts on the medial tibial surface 5 to 7 cm below the joint line. They function as internal rotators and flexors of the knee.

The iliotibial band laterally arises from the iliac crest and inserts on Gerdy's tubercle on the tibia. It functions as both a secondary extensor and flexor of the knee as it shifts anterior to posterior to the axis of the knee rotation during flexion and extension.

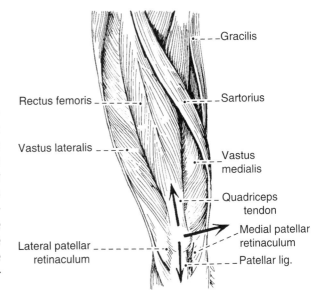

FIGURE 8-4. The quadriceps: The rectus femoris conceals the vastus intermedius. Note the insertion of some fleshy fibers of the vastus medialis into the medial side of the patella, which helps balance the pull on the patella by the quadriceps tendon and the patellar ligament. *Arrows* indicate directions of pull.

The popliteus muscle is deep on the posterior lateral corner of the knee with its origin on the femur and insertion on the posterior medial aspect of the tibia. The popliteus helps control external rotation of the femur on a fixed tibia and anterior displacement of the tibia on the femur when the lower extremity is fixed.

The most posterior muscles, the semimembranosus, semitendinosus and biceps femoris, are collectively called the hamstrings and are the major flexors of the knee. They also function to extend the hip and decelerate the knee during extension.

The semimembranosus dynamically stabilizes the posterior medial corner of the knee and therefore prevents excessive rotation of the tibia on the femur.

The biceps femoris has two origins—the long head from the ischial tuberosity and the short head from the lateral femur. It inserts on the fibular head posteriorly and has a secondary function of stabilizing the lateral aspect of the knee during flexion. Medially, adductor magnus, brevis, longus, and gracilis (the adductor group) rise in the pubic ramus and insert along the medial aspect of the distal femur with the gracilis attaching in the pes anserine complex medial on the tibia. These muscles adduct the hip and are hip and knee flexors. The hip abductors are the tensor fascia and the gluteus medius muscles that originate from the crest of the ilium. The gluteus medius inserts on the greater trochanter, and the tensor fascia lata travels laterally over the thigh to insert on the lateral aspect of the tibial and femoral condyle. These muscles cover the longest and strongest bone in the body, the femur.

Bursae

There are numerous bursae about the knee (Fig. 8-5). These function to reduce friction between structures that glide past one another. They are usually thin, but with repeated stress or direct trauma they may become thickened and fluid filled secondary to inflammation.

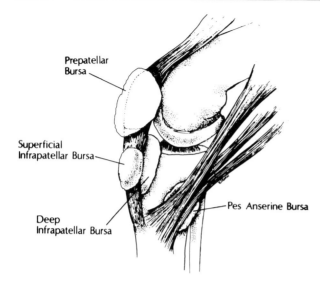

Prepatellar Bursa

Superficial Infrapatellar Bursa

Deep Infrapatellar Bursa

Pes Anserine Bursa

FIGURE 8-5. The bursae of the knee.

The prepatellar bursa (bricklayer's or housemaid's knee) is most commonly involved. It presents with soft tissue swelling localized anterior to the patella. It may become acutely inflamed with bleeding into the bursa with knee-loading activities.

The Painful Thigh

Physical Examination

Inspection

The patient should be examined appropriately exposed. This usually requires complete removal of clothes to allow exposure of both legs. The patient is inspected in the standing position and is viewed from all directions. This allows the examiner to evaluate alignment of the femur and to look for areas of ecchymosis or swelling. Muscle bulk and symmetry are noted. Attention should be paid to standing postures. If the patient is unable to fully extend the knee, there may be a problem with the hamstring or a chronic knee flexion contracture. Observation of the asymmetry of anterior musculature is facilitated by asking the patient to kneel with the buttocks on the heels.

Palpation

The patient is examined with systematic palpation of the origins and insertions of the thigh musculature as well as palpation of the muscles for enlargement, tenderness or defects.

The patient is asked to gently contract the quadriceps and hamstrings so the examiner can feel for areas of defects or tenderness. With the patient supine, range of motion of the hip and knees is evaluated. Determination of full range of motion is essential. Hamstring tightness is evaluated by lifting the legs off the examining table by the heels with the knees extended. The hips should flex at least 60 degrees before any knee flexion occurs. Early knee flexion is indicative of a hamstring contracture. The patient then is placed in the prone position, and the posterior structures of the thigh are examined from the gluteal fold with careful palpation of both the medial and lateral hamstrings. With active knee flexion, the hamstring muscles are brought into tension and the examiner may apply resistance to evaluate for muscle defects or tenderness with motion. Palpation in the medial and lateral aspects of the popliteal fossa will allow for palpation of the medial and lateral hamstring tendons. Range of motion is evaluated. Limitation of flexion is indicative of contracture of the anterior thigh musculature. The lateral aspect of the leg is palpated from the iliac crest along the fascia lata to its insertion on the tibia. Tenderness over the greater trochanter may be indicative of trochanteric bursitis or snapping iliotibial band (Fig. 8-6).

The Ober test is used to determine tightness of the iliotibial band. Tightness in the iliotibial band may also produce pain over the lateral joint line and lateral flair of the femur. Most complaints of thigh pain will be the result of direct trauma although sources of referred pain from back, hip, knee should always be excluded.

Contusions

Contusions are a result of direct trauma and are common sequelae of sporting activity. Proper treatment of these injuries is imperative to prevent serious impairment of athletic performance. After a direct blow to the thigh, there is local damage to blood vessels and muscle. The athlete may continue to play, but as bleeding and

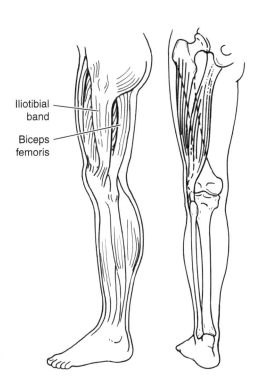

Iliotibial band

Biceps femoris

FIGURE 8-6. The iliotibial band.

swelling continue the thigh begins to get stiff with loss of full knee motion. Treatment consists of ice and compression to control swelling and bleeding. This early therapy is essential to promote painless range of motion. Rehabilitation begins with establishing painless range of motion, followed by flexibility and strengthening exercises. Return to sport is allowed when full painless range of motion and strength equal to the unaffected extremity are obtained. Do not use heat on a contusion acutely. Padding to prevent knee reinjury is indicated in at-risk collision sports (eg, football, soccer, field hockey).

Myositis ossificans or calcification of muscle at the site of injury is a late sequela of a severe blow to the thigh. Its occurrence is associated with repetitive reinjury before primary healing occurs and when heat is used to treat an acute hematoma.

Treatment consists of excision of the mass after it is mature.

Muscle Strains

Quadriceps

Quadriceps strain usually involves the rectus femoris, but may involve the vastus medialis and vastus lateralis. Injury most commonly occurs during rapid acceleration while running, or when a kick is mistimed or blocked. The most common predisposing factor is lack of adequate stretching or warm-up before initiation of the activity. Excessively tight quadriceps, short legs, or significant muscle imbalance can also be predisposing factors.

The clinical presentation is usually of pain over the anterior thigh, localized tenderness and an associated limp. Treatment consists of ice, compression, and rest followed by stretching exercises to restore painless range of motion. The athlete returns to sports when there is equal flexibility in both quadriceps, full painless range of motion, and restoration of strength and endurance strength in the injured muscle. A compression sleeve may facilitate an earlier return to sports.

Hamstring Strain

This injury is the most common of the lower extremity muscle injuries. It is usually a direct result of lack of flexibility in these muscles and lack of appropriate warm-up. Other factors that have been implicated include hamstring/quadriceps imbalance, imbalance between medial and lateral hamstrings, poor running mechanics, overstriding, and too rapid a deceleration during running activities.

This injury presents as sudden onset of pain in the posterior thigh, and often the athlete "pulls up lame." Swelling may occur immediately after injury or be delayed. Delayed ecchymosis is common and is often extensive. Treatment consists of ice, compression, and support. Rehabilitation begins after pain subsides with the goal of establishing full painless range of motion before strengthening and endurance strengthening exercises.

Iliotibial Band

Lateral thigh pain, especially in a runner, may be due to an irritation of the iliotibial band. This presents as pain over the lateral aspect of the leg and is commonly aggravated by running down hills. Pain may be present over the knee, at 30 degrees of flexion during full weight bearing. This pain pattern is due to a tight iliotibial band and is demonstrated by the positive Ober test and is also associated with inadequate shock absorption in the shoes, poor running mechanics, and with leg length inequality.

The Painful Knee

History

When a patient presents with a knee complaint, one should not limit oneself to the knee. A precise review of systems and evaluation of the hip and back will prevent one from overlooking patterns of referred pain from discogenic disease or hip fracture. A review for systemic illnesses such as rheumatoid arthritis, systemic lupus, and Lyme disease also needs to be performed as well as taking a sexual history to evaluate for risk of gonococcal arthritis.

Determine if the problem is acute or chronic. How, what, when, and where are essential questions. In the acute injury, determine the mechanism of injury (how). If it is subacute or chronic, how did the symptoms develop? Were there any changes in the training regimen, activity levels, or work requirements (eg, did the patient recently increase stair climbing, squatting, lifting activities) before the onset of pain? These activities are often associated with an increase in patellofemoral pain, especially in women.

When did symptoms begin? At the time of injury or later? Was the patient able to continue the sport? A tear of the anterior cruciate ligament usually presents with an acute hemarthrosis and inability to continue activity. A meniscus tear may present with an acutely locked knee but may present as a delayed onset of swelling with intermittent catching or giving-way episodes associated with joint line pain after a twisting episode to the knee.

What are the specific complaints? Is there swelling, locking, giving way, pain weakness, numbness, or sensation of instability? What activities aggravate the symptoms? Walking down stairs and prolonged sitting may bring out symptoms associated with patellofemoral disorders. Instability with cutting, twisting, and turning is associated with anterior cruciate lesions and meniscal pathology. Determine the severity of the disability. Are there difficulties with activities of daily living, light sports, or sports requiring vigorous cutting, twisting, and turning activities?

Determine the location of the pain (where). Meniscus pain will be localized to the joint line, but pain of a medial collateral ligament (MCL) injury will be diffuse along the medial aspect of the knee along the path of the MCL. The pain of patellar subluxation or dislocation will be localized to the retinacular structures about the patella.

Physical Examination

Observation

The physical examination begins with observation. Does the patient walk with an antalgic gait? Does the patient sit with the knee extended? If so, there may be a knee effusion.

Inspection

Inspection begins with the patient erect with the legs exposed to midthigh. Note the alignment of the knee. Eight to 12 degrees of valgus (knock knees) is normal. Make note of any excess valgus or varus (bowed legs; Fig. 8-7). Note the location and position of the patella; they should face anteriorly and be at the same level. A medially positioned patella or squinting patella is associated with patellofemoral pain syndromes. Inspect the symmetry of the quadriceps; note any muscle atrophy. The vastus medialis oblique is the first muscle to show muscle atrophy. With the knee in full extension, measure the circumference of the thigh at a point 5 cm above the superior pole of the patella. Measure leg lengths. Inspect for soft tissue fullness. Loss of soft tissue dimples about the knee is an indicator of a knee effusion. A knee effusion may give one a false circumferential measurement because the suprapatellar pouch may extend significantly proximal to the superior pole of the patella.

Inspection of the bony insertion of the patellar tendon may reveal an enlargement that in the adolescent may indicate Osgood Schlatter disease. Examine the patient's gait. Antalgic gait (avoidance of putting full weight on the painful leg) may represent painful arthropathy. The inability to gain full knee extension at heel strike usually represents intra-articular pathology, meniscus tear, arthritis, loose body, or large effusion. An abnormal lateral or medial thrust may indicate ligamentous instability or advanced joint arthritis with joint collapse. Back kneeing, or genu recurvatum, may be an indication of hypermobility syndrome or a posterior cruciate ligament injury. Excessive foot pronation and interior tibial torsion are associated with patel-lofemoral pain syndromes (Fig. 8-8). Observation of the inability to duck walk or walking in a squatting position is associated with meniscal injury.

Palpation

Look first for a knee effusion, then gently palpate the knee. A large effusion is seen with a ballottable or floating patella. With the patient's knee extended, depress the patella into the trochlear groove and gently tap; the patella will bounce back

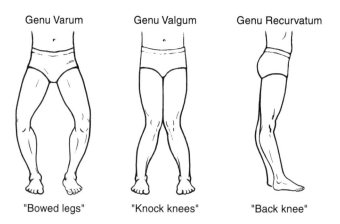

Genu Varum   Genu Valgum   Genu Recurvatum

"Bowed legs"   "Knock knees"   "Back knee"

FIGURE 8-7. Common knee deformities.

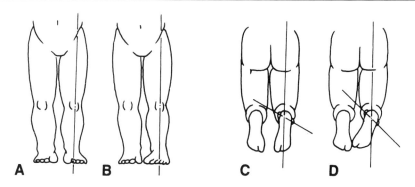

FIGURE 8-8. Examining for tibial torsion. (**A** and **B**) Child supine: (**A**) normal, (**B**) internal tibial torsion. (**C** and **D**) Child prone, knee flexed 90°: (**C**) normal, (**D**) internal tibial torsion. (Steinberg, G. et al. [1992]. *Ramaturi's orthopaedics in primary care.* Baltimore: Williams & Wilkins)

with a large effusion. An effusion may also be demonstrated by tapping the lateral retinaculum with a palpable fluid wave appreciated on the medial side. A small effusion may be demonstrated by milking the superior patellar pouch inferiorly to force fluid into the knee joint. This will result in a ballottable patella. Palpate the prepatellar bursa. If it is swollen, there may be bursitis; however, the bursa often communicates with the knee joint and may be present with a concomitant knee effusion.

The precise localization of pain in the evaluation of the knee is helpful in defining the pathology (Fig. 8-9). In general, it is best to palpate areas of tenderness last because provocation of pain early in the examination may cause anxiety and the patient may become unable to relax and cooperate fully.

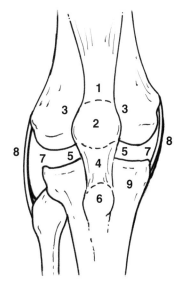

FIGURE 8-9. Palpation of pain in the knee. *1,* quadriceps tendinitis; *2,* prepatella bursitis, patella pain; *3,* retinacular pain after patella subluxation; *4,* patella tendinitis; *5,* fat pad tenderness; *6,* Osgood-Schlatter disease (tibial tubercle pain); *7,* meniscus pain; *8,* collateral ligament pain; and *9,* pes anserine tendinitis bursitis.

Palpate the patella and extensor mechanism; palpate the superior pole. Feel for defects in the muscle attachments over areas of pain. This is consistent with rupture or avulsion from the patella. Pain at this location is seen with quadriceps tendinitis. Palpate the anterior patella for warmth, redness, and swelling. Increased warmth, redness, and swelling are found with prepatellar bursitis (housemaid's or bricklayer's knee).

Palpate the medial and lateral retinaculum and the medial and lateral facets of the patella. Tenderness over the retinaculum is seen with patellar subluxation and dislocation, and facet discomfort is seen with patellofemoral pain syndrome. The patella should be gently pushed from medial to lateral to test its intrinsic stability. The patella should not sublux more than 50% of its width.

The Q angle or the angle of the patellar tendon with the quadriceps is measured. Increased Q angles greater than 20 degrees are associated with patellofemoral pain syndromes (Fig. 8-10). Palpate the inferior pole of the patella. Pain at this location is seen with jumper's knee or inferior patellar tendinitis. The patellar tendon is palpated with the accompanying fat pads and bursae. In blunt trauma to the anterior knee, these structures may remain painful for many months. Excessive kneeling may also cause infrapatellar bursitis. The insertion of the tendon in the tibial tubercle is palpated next. Pain at this location in an adolescent is the hallmark of Osgood Schlatter disease. The adult who has had Osgood Schlatter disease as a child may

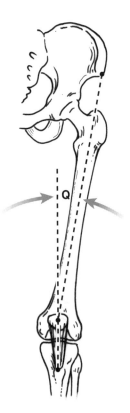

FIGURE 8-10. "Q" or quadriceps angle is formed by the intersection of lines between the anterior superior iliac spine and the mid-portion of the patella and the tibial tubercle. It is the angle formed by the quadriceps muscle and the patellar tendon.

experience discomfort with repetitive kneeling activities over this bony prominence. Palpate the medial and lateral aspects of the knee.

Examination of the medial aspect of the knee is performed with the knee in extension and in flexion. A repeat examination of the retinacular structures is performed followed by a careful palpation of the femoral condyle and tibial plateau. In the adolescent, pain along the femoral or tibial epiphysis after trauma may represent a nondisplaced fracture through the epiphysis. In the adult, painful osteophytes of arthritis may be palpated. In the elderly, pain over the tibial flair or femoral condyle may be seen with osteonecrosis. In the adult or adolescent with an osteochondritis lesion, pain may be palpated over the involved compartment.

Carefully palpate the joint line. The anterior soft spot between the femoral condyle and the tibial plateau allows one to quickly localize the joint surface. Pain along the joint line is indicative of meniscus pathology. Flex the knee to 90 degrees to allow the pes anserine complex to displace posteriorly. This allows for palpation of the joint line and the MCL. Pain along the course of the MCL from the femur to tibia is seen with injury. Palpation of the MCL should include origin, midsubstance, and insertion. Palpate the pes anserine complex, and look for tenderness associated with bursitis or tendinitis.

Examine the lateral aspect of the knee from proximal to distal, palpate the lateral femoral condyle, lateral tibial plateau, and lateral joint line. Lateral joint line pain is synonymous with meniscal pathology.

Examine the lateral collateral ligament with the knees crossed or in the figure-four position. This puts stress on the lateral collateral ligament and allows easier palpation of its origin from the femoral condyle to its insertion on the fibular head. The iliotibial band is palpated along its course over the lateral thigh and knee to its insertion on Gerdy's tubercle on the anterior lateral aspect of the tibia. Pain is often seen in runners with a contracted iliotibial band and is a result of friction as the band is rubbed over the lateral knee structures.

The tightness can be demonstrated with the Ober test (Fig. 8-11). Ask the patient to lie on the side with the leg to be tested up. Flex the opposite leg (away from the body) to stabilize the pelvis. Abduct (away from the body) as far as possible and then flex the knee to 90 degrees. The symptomatic leg is allowed to be adducted (toward the body). If the iliotibial band is normal, the thigh should drop to the adducted position. If there is a contracture of the iliotibial band, the thigh will remain in the abducted position when the leg is released (positive Ober test). If there is inflammation, this test will illicit discomfort over the iliotibial band.

Next, palpate the posterior aspect of the knee. Fullness may indicate a popliteal cyst. Pain over the medial and lateral heads of the gastrocnemius may represent tendinitis or a muscle injury. Palpate the posterior tibial pulse. In a patient with acute multiplanar instability, a knee dislocation should be assumed and an appropriate vascular assessment should be obtained.

Stability Testing

Stability testing is performed in the anterior/posterior/medial-lateral (varus/valgus) and rotational planes. The ability to assess the anterior/posterior, varus/valgus planes of instability is essential to the basic knee examination.

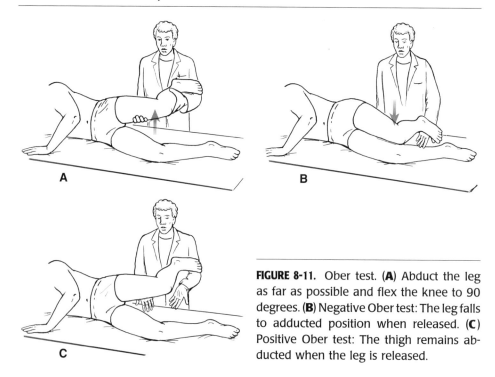

FIGURE 8-11. Ober test. (**A**) Abduct the leg as far as possible and flex the knee to 90 degrees. (**B**) Negative Ober test: The leg falls to adducted position when released. (**C**) Positive Ober test: The thigh remains abducted when the leg is released.

With the knee in full extension and in 30 degrees of flexion, test for medial collateral stability by placing the ankle in one hand, or cradled on your hip, while the other hand is placed over the lateral joint line. Apply a gentle valgus force to the joint line (if the MCL is torn); this will open up the medial joint line. If there is instability in full extension, then the MCL and secondary stabilizers of the capsule are completely disrupted and this usually represents a surgical problem. Next, examine the knee in 30 degrees of flexion. If instability is only present at 30 degrees of flexion, the capsule is intact and there is only a partial injury to the medial collateral or an isolated MCL injury.

Reverse the test to evaluate the lateral collateral ligament with a varus force applied to the medial joint line at both full extension and 30 degrees of flexion. Anterior and posterior displacements evaluate the anterior and posterior cruciate ligaments. The anterior cruciate ligament resists anterior displacement of the tibia on the femur, and the posterior cruciate resists posterior displacement.

The anterior and posterior drawer test is performed with the knee flexed to 90 degrees. The foot is kept in neutral rotation to relax the secondary stabilizers of the joint capsule and the collateral ligaments. The test is best performed with the examiner sitting on the neutrally aligned foot. Grasp the knee firmly with both hands as the index fingers palpate the hamstrings for relaxation.

The tibia is gently pulled anteriorly for the anterior drawer or pushed posteriorly for the posterior drawer. The degree of displacement from the neutral starting position is assessed as well as the character of the end point (ie, firm or soft). Comparison is made of the affected and unaffected knees. It is sometimes difficult to assess if the drawer is positive anterior or posterior because of the starting point. This may be evaluated with a drop back test. The test is performed with both knees flexed to 90 degrees, both hips flexed to 90 degrees and the legs supported only by the ankles and viewed from the side. In a posterior cruciate-deficient knee, this will show as a posterior sag or drop back of the tibia on the femur.

Secondary or rotatory instabilities may be assessed with the knee at 90 degrees and the foot rotated internally or externally and the drawer repeated. With internal rotation, the lateral structures are tightened. If a drawer is present, anterior lateral rotatory instability is present. Conversely, anterior medial instability is present if the anterior drawer is seen with the foot externally rotated, because this should tighten the secondary medial stabilizers of the knee. Similar evaluation for posterior rotatory instabilities may be performed (Table 8-1).

Multiplanar instability in the acutely injured knee is a sign of a serious knee injury. All patients with this injury pattern should be presumed to have a knee dislocation. This injury often has associated vascular injury and requires close monitoring and an arteriogram to evaluate the vascularity to the leg.

The patella is examined for stability with the knee in extension and slight flexion. Medial and lateral displacement forces are applied to evaluate stability. "Positive apprehension" may be elicited with existing patellofemoral disease. The position of the patella is palpated during passive flexion extension to evaluate its tracking.

TABLE 8-1
*Knee Ligament Instabilities**

Clinical Instabilities†	Laxity Tests
Single-plane instabilities	
Medial	Valgus stress at 0 degrees and 30 degrees of flexion
Lateral	Varus stress at 0 degrees and 30 degrees of flexion
Anterior	Anterior drawer at 90 degrees of flexion Lachman test
Posterior	Posterior drawer at 90 degrees of flexion
Rotatory instabilities‡	
Anteromedial	Anterior drawer with foot in external rotation at 90 degrees of flexion
Anterolateral	Anterior drawer with foot in internal rotation at 90 degrees of flexion Pivot shift test
Posterolateral	Hyperextension of leg Posterior drawer with foot in internal rotation at 90 degrees of flexion
Posteromedial	Posterior drawer with foot in external rotation at 90 degrees of flexion (rare)

*Note: Classification of instabilities was adapted from the Research and Education Committee of the American Orthopaedic Society of Sports Medicine. From Roy, S., & Irvin, R. (1983). *Sports Medicine. Prevention, Evaluation, Management, and Rehabilitation.* Englewood Cliffs, NJ: Prentice-Hall, p. 310.
†Movement of the tibia in relation to the femur. Medial means the tibia is moving away from the femur on the medial side.
‡Movement of the tibia in relation to the femur. Anteromedial rotatory instability means the tibia is rotating anteriorly and moving away from the femur on the medial side.

It is examined to see if it remains centered within the trochlear groove or subluxes laterally. The character of joint motion is also assessed while feeling for crepitus associated with patellofemoral pain syndromes.

Provocation testing for patellofemoral pain is also performed. The knee is extended, and the patella is gently depressed into the trochlear groove as well as slightly inferiorly. The patient is then asked to maximally contract the quadriceps. The location of pain similar to the complaints confirms the diagnosis of patellofemoral pain syndrome.

The final provocation testing is for the evaluation of meniscus pathology. The McMurray test is performed with the knee in full internal or full external rotation. The knee is flexed fully, and a rotational force is applied. The knee is then gently brought out into full extension. The presence of pain localized to the joint line or a palpable joint line click is strongly suggestive of meniscus pathology.

The Apley compression test may also be performed. This test is done with the knee flexed 90 degrees while the patient is prone. Axial pressure is applied to the foot during internal and external rotation. The elicitation of pain along the joint line is positive for meniscal pathology (Fig. 8-12).

The inability to gain full extension in conjunction with joint line pain is also highly suggestive of a displaced torn meniscus. An intra-articular loose body also needs to be considered.

Manual muscle testing may be performed, but it is difficult to assess subtle differences in strength in the lower extremities. Profound atrophy is usually appreciated on inspection. Diffuse atrophy and weakness seen with muscle degeneration and neurologic disorders will be appreciated on manual muscle testing.

Diagnostic Guidelines

Radiographic Evaluation of the Knee

Radiographs are almost always needed to completely evaluate knee complaints. Obtain a standing anterior-posterior view of both knees on a single cassette with a lateral of the affected knee. This will allow for the determination of most fractures, loose bodies, arthritis, chondrocalcinosis, and osteochondritis dessicans. The presence of joint space narrowing in one compartment is seen with early osteoarthritis. If tricompartmental disease is seen, a pansynovial process such as is seen in gout, rheumatoid arthritis, pigmented villonodular synovitis, or chondrocalcinosis should be considered. This finding is also seen in the late stages of osteoarthritis. Obtain a tunnel view to evaluate for flecks of bone off the tibial spine. This is useful to evaluate for acute anterior cruciate injury. Obtain oblique views to evaluate for an avulsion fracture of the lateral tibial attachment of the lateral collateral ligament. This finding, "lateral capsular sign," is strongly suggestive of an anterior cruciate injury with anterior lateral rotatory instability. Calcification in the MCL is seen as a late finding after MCL injury.

Obtain sunrise views of the patella to evaluate patellofemoral tracking and subluxation. Obtain a lateral x-ray to assess the presence of a low-riding or high-riding patella and possible extensor dysfunction. In the skeletally immature adoles-

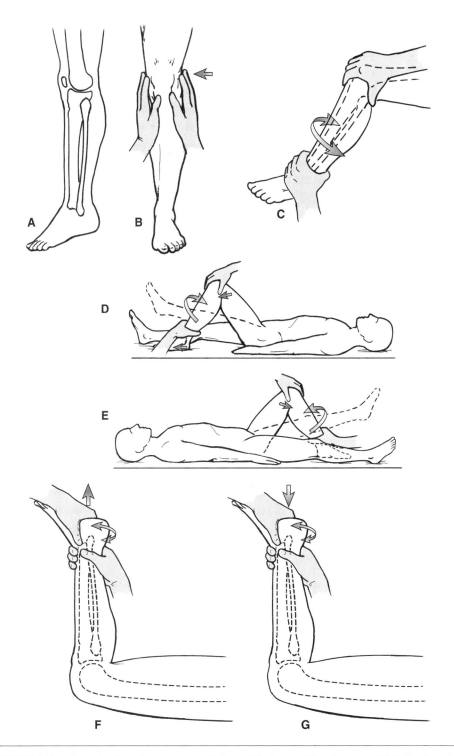

FIGURE 8-12. Examination for meniscus injury. (**A**) Area of tenderness. (**B**) Palpation for tenderness. (**C**) Palpation for "click" during alternate internal and external rotation of the leg. (**D** and **E**) McMurray's maneuver. (**F**) Apley's distraction maneuver; pain is compatible with ligament injury. (**G**) Apley's compression maneuver; pain is compatible with meniscus injury.

cent, the epiphysis should be examined for evidence of fractures. Stress views are sometimes useful to confirm epiphyseal injury.

Obtain a magnetic resonance image (MRI) or arthrogram to evaluate intra-articular soft tissue injuries of the meniscus, and anterior and posterior cruciate ligaments. Obtain an arteriogram when multiplanar instability is present in an acutely injuried knee. Obtain a bone scan or MRI to confirm epiphyseal injuries, avascular necrosis lesions, early osteochondritis lesions as well as stress fractures.

Synovial fluid analysis should be performed in all knees with an effusion (Table 8-2). Sterile aspiration is easily performed through medial or lateral patellar retinac-

TABLE 8-2
Clinical Diagnosis of Ligament Injuries

	First-Degree Sprain	Second-Degree Sprain	Third-Degree Sprain
Synonym	Mild sprain	Moderate sprain	Severe sprain
Etiology	Direct or indirect trauma to the joint	Direct or indirect trauma to the joint	Direct or indirect trauma to the joint
Symptoms	Pain and mild disability	Pain and moderate disability	Pain and severe disability
Signs and symptoms	Tenderness over the collateral Stable joint examination with no abnormal motions Little or no swelling	Point tenderness over collaterals, swelling, may have localized hemorrhage; loss of normal joint function with laxity tested in 30 degrees flexion; no instability in full extension	Loss of function, marked instability, unstable in full extension
Pathology	Minor tissue tearing Continuity of ligament is intact	Partial tearing with partial loss of ligamentous support	Complete disruption of ligament; no remaining tensile strength
Treatment	Rest, ice, compression, elevation, quadriceps-strengthening exercises	Rest, ice, compression, elevation, immobilization, muscle-strengthening activities, protective bracing, fracture brace for 6 to 8 weeks	Rest, ice, compression, elevation surgery is generally required
Complications	Tendency to recur or be aggravated	Persistent instability, traumatic arthritis	Persistent instability, traumatic arthritis
Prognosis	Normal function, no laxity	Good function, good stability if adequate healing occurs with good bracing	Generally better with primary reconstructive surgery than with casting or fractures bracing

ular portals with a large-bore needle (18 gauge). Aspiration of blood is consistent with an anterior cruciate ligament injury or other major injury such as osteochondral fracture or retinacular tears or capsular tears. Fat cells may be present with a fracture but are also seen with acute cruciate insufficiency. The fluid should be examined for crystals, looking for both gout and pseudogout. A cell count with differential should be obtained. Routine cultures should be sent along with cultures for gonococcus, especially in the absence of trauma history.

Arthroscopy allows for direct visualization of the intra- articular structures; it may be performed under local anesthesia to complete a diagnostic evaluation of the knees.

Injuries to the Knee

Meniscus

ETIOLOGY. A meniscus injury occurs as an acute injury or as a result of repetitive stresses over a period of time (degenerative tears). Injury to the meniscus is commonly the result of knee rotation on a partially flexed knee (Fig. 8-13). Sports injuries are well documented, but simple activities such as getting out of a bucket seat of a car or getting lettuce out of the hydrator of the refrigerator can precipitate an acute meniscus tear. The patient may or may not be able to give a precise mechanism of the injury, especially the older patient with a degenerative meniscus.

SIGNS AND SYMPTOMS. The signs of meniscus pathology are pain at the joint line, swelling, and giving-way episodes or a sensation of instability. If the meniscus

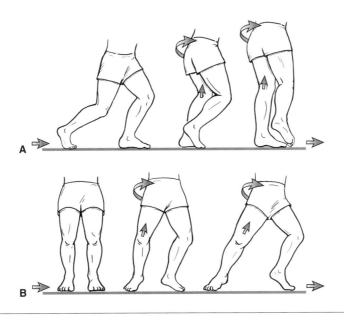

FIGURE 8-13. The damaging forces acting on the menisci of the knee. (**A**) Forces that damage the lateral meniscus. (**B**) Forces that damage the medial meniscus.

is displaced, it may create a mechanical block to knee motion and may result in a locked knee. The physical examination usually reveals an effusion with joint line tenderness. McMurray's and Apley's provocation testing usually produces pain. Clicking may or may not be present and is nonspecific.

DIAGNOSTIC TESTING. Diagnostic tests include aspiration and routine x-rays to exclude other causes of symptoms (loose bodies, osteochondritis dissecans). MRI and arthrograms may be obtained to define the pathology before treatment.

TREATMENT. Initial treatment of the patient with a painful knee that is also suspected of having meniscal pathology should be to control the inflammation with ice and anti-inflammatories and to rest the knee with immobilization in a position of comfort. Patients with a locked knee should be referred to an orthopedic surgeon for immediate evaluation, and those presenting with joint line pain and mild meniscal symptoms may have the appropriate tests ordered and may be referred to an orthopedic surgeon for definitive therapy. Arthroscopic repair or resection is the treatment of choice in the symptomatic patient. In the older patient with presumed early degenerative arthritis, care should be taken to preserve the meniscus in its entirety or resect as little as possible. Excision of the entire meniscus leads to an acceleration of the degenerative arthritis in the knee. In the elderly, AVN needs to be excluded because resection of a degenerative meniscus will often lead to a severe increase in symptomatology. MRI is highly diagnostic.

Acute Ligamentous Injuries

Ligamentous injuries are always the result of direct trauma and depend on the direction of the applied forces and the position of the knee (Fig. 8-14).

A valgus-directed force will put the medial collateral, medial meniscus, posterior medial capsule, and anterior cruciate ligament at risk for injury. It is also a commonly encountered injury pattern. Hyperextension results in stresses on the cruciate and may result in the anterior cruciate or posterior cruciate injury. A varus force (being struck in the medial side of the knee) will put the lateral collateral, posterior oblique ligamentous complex at risk. An injury that results in an immediate effusion is probably due to a hemarthrosis and usually means an anterior cruciate ligament tear or an osteochondral fracture.

Physical examination is best performed acutely before swelling occurs. Localization of the pain and stability testing dictate treatment.

Treatment is based on the instability patterns that are appreciated.

Chronic Ligamentous Injury

Often a serious injury is overlooked. The patient experiences a 2- to 3-week disability and resumes a normal lifestyle. Over the next 5 to 10 years, the patient develops secondary instability of the knee. This allows increased rotation of the femur on the tibia. These abnormal rotational forces result in medial or lateral meniscus tears, and degenerative changes develop in the knee. Treatment for chronic rotatory instability is based on the functional levels of the patient. Quadriceps and hamstring rehabilitation are the base for conservative treatment and allow many patients to continue sporting activities with a brace. Surgery is the treatment of choice for

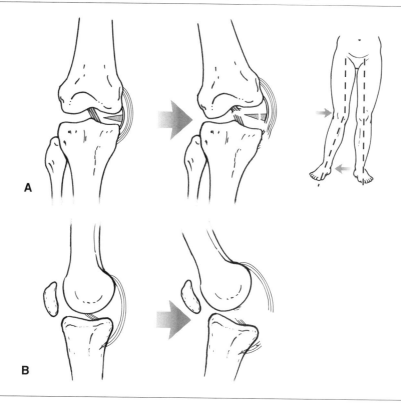

FIGURE 8-14. *Severe ligamentous sprain* (the unhappy triad). (**A**) Lateral (valgus) stress caus-ing disruption of the medial collateral ligament, the medial meniscus, and the anterior cruciate ligament (the unhappy triad). (**B**) Lateral view of a severe anterior stress causing hyperextension of the joint and disrupting both anterior and posterior cruciate ligaments and the posterior capsule. Clinically, it has a positive drawer sign.

high-performance athletes and individuals who remain symptomatic during activities of daily living.

Tendon Injuries

Tendinitis

ETIOLOGY. Tendinitis is a common complaint and is a result of inflammation secondary to macrotrauma or repetitive microtrauma. Tears in the collagen structure cause inflammation and scar deposition. Persistent tendinitis can lead to weakening of the tendons and ultimate failure. Tendinitis may affect the quadriceps at its insertion into the patella, the patellar tendon, the biceps tendon, the popliteus, or iliotibial band.

SIGNS AND SYMPTOMS. These present as localized pain over the affected tendon. Localized soft tissue swelling may be present. Pain is aggravated by activity and relieved with rest.

DIAGNOSTIC TESTS. Radiographs are usually normal. With persistent inflammation, calcific degeneration of the involved tendon may sometimes be seen. Three-phase bone scanning may show increased activity in the first two phases of the scan. Blood work to evaluate for an underlying collagen vascular disease may be useful in patients who do not respond to treatment.

TREATMENT. Primary treatment is rest with treatment of the localized inflammation with ice and anti-inflammatory medication. Supportive bracing may be helpful in controlling the acute phase of inflammation and in preventing repetitive episodes.

Quadriceps Tendinitis

Presents as pain localized over the superior pole of the patella. It is seen in patients whose sports or jobs require quick acceleration or quick deceleration movements. Treatment is ice, rest, restoration of flexibility, strength, and endurance and a return to sport. A patellar stabilizing brace may be useful in unloading these areas in the rehabilitation phase.

Patellar Tendinitis ("Jumper's Knee")

"Jumper's knee," or infrapatellar tendinitis, is the most common tendinitis of the knee. It is the result of repetitive microtrauma concentrated at the inferior pole of the patella. Chronic inflammation may result in the rupture of the tendon at its insertion into the patella. It is most commonly found in dancers, basketball players, and other athletes who perform jumping activities. The condition may become chronic and not respond to conservative care.

TREATMENT. If diagnosed early (within the first 3 weeks), rest, ice, anti-inflammatory medication coupled with activity modification and progressive return to sports may be all that is needed. If the condition has become chronic, complete restriction of activity may be necessary with possible casting. Referral to an orthopedic surgeon for injection of steroids may be useful in these cases, but great caution should be taken to avoid injection into the tendinous structure. Injections of steroids into the tendon significantly weaken the collagen structure and have been associated with tendon rupture. Nonsteroidal anti-inflammatory drugs (NSAIDs), ice after sports, and compression strapping or bracing of the area may be of benefit in controlling symptoms and allowing for early return to sporting activity. If the knee is completely nonresponsive to rest, surgery may be necessary.

Tendon Rupture

ETIOLOGY. Chronic inflammation leading to decrease in collagen strength of the tendon is followed by a load that exceeds the strength of the tendon, resulting in failure.

SIGNS AND SYMPTOMS. Acute loss of the ability to extend the knee against gravity as well as pain and swelling. Localized ecchymosis may be present. The patella will be high riding with a complete infrapatellar tendon rupture and low riding with a quadriceps tendon rupture. Partial tears may present as localized pain and swelling with weakness in knee extension. A palpable defect in the tendon may be appreciated on physical examination.

DIAGNOSTIC STUDIES. Radiographic evaluation of the knee may show an altered position of the patella. Careful observation for bony avulsion fractures from the patella should be performed. Calcific deposits within the substance of the tendon may be observed and are indicative of chronic inflammation.

Osgood Schlatter Disease

In the adolescent, Osgood Schlatter disease presents as pain at the insertion of the tendon into the tibial tubercle. This represents an apophysitis of the tibial tubercle.

ETIOLOGY. Robert B. Osgood first described partial avulsion of the tibial tubercle that caused painful swelling in the knee of the adolescent in 1903. Carl Schlatter, some months later, described the same condition and concluded that it was an apophysitis of the tibial tubercle rather than a true avulsion fracture. The argument has never been settled. It occurs in the age of rapid growth and is more common in boys than girls. Bilateral involvement is noted in some 20% to 30%.

SIGNS AND SYMPTOMS. The disease is characterized by painful swelling over the tibial tuberosity that is exacerbated by activity, relieved by rest, and usually of several months' duration. Tenderness is most marked at the insertion of the patellar tendon. In the adolescent, an acute fracture may occur at this region and present as an acute loss of ability to extend the knee.

DIAGNOSTIC IMAGING. X-rays may show an irregularity or fragmentation of the tibial apophysis. Fragmentation can also be seen in adolescents with no symptoms. In the occasional acute case, a flake of bone can be detected that suggests an avulsion fracture.

TREATMENT. The treatment of Osgood Schlatter disease is purely symptomatic. In persistent or moderately painful knees, one restricts physical activity. When there is a suggestion of a recent acute episode or evidence of a flake fracture, the knee may be immobilized in a plaster cast for 4 to 6 weeks. Knee pads are used to avoid contusions to the prominent tibial tubercle. A Chopat strap may be used to unload the tendon insertion. Symptoms stop after growth ceases. However, the bony prominence will remain throughout life. On occasion, an isolated or separated ossicle may be symptomatic. If it persists in being painful, excision of the ossicle may be necessary. In the case of fracture, if there is significant displacement, open reduction and internal fixation may be required.

Biceps Tendinitis

Biceps tendinitis presents as localized pain over the posterior fibular head. It is most commonly seen in patients with tight hamstrings.

Treatment consists of ice, rest, and NSAIDs, as well as stretching and strengthening exercises, with return to sporting activities as symptoms resolve.

Popliteus Tendinitis

Popliteus tendinitis presents as pain in the posterior lateral corner of the knee and is often accentuated by running downhill and descending stairs, as well as prolonged ambulatory activity. The pain is commonly mistaken for a lateral meniscus tear. Treatment is the same as for all inflammatory lesions.

Iliotibial Band Tendinitis

Iliotibial band tendinitis presents as lateral knee pain over the fibular collateral ligament. It is a result of inadequate stretching and results in a tight iliotibial band that then rubs over the posterior lateral corner of the knee, which results in inflammation and pain.

Physical examination reveals localized pain over the posterior lateral corner of the knee, and the iliotibial band is seen to tighten (a positive Ober test confirms the diagnosis). The treatment is conservative—stretching, strengthening, and return to sports.

Patellofemoral Pain Syndrome

Anterior knee pain is often vague in its history and common in its presentation. It may result from the sequelae of direct trauma, chronic overuse, or patellofemoral malalignment. Patellar complaints are more common in women due to the increase in the Q angle secondary to increase in the pelvic flair.

ETIOLOGY. This increase in Q angle leads to a tendency for the patella to tilt laterally or sublux laterally during activity. With any injury that limits knee activity, quadriceps strength is lost, and the medial dynamic stabilizers of the knee, the vastus medialis obliquus, undergo atrophy. This relative muscle imbalance allows for lateral subluxation of the patella resulting in patellofemoral discomfort. Acute dislocations may also result in a lax medial retinaculum and lateral tracking of the patella.

Patellofemoral pain may also be a direct result of a repetitive trauma such as long distance running that leads to chronic inflammation. Direct trauma to the patella may result in a chondral fracture with resulting anterior knee pain. This is often seen when the knee strikes the dashboard during a motor vehicle accident or as a sequela of a dislocated patella.

SYMPTOMS. Hallmarks of this problem are pain on rising from sitting, pain on stair climbing, and aches at the end of the day. This pain is often dull and poorly localized and may be referred to posteriorly in the popliteal recess.

SIGNS. A sensation of instability with twisting activities may also accompany the syndrome. The diagnosis is made on physical examination with positive patellofemoral provocation testing with or without a subluxable patella.

DIAGNOSTIC STUDIES. X-rays to assess patellofemoral congruency and tracking are useful. A bone scan or MRI with normal x-rays is useful to evaluate whether osteochondral injury has taken place. Arthrograms are not usually useful in this syndrome. Diagnostic arthroscopy may be useful, but clinical symptoms do not correlate to the degree of articular softening or chondromalacia found at surgery.

TREATMENT. Treatment is conservative with quadriceps setting exercises and patellofemoral support. If after 6 months symptoms persist and quadriceps are strong, surgical intervention may be considered. Eighty-five percent of patients show improvement with conservative treatment. Surgery is performed to correct the abnormalities of patellofemoral tracking. For severe patellofemoral arthritis, tibial tubercle elevation to decrease the patellofemoral joint reactive forces may be helpful.

Osteonecrosis

Osteonecrosis is an acute vascular insufficiency of the tibial plateau or femoral condyle. It presents in the fifth to eighth decade as spontaneous onset of severe pain.

ETIOLOGY. The etiology is unknown.

SIGNS AND SYMPTOMS. It may be accompanied by an effusion and loss of joint motion. The physical examination reveals point tenderness over the involved femoral condyle or tibial compartment.

DIAGNOSTIC STUDIES. X-rays performed at the onset of symptoms are usually normal, and the diagnosis is confirmed with technetium bone scanning, with increased activity noted. MRI is also diagnostic of an acute osteonecrosis. The most common sites are the medial femoral condyle and the medial tibial plateau. X-ray changes occur late and appear as collapse of the osteochondral surface.

TREATMENT. Treatment is symptomatic with rest and protected weight bearing, with support, ice, and NSAIDs. Core decompression has been reported to relieve pain. If arthritis develops, surgical reconstruction of the knee is the treatment of choice.

OUTCOME. The outcome depends on the percentage of the weight-bearing surface involved with the process. Those patients who have more than 50% involvement of the involved compartment usually require some form of reconstructive surgery (knee replacement).

Traumatic Conditions

Fractures

ETIOLOGY. Fractures are usually the result of trauma but may occur as a result of bone failure secondary to osteoporosis.

SIGNS AND SYMPTOMS. Fractures usually present with the acute onset of pain and swelling. Ecchymosis develops secondary to the fracture hematoma. Inability to bear weight is often present. Pain is usually increased with weight bearing. Obvious angular deformity of the extremity may be present.

Femur Fractures

ETIOLOGY. Femoral shaft fractures are often caused by direct blows or by rotary forces.

SIGNS AND SYMPTOMS. Pain and inability to bear weight on the involved extremity. Swelling may be rapid, and blood loss may be substantial. Shortening of the extremity with angular deformity is often present.

DIAGNOSTIC EVALUATION. AP and lateral radiographs of the entire femur are necessary to define the fracture geometry.

TREATMENT. Primary treatment is to stabilize the extremity in a splint. Definitive treatment will be traction, plate fixation, or intramedullary nailing of the femur. Fracture bracing may be used to facilitate early mobilization of the patient.

Supracondylar Femur Fractures

ETIOLOGY. Supracondylar femur fractures are common in the elderly and usually result from direct trauma.

SIGNS AND SYMPTOMS. Pain and swelling immediately above the knee and an inability to bear weight. A gross deformity of the knee may be present. With fractures that extend into the joint, a tense hemarthrosis may be present.

DIAGNOSTIC EVALUATION. Radiographs are needed to define the extent of the fracture and the fracture geometry. AP, lateral, obliques, and tunnel views are usually necessary. Tomography or CT scanning will allow for greater three-dimensional visualization of the fracture geometry.

Treatment. For a nondisplaced fracture, a fracture brace is the treatment of choice. For a displaced fracture, some form of operative stabilization with restoration of joint congruency is advocated.

Epiphyseal Femur Fractures

Epiphyseal fractures of the distal femur are common in the adolescent.

ETIOLOGY. These fractures are the result of varus or valgus stress applied to the knee.

SIGNS AND SYMPTOMS. The adolescent complains of pain over the epiphyseal line and loss of joint motion. Swelling and ecchymosis may be present. Pain is increased with direct palpation of the epiphysis and with stress testing.

RADIOGRAPHIC EVALUATION. X-rays are often negative; stress films may be useful in defining pathology. A bone scan or MRI is often diagnostic and reveals increased activity at the epiphyseal line.

TREATMENT. Treatment is a cast with conversion to a fracture brace to allow for early motion. Epiphyseal injuries have great potential for growth arrest. Patients need be monitored closely after injury to ensure that growth injury does not occur. For those patients with displacement of the epiphysis, anatomic reduction is required either through closed or open means. Displaced fractures should be closely observed for neurovascular injury.

Tibial Plateau Fractures

ETIOLOGY. Plateau fractures are the result of direct trauma and are extremely common. They are secondary to osteoporosis or significant trauma.

SIGNS AND SYMPTOMS. Plateau fractures present with pain and swelling below the joint line. Ecchymosis usually develops. Bleeding into the fascial compartments of the leg may result in the development of a compartment syndrome and require fasciotomy. Angular deformity may or may not be present depending on the degree of displacement. Pain is increased with weight bearing.

RADIOGRAPHIC EVALUATION. AP, lateral, and obliques are necessary to define the injury. Plain radiography tends to underestimate the degree of articular surface depression, and tomography or CT scanning is indicated to define the full extent of the injury.

TREATMENT. Treatment is restoration of joint congruity with elevation of the articular defects and support with bone grafting and internal fixation. Nonweight-bearing ambulation for 12 to 16 weeks is required. For minimally displaced fractures, a fracture brace and nonweight-bearing activity is the treatment of choice. Follow-up treatment modalities should be aimed at restoring joint motion as quickly as possible.

Patellar Fractures

ETIOLOGY. Patellar fractures in an adult are usually secondary to a direct trauma or from an avulsion of muscle tendon units. Chondral fractures of the patella are secondary to dislocations.

SIGNS AND SYMPTOMS. Patellar fractures present as pain and swelling localized over the patella. Pain is accentuated with active knee extension; the position of comfort is full knee extension. A hemarthrosis of the knee may be present as well as loss of active knee extension.

RADIOGRAPHIC EVALUATION. AP, lateral, and sunrise views are usually adequate. The geometry of the fracture and degree of displacement define the treatment modality.

TREATMENT. If the fracture is nondisplaced, cylinder cast immobilization is the treatment of choice. For displaced fractures, open reduction internal fixation with tension banding technique is preferred. Avulsion fractures of the patella usually require operative stabilization when an extensor lag is present.

Patellar Dislocation

ETIOLOGY. Patellar dislocations are common and may recur as the result of direct trauma or as a result of a contraction of the quadriceps in conjunction with valgus and external rotation of the leg. Dislocations are more common in females secondary to the valgus alignment of the lower extremity.

SIGNS AND SYMPTOMS. The patient often complains that the knee went out of joint. There is usually immediate onset of intense pain and inability to move the knee.

If the patella is still dislocated, it will appear as a gross deformity on the lateral aspect of the knee. However, spontaneous reduction often occurs, and pain over the medial and lateral retinacular structures may be the only presenting signs in conjunction with a hemarthrosis.

RADIOGRAPHIC EVALUATION. AP, lateral, obliques, and sunrise views are obtained and evaluated for displacement of the patella as well as for any evidence of a fracture from the patella or the trochlea of the femur or for an osteochondral loose body.

TREATMENT. Initially, the patella should be gently reduced, iced, and placed in an extension splint. The limb should be held in a cast for 4 to 6 weeks, followed by a full patellar rehabilitation program. In a patient with a patella that can easily be dislocated again, consideration for repair of the medial retinaculum is important. Osteochondral fractures should be repaired or excised depending on their size and location.

Patellar Subluxation

ETIOLOGY. Patellar subluxation is a common finding in the female athlete. It is due to a number of causes including increased Q angle with excessive femoral anteversion, excessive knee valgus, external tibial torsion, and vastus medialis dysplasia or acquired atrophy.

SIGNS AND SYMPTOMS. Usually presents as a sensation of instability associated with cutting, twisting, and turning activities. Discomfort is usually present over the anterior aspect of the knee. It is brought out with flexion, valgus, and external rotation motions on the knee. The patient may complain of sudden giving way or buckling or popping with these activities.

With a subluxing patella, there is often a small joint effusion, but this may be absent with a relatively normal examination. Physical signs include a lateral squinting patella or lateral tilt, often with a high-riding patella. An increased Q angle may be present with external tibial torsion and genu valgum often seen.

On physical examination, tenderness may be elicited along the medial retinaculum and the medial facet of the patella. The patella should be examined for hypermobility with the knee in full extension and 30 degrees of flexion. After an acute subluxation, this provocation testing may be extremely painful. With provocation testing, a positive apprehension may be evident with the patient unwilling to undergo further testing.

DIAGNOSTIC EVALUATION. X-rays of both knees are useful in the evaluation of this patient. Sunrise views may show the lateral squinting of the patella. Careful observation should be made to look for osteochondral avulsions from the medial facet of the patella or off the femoral trochlear groove.

TREATMENT. Treatment should consist initially of ice, compression, and elevation with the knee splinted in full extension. Rehabilitation should then be used to reestablish quadriceps strength, especially the vastus medialis. A neoprene patellar stabilization brace with lateral horseshoe may be useful in providing stability during sporting activities. Surgical intervention is reserved for the patient with functional impairment after adequate rehabilitation.

Tibial Tubercle Avulsion Fractures

ETIOLOGY. The adolescent tibial tubercle avulsion fracture occurs as a hyperflexion injury.

SIGNS AND SYMPTOMS. Pain and swelling over the tibial tubercle and loss of active knee extension.

RADIOGRAPHIC EVALUATION. The lateral x-ray is usually diagnostic. Displacement or widening of the apophysis is seen.

TREATMENT. Treatment for a nondisplaced fracture is with a cylinder cast immobilization. A displaced fracture requires open reduction internal fixation with restoration of the epiphysis.

Tibial Spine Avulsion Fractures

Avulsions to the anterior tibial spine occur in early adolescence. The posterior spine injury is less common.

ETIOLOGY. Injury is secondary to hyperflexion and hyperextension injury to the knee.

SIGNS AND SYMPTOMS. These fractures usually present as swelling with a hemarthrosis.

RADIOGRAPHIC EVALUATION. AP, lateral and tunnel x-rays show a tibial avulsion.

TREATMENT. Treatment is to restore the anatomic position, either operatively or nonoperatively.

Osteochondritis Dissecans

ETIOLOGY. This injury is believed to be an avascular necrosis of the subchondral plate. It occurs most commonly in the nonweight-bearing portion of the medial femoral condyle. Approximately 70% of patients show bilateral knee involvement.

SIGNS AND SYMPTOMS. Patient presents with pain, limping, and giving-way episodes without history of trauma. A knee effusion may be present.

DIAGNOSTIC EVALUATION. Radiographs are usually diagnostic. The tunnel view x-ray is most useful in showing the pathology. A CT scan or arthrogram is useful to evaluate the integrity of the articular surface. Bone scanning may be useful in picking up the very early lesion.

TREATMENT. If the epiphyses are open, conservative treatment with protective weight bearing usually results in healing of the lesion. Once the epiphyses are closed, the prognosis for healing is guarded. If the fragment is detached, débridement of the bed, drilling, and possible replacement of the osteochondral lesion are preferred, especially if the fragment is in the weight-bearing area. For weight-bearing lesions, when acute reattachment is not possible, chondral resurfacing with osteochondral autologous grafts is now available. Protected range of motion with non-weight-bearing activity for 6 to 8 weeks is performed. For the patellar osteochondritis lesions, débridement, and lateral release are the preferred treatments.

Osteoarthritis

SIGNS AND SYMPTOMS. Pain is usually the presenting complaint of the patient and is usually aggravated with activity and relieved at rest; another complaint is morning stiffness that improves as the day progresses only to return later in the day. The pain is often aggravated by activities that require flexion and rotation of the knee, such as stair climbing and squatting. Associated complaints of locking, giving way, or a sensation of instability are often present. A knee effusion or history of knee effusions is usually present. A trauma history may be present. There is often a history of progressive development of bowed legs or knock knees.

The clinical examination may reveal a gross angular deformity—either genu valgum or genu varum. A fixed flexion contracture may be present. An antalgic gait with a lateral joint thrust and shortened stride may be present. Pain is usually present at the joint line of the involved compartment. Osteoarthritis may involve one or all of the compartments of the knee.

DIAGNOSTIC IMAGING. AP weight-bearing x-rays of both knees on a single cassette may demonstrate narrowing of the joint spaces, peripheral osteophyte formation, subchondral sclerosis, and cyst formation; they may also demonstrate angular deformity of the knee. Lateral and oblique films will demonstrate the presence of peripheral osteophytes and loose bodies. Sunrise views are needed to evaluate the patellofemoral joint for osteophytes, sclerosis, and maltracking. Tricompartmental disease suggests a panarticular synovitis process such as crystalline arthritis, rheumatoid arthritis, or chondrocalcinosis. Late presentation of osteoarthritis may also be seen as a tricompartmental phenomenon on x-ray.

TREATMENT. Initial treatment is rest, NSAIDs, with quadriceps and hamstring strengthening. Ambulatory assistance with a cane or walker is useful, unloading the affected extremity and providing relief of symptoms. Arthroscopic débridement may be useful, but meniscectomy in the presence of arthritis often leads to an acceleration of the degenerative process.

For varus knees with unicompartmental involvement, high-tibial osteotomy to shift the weight-bearing axis into the lateral compartment is useful in patients less than 65 years of age. For patients older than 65 years, hemiarthroplasty or total knee arthroplasty is used to relieve their symptoms. In the presence of tricompartmental disease, total knee arthroplasty gives excellent relief of pain with restoration of ambulatory functions. The young patient with severe tricompartment osteoarthritis, usually secondary to trauma, normally requires a fusion for relief of pain.

Popliteal Cysts

ETIOLOGY. Popliteal cysts are usually a symptom rather than an independent process. Popliteal cysts are an outpouching of synovial tissue in the posterior fossa and are a result of increased pressure within the knee secondary to recurrent effusions. This increased pressure results in the distention of a weakened area of the posterior capsule, usually medially with subsequent cyst formation.

SIGNS AND SYMPTOMS. Patients complain of a loss of motion, posterior knee pain, and a sensation of fullness in the popliteal space. There is often a history of knee joint effusions. Rupture of a cyst may mimic deep vein thrombosis with acute calf pain.

DIAGNOSTIC IMAGING. Confirmation of the popliteal cyst may be done with ultrasonography or arthrography to define the cyst and determine its location and origin. In the older patient, it is essential to exclude an aneurysm in the popliteal space. This may be done with ultrasonography or digital subtraction angiography if clinically suspected.

TREATMENT. Treatment is directed at determining and treating the underlying source of the knee effusion (ie, crystalline arthropathy or meniscal tear). This will usually result in resolution of the popliteal cyst. Excision is necessary for a cyst that does not resolve. For a cyst that creates venous obstruction, excision needs to be performed. It is important to rule out popliteal aneurysm in the differential diagnosis of a cyst.

Bursitis

ETIOLOGY. Bursae are closed, minimally fluid-filled sacs lined with synovium similar to the lining of joint spaces. Their single function is to reduce friction between adjacent tissues. Bursae are subjected to a variety of conditions including trauma, infection, metabolic abnormalities, rheumatic afflictions, and neoplasms.

SIGNS AND SYMPTOMS. Acute bursitis presents as pain and localized swelling. Pain is aggravated by any motion that puts pressure on the bursa. Erythema and localized increased skin warmth may be present.

DIAGNOSTIC EVALUATION. Radiographic evaluation will show a soft tissue swelling but is usually normal. Aspiration of the bursa should be performed, and the fluid should be evaluated for crystals and signs of infection.

TREATMENT. In the acute phase, initial treatment should consist of ice and compression, as well as rest. It may be coupled with aspiration and the use of nonsteroidal medication. Padding is used to prevent recurrent trauma. Cortisone may be injected into the bursa once infection has been excluded from the differential diagnosis. It should be used when conservative means of treatment have been unsuccessful.

Stretching and strengthening exercises for the knee are needed to reduce the stress on the bursa interposed between moving tissue planes.

Clinically Relevant Bursae

The deep infrapatellar bursa is positioned beneath the patellar tendon below the infrapatellar fat pad on the anterior surface of the tibia. Localized pain and tenderness at this location are frequently due to Osgood Schlatter disease but can be due to a chronic bursitis. The diagnosis is made by palpation of the bursa.

The superficial infrapatellar bursa rests between the skin and the anterior surface of the infrapatellar tendon. Inflammation of this bursa may be induced by repetitive kneeling or by direct treatment.

The pes anserine bursa lies between the pes anserine tendons (sartorius, gracilis, and semitendinosus) and the MCL over the medial aspect of the tibia. Bursitis develops because of tendon friction or from direct injury. Pain and tenderness are localized at the anteriomedial aspect of the tibia. External rotation and contraction of the pes anserine muscles aggravate the symptoms. Pes bursitis must be distinguished from an injury of the MCL. This bursa lies about 3 cm distal to the medial joint line, and pain is localized to this location. Swelling and tenderness may be palpated distal to the semitendinosus tendon.

The lateral aspect of the knee contains many small bursae that are somewhat inconstant. The biceps bursa, however, consistently lies between the lateral collateral ligament and the fibular attachment of the biceps tendon. Inflammation ensues after overactivity. Diagnosis again rests with excluding ligamentous and meniscal injuries. Local swelling is the only real sign, and such swelling includes the differential of cystic degeneration of the meniscus.

Recommended Readings

Arrington, E. D., & Miller, M. D. (1995). Skeletal muscle injuries. *Orthopaedic Clinics of North America, 26*(3), 411.

Blackburn, T. A., & Craig, E. (1980). Knee anatomy: a brief review. *Physical Therapy, 60*(12), 1556.

Carson, W. G., Jr., James, S. L., Larson, R. L., Singer, K. M., & Winternitz, W. W. (1994). Patellofemoral disorders: physical and radiographic evaluation. Part I: physical examination. *Clinical Orthopaedics, 185,* 178.

Carson, W. G., Jr., James, S. L., Larson, R. L., Singer, K. M., & Winternitz, W. W. (1994). Patellofemoral disorders: physical and radiographic evaluation. Part II: radiographic examination. *Clinical Orthopaedics, 201*(85), 178.

Colosimo, A. J., & Bassett, F. H., 3rd. (1990). Jumper's knee, diagnosis and treatment. *Orthopaedic Review, 19*(2), 139.

Dandy, D. (1993). *Essential orthopaedics and trauma.* New York: Churchill-Livingstone.

DiStefano, V. J. (1980). Function, post-traumatic sequelae and current concepts of management of knee meniscus injuries: a review article. *Clinical Orthopaedics, 201*(51), 143.

Drongowski, R. A., Coran, A. G., & Wojtys, E. M. (1994). Predictive value of meniscal and chondral injuries in conservatively treated anterior cruciate ligament injuries. *Arthroscopy, 10*(10) 97.

Dye, S. F., & Cannon, W. D., Jr. (1988). Anatomy and biomechanics of the anterior cruciate ligament. *Clinical Sports Medicine, 7*(4), 715.

Feagin, J. A., Jr. (1989). The office diagnosis and documentation of common knee problems. *Clinical Sports Medicine, 8*(3), 453.

Gerosff, W. K., & Clancy, W. G. (1988). Diagnosis of acute and chronic anterior cruciate ligament tears. *Clinical Sports Medicine, 7*(4), 727.

Gross, J., Fetto, J., & Rosen, E. (1996). *Musculoskeletal examination.* Oxford: Blackwell.

Hardin, G. T., Farr, J., & Bach, B. R., Jr. (1992). Meniscal tears: diagnosis, evaluation and treatment. *Orthopaedic Review, 21*(110), 1311.

Henderson, R. C. (1992). Tibia vara: a compilation of adolescent obesity. *Journal of Pediatrics, 121*(3), 482.

Hershman, E. B., Lombardo, J., & Bergfield, J. A. (1990). Femoral shaft stress fractures in athletes. *Clinical Sports Medicine, 9*(10), 111.

Herzog, R. J. (1992). Imaging of the knee. *Orthopaedic Review, 21*(12), 1409.

Hoppenfeld, S. (1976). *Physical examination of the spine and extremities.* East Norwalk, CT: Appleton-Century-Croft.

Install, J. N. (1981). Patella pain syndromes and chondromalacia patallae. *Instructor Course Lectures, 30,* 342.

Johnson, A. W., Weiss, C. B., Jr., & Wheeler, D. L. (1995). Stress fractures of the femoral shaft in athletes more common than expected. A new clinical test. *American Journal of Sports Medicine, 22*(2), 248.

Johnson, D. L., & Warner, J. J. (1993). Diagnosis for anterior cruciate ligament surgery. *Clinical Sports Medicine, 12*(4), 671.

Martin, D. F. (1994). Pathomechanics of knee osteoarthritis. *Medicine and Science of Sports and Exercise, 26*(12), 1429.

McLatchie, G. R., & Lennox C. M. E. (1996). *The soft tissues: trauma and sports injuries.* London: Butterworth-Heinemann.

Mellon, M. B. (1994). *Sports medicine secrets.* Philadelphia: Hanley & Belfus/Mosby.

Nichols, C. E. (1992). Patellar tendon injuries. *Clinical Sports Medicine, 11*(4), 807.

Norden, M., Gunnar, A., & Pope, M. (1997). *Musculoskeletal disorders in the work place: principles and practices.* St. Louis: Mosby.

Norris, C. M. (1993). *Sports injuries: diagnosis and management for physiotherapists.* London: Butterworth-Heinemann.

Noyes, F. R., Mooar, L. A., & Barber, S. D. (1991). The assessment of work-related activities and limiations in knee disorders. *American Journal of Sports Medicine, 19*(2), 178.

Renstrom, P., & Johnson, R. J. (1986). The anatomy of the iliopatellar band and illiotibial tract. *American Journal of Sports Medicine, 14*(1), 39.

Rothenberg, M. H., & Graf, B. K. (1993). Evaluation of acute knee injuries. *Postgraduate Medicine, 93*(3), 75.

Rovere, G. D., & Adair, D. M. (1983). Anterior cruciate-deficient knees: a review of the literature. *American Journal of Sports Medicine, 11*(6), 412.

Ryan, J. B., Wheeler, J. H., Hopkinson, W. J., Aciero, R. A., & Kolakowski, K. R. (1991). Quadriceps contusions. *American Journal of Sports Medicine, 19*(3), 299.

Smith, A. D., & Tao, S. S. (1995). Knee injuries in young athletes. *Clinical Sports Medicine, 14*(3), 629.

Smith, B. W., & Green, G. A. (1995). Acute knee injuries: part I. History and physical examination. *American Family Physician, 51*(3), 615.

Snider, R. (1997). *Essentials of musculoskeletal care.* Rosemont, IL: American Academy of Orthopaedic Surgeons. American Academy of Pediatrics.

Weissman, B. N., & Hussain, S. (1991). Magnetic resonance imaging of the knee. *Rheumatologic Disease Clinics of North America, 17*(3), 637.

Chapter 9

The Lower Leg, Ankle, and Foot

James E. Nixon, MD

Anatomy

The tibia is the second largest bone in the body. It is slightly cup-shaped proximally and is generally cylindrical through most of the shaft. The distal end widens to establish the ankle mortise. Posteriorly and laterally, it is covered by musculature. Anteriorly, the tibia is subcutaneous through most of its length.

The fibula is a slender bone lying laterally to the tibia. It forms an arthrodial joint proximally and a syndesmosis distally with the tibia. It serves primarily for muscle attachment and is the lateral buttress of the ankle joint.

The muscles of the leg are divided into four distinct compartments separated by thick fascial planes (Fig. 9-1). The anterior compartment contains the anterior tibia, extensor hallucis longus, and the extensor muscles to the toes as well as the deep peroneal nerve and anterior tibial artery. The superficial posterior compartment contains the gastrocnemius, soleus, and sural nerve. The deep posterior compartment contains the posterior tibial, flexor digitorum longus, and flexor hallucis muscles. The lateral compartment contains the peroneus longus and brevis muscles, as well as the superficial peroneal nerve. The posterior compartment muscles are innervated by the tibial nerve, whereas the anterolateral compartments are innervated by the peroneal nerve.

History

The history of the subjective complaint is no more than the identification of a temporal period in which symptoms were initiated, evolved or modified. Complaints should be sharply defined as to onset, frequency, duration and ameliorative or exaggerating factors.

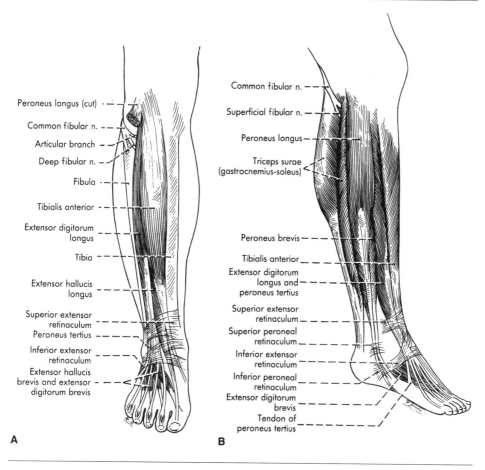

FIGURE 9-1. **(A)** Anterior muscles of the leg; **(B)** muscles of the lateral or peroneal compartment in relation to the anterior and posterior musculature.

With disabling symptoms, one works through onset or mechanisms of injury. One evaluates the duration, frequency, and intermittence. One ascertains symptomatic modification by treatment, medication, and rest. The examiner seeks to understand restrictions in functions, as well as anatomic localization. In a sense, the examiner is attempting to experience what the patient is experiencing.

Physical Examination—Background

The physical examination must be systematically organized to minimize the risk of overlooking something important.

One may begin with the screening procedure that includes observation of gait and station. The patient is asked to cross the room. Observe the posture, balance, the swing of the arms and movement of the legs. If balance is easy, the arms swing at the side, turns are smoothly accomplished with no change in periodicity, and satisfactory function is appreciated. In examining a reasonably healthy, ambulatory patient, one may ask the patient to hop in place on each foot in turn. The ability to do this indicates an intact motor system for the legs, normal cerebellar function and a good position sense as well as acceptable muscle strength. If one detects abnormal findings or indications in the screening of patients, a more specific examination is indicated that targets an anatomic area.

The underlying organization of the assessment is inspection, palpation to include that of muscle tone, testing of the muscle strength, and assessment of coordination. One may simply screen the sensory system, especially if there are no neurologic symptoms. This screening includes an evaluation of vibration in the lower extremities, a brief comparison of touch over the leg and foot, and an assessment of coordination by point-to-point testing. Point-to-point testing consists of placing the patient's foot on the opposite knee and having the patient run it down the shin to the big toe. If there are tremors or awkwardness, this may suggest cerebellar disease or loss of position sense. Vibration sense is often the first sensation to be lost in peripheral neuropathy. The common cause for peripheral neuropathy is diabetes.

A parallel placement of the standing feet may be coupled with a request to squat while maintaining the foot posture. This will give an indication of full joint motion in the lower extremities and may indicate restriction to the joint or musculotendinous unit traversing them. The short sural muscles require rising on the toes to carry out the request.

One should not jump at the obvious or concentrate all attention on the patient's presumed area of pathology. Establish a progressive system that will define the musculoskeletal unit: limb alignment and symmetry, joint motion, muscle mass, and neurologic as well as vascular integrity. One inspects for alignment, length, color, texture, swelling and posturing and asymmetric differences. One feels for heat, swelling, induration, joint fluid, thickening, edema, tenderness, mass and appreciative sensation. Initially, the effort is gentle and rapid, storing the need for later selectivity. The process is not one of "attack" but gentle, concerned tactile communication.

A sensibly complete assessment and a derivative, data-based diagnosis, leading to a logical treatment plan, is the overall purpose when one employs a physical examination. Assessment does not necessarily demand absolute determination as abnormality is encountered. It is the acquisition of descriptive data that logically and creatively leads to more sharply defined systems of investigation and, happily, a rational explanation or diagnosis. The more intrusive or evidently symptomatic the testing, the more it should be delayed to the end of the process.

Physical Examination—General

The aging process may be associated with a decreased vibratory sense. Loss of position and vibration senses suggests posterior column disease. Obviously, one needs to examine in special detail those areas where (1) there are symptoms such as numbness or pain, (2) there are reflex abnormalities, and (3) there are atrophic changes, absent or excessive sweating, atrophic skin, or cutaneous ulceration.

Leg length discrepancy should be noted in particular because this is frequently associated with overuse syndromes (the shorter leg usually being the injured leg).

Other subtle anatomic abnormalities that may lead to overuse syndromes are femoral anteversion with excessive internal rotation of the hips, tight hamstrings, genu varum or valgum, excessive Q angle of the patella, tibial varum (bowed legs), functional shortening of the gastrocnemius-soleus, and functionally pronated feet. All can produce distal symptomatology of overuse.

With observation, one may note limping, atrophy, swelling, and bruising as evidence of objective differences between the limbs.

Vascular Examination

Because venous disease most commonly affects the legs, special attention should be paid to the structure and function of the leg veins. Superficial veins are located subcutaneously where they are supported relatively poorly. Anastomotic channels join the deep and the superficial systems as communicating or perforating veins along the entire course. Aging alone brings relatively few clinically important changes to the peripheral vascular system. Although arterial and venous disorders (especially atherosclerosis) do affect older people more frequently, these disorders cannot be considered part of the aging process. Age may make tortuous or typically stiffen arterial walls, but these changes develop with or without atherosclerosis and therefore are not diagnostically specific. Loss of arterial pulsation is not part of normal aging and demands careful evaluation. The skin may get thin and dry with age. Nails may grow more slowly, and hair on the legs often becomes scant. These are not specific for arterial insufficiency. Diminished or absent posterior tibial, popliteal, or femoral pulse suggests occlusive arterial disease. The dorsalis pedis pulse, however, may be congenitally absent. Its absence is not diagnostic of occlusive arterial disease.

With the patient standing, inspect the saphenous system for varicosities. They may be easily missed when the patient is supine. Look for edema of the legs and check for pitting edema. Look for an increase in the venous patterns of the leg or diffuse red cyanosis of the leg. Feel for increased firmness or tension in the calf muscles. Superficial phlebitis may be characterized by redness or discoloration overlying the saphenous system. Palpate for tenderness or cords. Competency of the venous valves in varicose veins may be assessed by manual compression tests. With the fingertips of one hand, feel the dilated vein. With your other hand, compress the vein firmly at a place at least 20 cm higher in the leg. Clear the vein, then release compression. Feel for an impulse transmitted to your lower hand. Competence of the saphenous valves should block the transmission of any impulse. With a history of chronic pain and swelling, more particularly with dermatologic changes and ulcerations, the advances in noninvasive directional and volume ultrasound have advanced specific diagnosis and treatment.

If one suspects chronic arterial insufficiency, elevate the patient's leg approximately 12 inches and have the patient move the feet up and down at the ankle for approximately 60 seconds. The maneuver drains the feet of venous blood, unmasking the color produced by arterial supply. Relative pallor is normal. Increased or deathly pallor is arterial insufficiency. After this, have the patient sit promptly at the edge of the examining table with the legs dangling. The color should return in about 10 seconds, and filling of the veins of the feet and ankle should occur normally in about 15 seconds. If there is delay in color or venous filling return, there is arterial insufficiency. A Doppler in the office is a useful extension of the palpating finger.

Neurologic Examination

Peripheral neuropathy is an acute or chronic degenerative condition of either the peripheral nerves, the autonomic nervous system, or the central nervous system. Diabetes mellitus is, by far, the most common cause of peripheral neuropathy. Among other etiologic agents are toxic substances (eg, alcohol, lead, mercury, arsenic, methyl-n-butyl ketone, thallium, n-hexane [an organic compound in glues]) as well as therapeutic drugs.

The toxicity of the workplace is increasing. Diagnosis may rest on an index of suspicions. Symptoms are characterized by complaints located in the distal portions of the limb, particularly the digits, and the symptoms range from paresthesias such as numbness, tingling, and prickling to burning, aching, or sharp intense pain. Frequently, tenderness is present along the course of the nerves. The objective findings consist of impairment of touch, vibration, position, and temperature sense. There may be hyperesthesia present. If the condition has progressed to the point of complete functional severance, pain is absent and loss of sensation is complete. Nutritional neuropathy is found most often in the chronic alcoholic as a result of folate and niacin deficiency.

Generalized conditions can produce localized neuropathy. It is found in polyarteritis nodosa, rheumatoid arthritis, Sjögren's syndrome, or, in a sense, any condition in which the ischemia due to a vasculitis may affect several or more peripheral nerves. Trauma or compression of peripheral nerves may lead to a neuropathy.

Peripheral neuropathy must be differentiated from ischemic neuropathy, which is due to a severe degree of ischemia of the peripheral tissues including the mixed nerves. It is produced by chronic occlusive arterial disease, generally arteriosclerotic obliterans of the lower extremity. Although the symptoms of the two conditions are frequently similar (sense of coldness, numbness, or burning in the feet, paresthesia of the toes, and shooting, lancinating pain), the complaints of ischemia appear soon after the patient lies in bed in preparation for sleep and are immediately alleviated by placing the lower limbs over the edge of the bed, sitting up, or standing. This particular posturing may be found in entrapment neuropathies, although in general these positions have no eliciting or controlling effect on the symptoms of peripheral neuropathy.

As one regards the physical findings, ischemic neuropathy is always associated with signs of markedly reduced arterial circulation (absent pulses). The final insult may occur suddenly.

Gait Abnormalities

Both upper and motor neuron disease, as well as peripheral nerve disease, are evident with ambulation, and they demonstrate characteristic gaits.

1. Ataxic: There is loss of proprioceptive sense in the extremities.
    a. Wide base with slapping feet while watching the leg and surface

    b. Clumsiness and uncertainty are characteristic. There is abnormal height elevation of the extremities lowered with the slapping of the foot. There is uneven spacing of the steps.

2. Hemiplegic (upper motor neuron): The affected leg is rigid and is swung from the hip in a semicircle by movements of the trunk. The patient leans to the affected side. The arm on the affected side is held in a rigid, semiflexed position. The spastic lower limb is moved forward with difficulty, and the toes of the lower limb tend to be forced down, demanding abduction and circumduction to afford forward motion.

3. Scissors gait: spastic paraplegia. The legs are adducted, crossed alternately in front of the contacting flexed knees. Progress is labored, with compensatory rotation motions of the trunk and upper extremities.

4. Waddling: muscular dystrophy with involvement of the pelvic girdle. The weakness of the hip musculature results in the pelvic tilt and exaggerated compensatory sway of the trunk toward the weight-bearing side. It produces a swaybacked, potbellied posture and a waddling gait.

5. Propulsion or festination: parkinsonism produces a forward-leaning posture and short, shuffling steps, beginning slowly at first and becoming more rapid.

6. Steppage gait: paralysis of the anterior tibial muscle group (peroneal nerve injury, polio, toxic neuritides, and so forth) is productive of high knee action, a dragging toe, and a flopping of the foot on placement.

With specific reference to the lower extremities for conditions that manifest muscle or sensory disturbances below the knee, there are a group of conditions called peripheral neuropathy or a polyneuritis that can be categorized, etiologically, into four general groups.

1. Intoxicants: alcohol, heavy metals such as arsenicals and lead, carbon disulfide, benzene, phosphorous compounds, insecticides, as well as medications that include antibacterial, antitubercular and antidepressant drugs

2. Infections: syphilis, diphtheria, Guillain-Barré syndrome, herpes zoster, varicella

3. Metabolic: diabetes mellitus, hyperthyroidism, pregnancy

4. Nutritional: B-complex deficiency, pernicious anemia, beri-beri, pellagra

The history, coupled with that of the neuromuscular evidence in the physical examination, should point the way to identification of intoxicants. The major complication of pernicious anemia is posterolateral sclerosis. On the other hand, the onset clinically is characterized by tingling, numbness and "pins and needles." With more pronounced peripheral involvement, there may be calf tenderness, stocking distribution of impaired sensation, weakness and depression or absence of the ankle jerk. The early neurologic findings are reversible with vitamin B_{12}. The subtleties of hyperthyroidism may be reflected by paresthesias and pain in the extremity with "burning" of the feet. The symptoms are generally out of proportion to the findings. Diabetes mellitus, on the other hand, may present with initial clinical manifestations of a neuropathy. Sensory involvement is usually symmetric and more common in the lower extremities. Pain is an outstanding symptom. An early finding is an impaired vibratory sense, often with diminished or absent deep tendon reflexes.

The isolated absence of the Achilles reflex is present in approximately 50% of diabetic patients. Motor involvement is generally unilateral. Foot drop can be present. There may be asymmetric muscle weakness and wasting.

Adolescents With Leg Pain

The young, although not subject to the rigors of the workplace and functioning, may still present with problems related to the skin, vascular, and musculoskeletal structures.

Common nontraumatic problems found in this age group are contact dermatitis from substances used in the manufacture of uniforms, shoes, and protective equipment. Tincture of benzoin used as a tape adherent is a potential sensitizer. The "neoprene brace" or encasement, when combined with chronic aquatic use, can produce fungal growth, especially in the seam area. The environment is a source of contact dermatitis from such elements as poison ivy. Tick-borne disease with both skin and arthralgia complaints is to be considered in this age group.

Dermatitis

The diagnosis of contact dermatitis is found in a history of the recent purchase of an item of clothing, footgear or a uniform. Look for localized responses, particularly those that follow the outline of the object. It is noted that some of the cream bases used as vehicles for cortisone preparation may be sensitizers. The logical treatment is avoidance of the suspected object. Contact dermatitis affects the dorsum of the toes and foot and spares the toe-webs and sole. *Tinea pedis* has the opposite distribution. Identification of the agent is acquired with a shoe screening patch-test kit. When the dermatitides are secondarily invaded or infected, they present as increasing problems in treatment and diagnosis.

In addition to housing vermin and irritants, the environment is a potential source of nontraumatic consequence on the lower extremity.

On the feet, contact dermatitis is commonly caused by four major groups of materials: (1) components of shoes and stockings, (2) applied medications, (3) appliances used on the feet, and (4) substances encountered in occupational exposures. In the classic case, shoe dermatitis presents as an eczematous dermatitis beginning on the dorsal aspect of the big toe with eventual extension to other toes, sparing the toe webs and soles. Climatic and environmental factors play a role in the development of some occupational skin diseases. The predominant cause of industrial dermatitis is leakage of chemical agents that spill on the shoes and feet. Cement, for instance, can cause contact dermatitis through the corrosive action of the cement and/or allergic reaction from the chromates in the cement. Another type of exposure may arise from the components of specially designed work shoes or rubber boots worn in various occupations.

The diagnosis of allergic contact dermatitis depends on history and eczematous eruption and its localization. Special patch testing is valuable in defining the causative agent.

Heat Cramps

This condition is due to excessive salt loss under conditions of high ambient temperature and may be prevented by adequate salt and water intake. Heat exhaustion is due primarily to loss of body water. Peripheral vasodilation and pooling of blood in the lower extremities due to standing may contribute to this condition as well as sustained muscular exercise with no regard for replacing lost water. Psychotropic drugs may have an atropinelike effect. These effects, when combined with high ambient temperatures, may produce symptoms in excess of those expected. Patients complain of painful gastrocnemius and soleus muscle contractions. Attention to the history of drug use in the process of supportive therapy may prove useful. Treatment consists of oral fluid and electrolyte replacement coupled with passive stretching. Instruct athletes to drink water at least every 20 minutes during endurance competition and to stop and stretch periodically.

"Night cramps" in the lower extremities have no good physiologic explanation but appear in the intensely used, gravity-resisted muscles of the leg. Although bothersome, they require no treatment at this age.

Frostbite

Prolonged exposure of the body to cold temperatures may produce frostbite that occurs from cooling of the skin and subcutaneous tissues. This cooling can be carried to the point at which circulation is closed off. If not rapidly corrected, the skin loses its vascularity. Additionally, frostbite can be found as a consequence of the injudicious use of cooling agents, ethyl chloride, and the prolonged use of ice. The clinical presentation consists of pain, loss of sensation, and a cold, white extremity.

The prophylaxis for frostbite is keeping exposed areas of skin covered, reducing local heat loss, and preserving local circulation by avoiding constrictive clothing. The treatment is rapid warming of the affected part and prevention of re-exposure.

Neuropathies

Neuropathies are usually the result of trauma to the nerve. Adolescents are not good historians. They do not necessarily consider "acceptable" strain as trauma. As a consequence, there may be "nontraumatic" entrapment neuropathy, in which various nerves of the legs may be involved.

Saphenous Nerve

Neuropathy of the saphenous nerve produces pain at or below the level of the knee with radiation downward to the medial side of the foot. The entrapment may be apparent while negotiating stairs, exaggerated with extension of the knee. Adduction of the thigh against resistance reproduces the symptoms by tensing the subsartorial fascia. The area of entrapment is at the site of exit from the subsartorial canal. The point of exit is approximately 10 cm proximal to the medial epicondyle. While palpating the anteromedial muscle (the vastus medialis), the examiner slides the hand posteriorly to the edge of the sartorius. The saphenous opening is beneath this point. Pressure at that point is painful and will cause radiation distally. There is a Tinel's sign.

Peroneal Nerve

The nontraumatic, noniatrogenic causes for involvement of the peroneal nerve are few. They are seen in patients with diabetes or herpes zoster. The common mechanism of damage to the peroneal nerve at the head of the fibula is acute compression. Compression is caused by prophylactic braces, stockings and garters, or sitting for a prolonged period, as during a card game with the leg resting against the side of the chair. Squatting or kneeling for extended periods may produce a sudden, painless foot drop. Compression may be produced by ganglia from the proximal tibiofibular joint. Pure entrapment of the fibular tunnel (against the roof of the peroneus longus) is rare.

L-5 radiculopathy may resemble peroneal palsy or entrapment of its branches. In the uncommon individual, there may be no back or thigh pain (Fig. 9-2). Observations that indicate an L-5 radiculopathy should be considered. Some observations include:

1. Weakness of inversion of the foot. The posterior tibialis is not innervated by the peroneal nerve.
2. The clear-cut lumbar L-5 lesion sensory loss that is well above the midpart of the calf.
3. Greater weakness in the extensor hallucis than in the anterior tibial. (The latter muscle receives L-4 innervation.) Complete paralysis of the dorsiflexors of the foot favor a peroneal palsy.

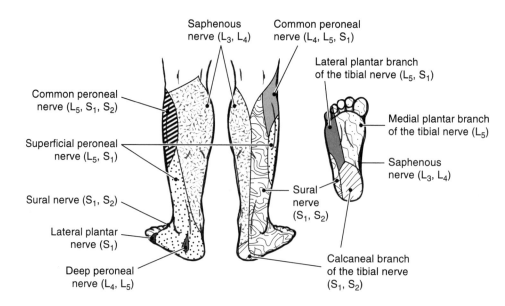

FIGURE 9-2. Distribution of the cutaneous nerves of the leg.

DIAGNOSTIC STUDIES. The electrophysiologic (EMG, nerve conduction) assessment of the peroneal nerve has several uses. It may be used in the differential diagnosis as well as to establish prognosis and identify early signs of recovery. Nerve conduction and EMG studies are employed. Although EMG is theoretically useful, clinically it may not aid in differential diagnosis. Sensory action potentials may identify entrapment of the cutaneous nerves. Prognosis may be suggested by conduction velocity studies. Normal or near-normal studies suggest an excellent prognosis. If slowed or undetermined, the prognosis is poor.

TREATMENT. Treatment for the lesions of the common peroneal nerve should consist of bracing. The usual appliance is a plastic orthosis extending from the posterior leg and encasing the plantar surface of the foot as a molded structure. A slowly progressive disturbance in peroneal nerve function, in which there is pain as well as motor and sensory loss, suggests an entrapment neuropathy. Ganglion cysts and other tumors should be suspected. In such patients, relatively early exploration is indicated. In entrapment neuropathies, decompression results in rapid and complete recovery in most patients. The conservation period is about 2 months.

The second portion of the superficial peroneal nerve is subjected to entrapment neuropathy in the distal portion of the leg. The usual suggested origin of the neuropathy is forced plantar flexion or an inversion twist of the ankle and foot. The nerve is tethered at the point of derivation at the fibular neck and distally at the subcutaneous exit. The foot–ankle inversion force applied will make a nerve taut against its opening and provide the initiating trauma. Occasionally, repetition of contact over the distal lateral portion of the leg will produce symptoms. Injury can occur from a tightly laced boot that ends at the level of the subfascial penetration by the nerve. In general, the pain is burning and superficial.

Because the pain distribution strongly resembles that produced by irritation of the L-5 root, the differentiation between the two conditions may be difficult. Adding to that difficulty is the fact that the irritated root can cause marked tenderness of the peripheral trunk extension.

Adults With Leg Pain

All of the problems found in adolescents, with the exception of overuse and trauma directed against the growth apophysis or epiphysis of growing bone, are found in adults. Musculoskeletal symptoms are frequently due to activity pattern changes.

Although overuse syndromes have been indicated in sports, they have also been present in the workplace for centuries. These syndromes may be characterized by the external manifestations in the skin. One can see the protective callus in those who kneel, such as a cement finisher, rug and floor layer or tile setters. Beneath the subcutaneous calluses, there is evident, chronic bursae formation. The incidental burns of the welder are examples of work-related trauma. The chronic joint and tendon problems related to the repetitive acts of the musician, dancer, factory and clothing worker lead over time to degeneration and disability.

Nontraumatic Problems

A change in usual or conditioned activities may produce inflammation. If, initially, these traumas are only awareness, stiffness, or temporary aching, there may be little concern. If the symptoms increase and linger, they may be brought to medical attention.

The entrapment syndromes enumerated above may evolve. Laying paving bricks may produce peroneal neuropathy. A change in shoe height, particularly in those with tight heel cords, may produce peroneal tendinitis. Standing on a ladder or shoveling may produce plantar fasciitis. Gardening may require crouching, squatting, digging with shovels and forks, as well as contact with fertilizers and insecticides, all of which can affect the lower extremity. The power lawn mower can damage a foot.

In evaluating nontraumatic complaints related to the lower extremity, the examiner should search for a change in pattern that may be the etiologic agent: a holiday, trip, prolonged plane flight, household chores induced by weather changes, and so forth.

Cramps

Lower extremity cramps are common in the gastrocnemius and soleus muscles of the calf. Individuals complain of either a sudden or gradual onset of incapacitating calf pain. This can be related to improper warm-up before sports activity, any sustained muscle activity, or salt depletion during an endurance activity. The exact physiology of muscle cramps is unknown.

The treatment consists of proper stretching before an activity as well as adequate salt and fluid replacement during athletic competition and passive stretching of the muscle to relieve the painful spasm.

Common Traumatic Problems

Contusions of the Tibia

Contusions over the anterior leg are very common in both sports and the work environment. The nature and severity of the injury depend on the site of the direct trauma. Much of the tibia is superficial and, therefore, has very little protective covering. As a consequence, rather deep abrasions, lacerations, and involvement of the venous structures are more evident over the anterior leg. The leg is prone to infection. Folliculitis and cellulitis can develop surrounding the more superficial wounds. Subcutaneous hemorrhage develops from contusion laceration of the superficial veins. This condition may be extensive, and the hematoma may become infected. The incidence of infection with surgery or trauma is highest in the lower extremity, more distally in the extremity and the ankle because of the anatomic fixation of the skin and limited subcutaneous tissue that buffers trauma and affords swelling without increased neurovascular damage.

TREATMENT. Cleansing, protection, and repeat observation are demanded by what initially, viewed from a functional standpoint, may be a relatively minor injury. Direct blows to the musculature of the lower leg may result in bleeding. If bleeding or reactive edema in the leg is present to any great degree, the limited expansion allowed within the compartments may cause ischemia. It is extremely important that severe contusions to the muscular areas of the leg be watched closely for increased swelling, increasing pain, changes in skin color and temperature, and loss of peripheral pulses as well as sensation. It may be necessary to restore perfusion with an immediate fasciotomy. To await the loss of peripheral pulses, as well as sensation, presages disaster. Compartment pressure measurements must be performed whenever there is disproportionate pain present or when there is significant pain on passive stretch of the muscles of the involved compartment. The change in pattern can occur late.

Contusions of the Fibula

Contusions over the proximal fibula may injure the peroneal nerve. More distally in the leg, the superficial peroneal nerve in the distal lateral aspect may be injured as it transverses the deep fascia to innervate the distal lateral portion of the leg, the dorsum of the foot, and the dorsum of the first four toes. The sensory alterations of the nerve distribution can range from hyperesthesia to hypoesthesia or analgesia. A complaint after resolution of the trauma can be burning in nature and is generally superficial. The neurologic findings with severe contusion are evident as weakness or paralysis of the dorsiflexors of the foot as well as first interspace anesthesia.

Strains/Sprains

Strains of the muscles and tendons of the leg are frequent in runners and jumpers. The diagnosis of a sprain to the muscle or tendon is based on the history of the mechanism, the site of point tenderness, and the degree of disability. Management is directed at reducing the inflammation with the use of rest, ice massage, and the use of oral anti-inflammatory agents. Rehabilitation is directed at increasing muscular endurance. Stretching exercises are begun slowly after resolution of the acute inflammation. Improving strength and endurance is essential before return to sports. A regimen of stretching before and after running coupled with the avoidance of running on hard surfaces, running downhill, running on uneven surfaces (eg, sand, grass, and so forth), and overtraining will decrease the chances of muscle injury.

Instruct runners in the importance of proper footwear. Shoes should be cushioned, especially at the heel, to absorb shock. Well-padded heel counters will support the heel and the Achilles tendon. Mesh uppers will allow the feet to breathe. Padded tongues will prevent irritation of the dorsum. The sole of the shoe should not be stiff because this may lead to lower leg strain. A flexible sole with an arch support that fits is essential. Instruct the athlete in the importance of regularly checking shoes for wear and replacing worn shoes.

Dislocation of the Head of the Fibula

This injury results from twisting forces applied to the knee that rotate it internally. At the same time, direct force is applied to the head of the fibula, levering it out of its shallow pocket. If the patient is seen immediately, reduction may be accomplished by closed manipulation. Frequently, the injury is missed and later is diagnosed with evidence of a painful luxating phenomenon manifest with traction of the hamstrings. If the joint remains unstable, the ligamentous structures may have to be repaired.

Shin Splints

"Shin splints" is an old catch-all term that includes tibialis posterior tendinitis, stress fractures, muscle tears and strains, periosteal strains, and certain chronic vascular disorders (compartment syndromes). This complex has, more appropriately, been characterized as a medial tibial syndrome or soleus syndrome. It must be differentiated from a more sharply defined, or concomitant, stress "fracture." The frequent cause is hyperpronation caused by forefoot varus.

Characteristic scintigraphic findings do not define the posterior tibial muscle origin. Abnormal tracer accumulation is localized to the middle and distal thirds of the posterior medial aspect of the tibial cortex on delayed images. A high-resolution gamma camera must be used to obtain both lateral and medial views. The pattern suggests that the soleus muscle margin is involved as opposed to the posterior tibial or other muscle tendon complexes of the leg. The patient presents with aching pain along the medial tibial border usually after a long run on uneven surfaces and with inadequate foot support.

TREATMENT. Management focuses on the cause of injury in the given patient. A collapsing medial arch should be supported with orthotics. Symptoms can be treated after the biomechanical cause of the injury is corrected. Strength and flexibility exercises can be instituted after pain subsides. Heel cord stretching is accomplished on an incline board.

Overuse Syndromes

Overuse syndromes generally present as leg pain without a history of specific injury. They are all associated with exercise. The overuse syndromes include acute muscle cramps, tenosynovitis of the anterior tibial, flexor hallucis longus, posterior tibial or Achilles tendon, periostitis of the tibia, stress fracture of the fibula or tibia, partial subcutaneous ruptures of the Achilles, tears of the musculotendinous junction of the medial head of the gastrocnemius, and chronic and acute anterior compartment syndromes.

Compartment Syndrome

Compartment syndromes may develop as the result of an acute injury or may be the result of muscle swelling in the encased compartment. Any of the four compartments of the lower leg may be involved. Because the compartments are bounded by tight fascial structures, swelling or bleeding within these compartments can raise the intercompartmental pressure, resulting in decreased profusion and relative anoxia of the muscle compartment. The initial presentation of this ischemia is pain that is disproportionate and is not relieved with minor analgesics. Pain is increased with passive stretch of the muscle of the involved compartment. With progression, paresthesias and paralysis develop. With the development of paresthesias and paralysis, the muscle compartments have usually undergone irreversible cell damage and death. The standard evaluation for pulses in this condition is not useful. The clinical sign of pain with passive stretching of the involved compartment should trigger automatic compartment pressure monitoring.

This condition is a surgical emergency and requires immediate referral for monitoring of compartment pressure and possible fasciotomies. Crush injuries of the lower extremities and tibial fractures are common etiologies for development of compartment syndrome. In a patient with head trauma or a polytraumatized patient, indwelling compartment pressure monitoring should be performed because symptomatic and neural assessment is not possible.

Acute and chronic exercise-induced compartment syndromes produce pain in the lower extremity but are due to muscle swelling within these compartments as a consequence of exercise and physical exertion. This can be demonstrated by increased compartment pressure after exercise. This syndrome presents predominantly as pain after a period of exercise. The acute condition may require immediate intervention. The chronic or intermittent stress-induced form may be improved with rest and modification of training programs, but in a high performance athlete this problem may require fasciotomy to obtain relief. These chronic exercise-induced compartment syndromes can be studied using treadmills and pressure catheterization techniques.

Gastrocnemius Tear

The medial head of the gastrocnemius can be ruptured. It occurs at the musculotendinous junction, usually in the deconditioned older age group, although it can occur in the hypertrophied muscle of the overdeveloped athlete. The postrupture state is characterized by an upward migration of the muscle with tenderness over the medial head. The junction of the musculotendinous area evidences swelling and ecchymosis with distal migration of subcutaneous blood in the more severe cases. Generally, the condition is caused by a sudden eccentric force on the muscle. The condition can be confused with deep thrombophlebitis, but in general the episode itself, the sudden onset, and the sharply defined anatomic location do not cause diagnostic problems.

TREATMENT. Treatment is directed at control of pain and inflammation, and restoration of normal motion and strength of the lower leg before return to sports. Conservative care generally suffices, although in the occasional case injury can recur. Pressure dressing, elevation, and icing are used early. A heel lift will relieve tension with ambulation. Crutches are used with weight bearing to tolerance. The healing phase requires not less than 6 weeks with subsequent rehabilitation. Early return to sports usually guarantees recurrence.

Achilles Tendinitis (Tendinosis)

Repetitive overextension or overuse of the Achilles tendon, such as jumping at basketball or distance running may cause the sheath to become inflamed and thickened. This results in chronic pain and tightness over the Achilles tendon. More frequently, it is insidious in onset. Incidence peaks in people in their midthirties. At times, the condition may become chronic and incapacitating, particularly to the competitive athlete. Examination may reveal a diffuse or localized swelling and tenderness to palpation over the tendon. The contour of the tendon should be smooth and even, and there should be no evidence of nodulations or scar formation.

In the more chronic tendinitis, nodulation or distortions in contour can occur, and these suggest degeneration within the structure of the tendon or partial subcutaneous tears.

TREATMENT. The initial treatment includes rest until acute inflammation subsides, ice to the affected area, and oral nonsteroidal anti-inflammatory drugs (NSAIDs). A heel lift may be useful to decrease tension on the tendon. Once the condition subsides, active stretching and strengthening of the gastrocnemius soleus complex can begin. If conservative treatment is not successful and the patient is disabled, consideration should be given to surgery.

Achilles Rupture

Acute Achilles tendon rupture occurs generally after a prodromal period of "tendinitis." The occurrence is usually 1 or 2 inches above the insertion of the tendon on the calcaneus. A palpable gap is apparent. There is a distinct history of a sudden, lancinating pain with loss of function and inability to stand on the toes.

Physical examination of the complete tear reveals swelling and ecchymosis over the posterior aspect of the leg and heel. This can be confused with an "ankle sprain." Generally, there is a palpable gap and the absence of active plantar flexion with good strength. Thompson's or Simond's test is performed by squeezing the calf musculature.

If there is no continuity between the gastrocnemius–soleus muscles and the Achilles tendon, the transmitted squeeze ("shortening" the muscle) will not produce plantar flexion of the foot (Fig. 9-3). Splinting and compression dressings with the foot in a relaxed plantar flexion mode with advised elevation and early icing can be useful in reducing the reaction about the area. In the young, active person, surgical repair is advised; the condition can also be treated in an equinus long leg cast.

Stress "Fracture"

The tibia, fibula and metatarsals frequently sustain stress fractures as a result of overuse. Although one tends to identify these strains with distance runners, they can be found in teenagers with "normal activity." The condition frequently occurs in the preseason training period during a rapid increase in activity. These fractures do not occur at any particular time, but rather are the end product of a failed reparative or adaptive process in which a bone attempts to remodel itself along the lines of increased stress. The bone becomes partially or completely disrupted by rhythmic, repeated subthreshold stress. Symptoms usually begin with a mild discomfort in the long shaft of the tibia or fibula after activity. Simple rest relieves the symptoms. With continued activity, the pain becomes more persistent, lasting from day to day. Ultimately, the pain is severe enough to prohibit activity.

Clinical examination may demonstrate localized tenderness to palpation directly over the fracture sites. There may be evident subcutaneous swelling. Early x-ray films may be negative or may reveal periosteal reactions or cortical thickening 2 to 4 weeks after the onset of symptoms. A bone scan will be positive before x-ray changes (Fig. 9-4). Bone pain may precede scintigraphic evidence of stress fracture, and repeat scanning may be necessary in people whose bone pain increases with

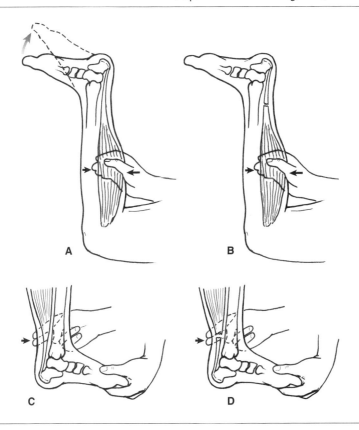

FIGURE 9-3. Diagnosis of the ruptured Achilles tendon. (**A**) Normal; (**B**) ruptured; (**C**) normal; (**D**) ruptured.

continued activity. Stress fractures are generally found in the lower third of each bone, and may be single or multiple.

Management of these fractures includes rest from the initiating stress. Generally no cast is required, and ordinary walking is allowed if it is not excessive. In some instances, a tibial Aircast fracture brace may be useful in decreasing symptoms and allowing earlier return to sports. It is to be noted that some patients require a cast primarily to induce rest. If the advice is ignored, the bone may completely fracture.

Fracture

Isolated fractures of the tibia and fibula occur but are not overly common in sports. Fractures of the neck of the fibula can occur with sudden turns in skiing as well as "cutting" in basketball. There may be secondary associated injuries due to bleeding that involve the peroneal nerve.

With fractures of the leg, the primary concern is restoring integrity of the tibia. The immediate management should be application of a splint and transportation to a facility where x-ray examination can be performed and more definitive care

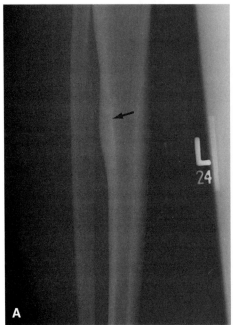

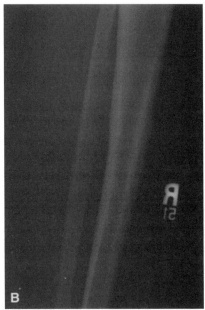

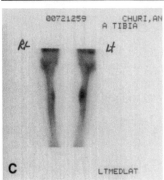

FIGURE 9-4. (A) X-ray of stress fracture in tibia. **(B)** X-ray of normal tibia. **(C)** Bone scan of stress fracture.

extended. Splinting, gentle compression, and external application of cold packs where feasible, as well as medication for relief of pain, should be routine. Trauma has the unfortunate consequence of inflammation, and this has little to do with distorted osseous anatomy. If the secondary inflammatory state is not treated immediately, the "disease" that ensues can seriously interfere with attempts to definitively treat the distorted anatomy. Definitive treatment requires restoration of length, alignment, and joint congruity by either closed or open means.

The Ankle

Anatomy

The ankle joint is formed by three bones: tibia, fibula and talus. The dome of the talus fits into the mortise (concavity) formed by the tibia and fibula. The medial and lateral malleoli project downward to articulate with the side of the talus. The ankle joint moves in one plane upward and downward with a central axis of rotation. As the ankle goes into plantar flexion, the more narrow posterior portion of the talus is brought into contact with the wider anterior portions of the joint. This permits a small amount of free play in the ankle joint that, in dorsiflexion, is lost. On the other hand, as the tibia is driven forward on the plantar flexed talus, the narrower portions of the tibia impinge on the wider anterior portions of the talus, stabilizing the tibia on the talus.

The relationship of these three bones is maintained by three groups of ligaments: the deltoid ligament medially, the lateral collateral ligaments, and the anteroposterior tibiofibular ligament and syndesmosis. The deltoid, the strongest of the three ligaments, has a broad triangular shape and is defined by the bony insertions on the navicular, the talus, and the calcaneus as it fans from the medial malleolus. The lateral collateral ligament of the ankle is T-shaped and consists of three distinct parts (Fig. 9-5). The posterior talofibular ligament arises from the posterior portion of the tip of the fibula and runs backward and slightly downward to attach to the lateral tubercle of the posterior process of the talus. This is essentially an interarticular ligament. It is the strongest of the three ligamentous elements and helps to resist posterior dislocation of the foot. The calcaneofibular ligament is the longest of the three and passes inferiorly in a posterior direction to insert on the lateral surface of the calcaneus. The ligament is extracapsular, but may be associated with the peroneal tendon sheaths. This ligament is completely relaxed when the foot is in a normal standing position. The anterior talofibular ligament arises from the anterior border of the lateral malleolus and passes forward somewhat medially to attach to the neck of the talus. Its direction corresponds to the longitudinal axis of the foot and is taut in all positions of flexion. The anterior talofibular ligament is the primary stabilizer of the ankle joint and is most commonly injured. The ligaments

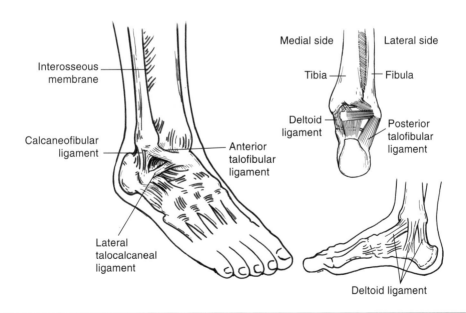

FIGURE 9-5. The ligaments of the ankle.

of the tibiofibular syndesmosis maintain the relationship of the distal tibia and fibula. The ligaments hold the fibula snug in the groove on the tibia where the fibula rotates around its longitudinal axis, as well as rising and falling with dorsi and plantar flexion of the ankle. The anterior tibiofibular and posterior tibiofibular ligaments blend into the interosseous membrane approximately 2 to 3 cm above the ankle joint.

Ankle Sprains

The best time for accurate assessment of the degree of damage is immediately after the injury when muscle spasm is absent, pain is not as severe, and swelling and hemarthrosis have not developed. Onset of swelling and hemarthrosis is extremely rapid after injury, and this appreciation is afforded to few other than team primary care providers. When subsequently seen, the ankle has reacted and is symptomatically resistant to stability testing. It is estimated that ankle injuries account for 20% to 25% of all lost time injuries in running and jumping sports.

In the workplace, ankle sprains can result from insecure footing secondary to slips or falls, dismounting from vehicles, and encounters with unexpected potholes.

MECHANISMS OF INJURY. Injuries to the ankle must be considered in relationship to the magnitude and direction of forces applied to the ankle. Once inversion is initiated, the ankle loses the bony stability of its neutral position. As inversion increases, the medial malleolus may lose its stabilizing function and begin to act as a fulcrum for further inversion. Because inversion injuries are the most frequent, sprains to the lateral collateral ligament are by far the most common ankle injury. The same mechanism of inversion and supination can lead to a fracture, usually an oblique fracture of the fibula with or without a fracture of the medial malleolus.

The other important mechanism of ankle injury is pronation and external rotation. This is rarely a pure ligamentous injury, and, when it does occur, the deltoid and anterior tibiofibular ligaments are torn. Usually, the deltoid ligament ruptures with the fracture of the fibula (Fig. 9-6).

Frequently, high fractures of the fibula can occur with sprains about the ankle as well as the associated injuries involving the interosseous membrane and the ligamentous structures of the medial ankle joint. Although the ankle may not be fractured, the evidences of trauma about the ankle, as well as the high fibular fracture, strongly suggest a transmitted disruption through the interosseous membrane across the front of the ankle and through the deltoid ligamentous structures. Thus, the high isolated fracture is associated with serious distal injuries.

DIAGNOSTIC GUIDELINES. It is estimated that there are approximately 27,000 ankle injuries per day in the United States. The diagnosis of sprain is established frequently by x-ray exclusion of a fracture.

Most patients return to normal activity within a month, leaving a residual of some 10% to 20% with persistent symptoms for months to years. When one couples the incidence with the percentage of residual problems, the need for continuing attention to this very common trauma is evident. The following grades have been defined:

Minor (grade I): No macroscopic tears, little swelling or tenderness, and no mechanical loss of stabilizing ligaments

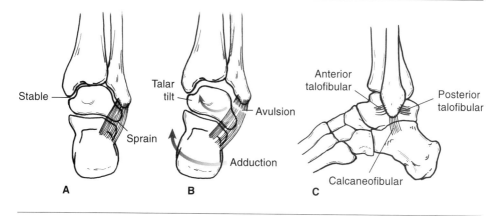

FIGURE 9-6. Lateral ligamentous sprain and avulsion. (**A**) Simple sprain in which the ligaments remain intact and the talus remains stable within the mortise. (**B**) Avulsion of the lateral ligaments; the talus becomes unstable and tilts within the mortise when the calcaneus is adducted. (**C**) Lateral ligaments of the ankle. The anterior talofibular and the calcaneofibular ligaments are the ligaments most frequently involved in inversion injuries.

Moderate (grade II): Partial macroscopic tear, mild to moderate pain and swelling and tenderness, loss of motion and possible mild clinical instability

Severe (grade III): Complete rupture of the ligamentous structure, severe swelling with evident hemorrhage and tenderness, loss of function and stability of the joint

The visual definitions of the grades of ankle sprain are related to the degree of swelling (none–slight–definitive) and the appearance of hematoma (none–slight–definitive).

PHYSICAL EXAMINATION. With serious ankle injuries, there may be a history of immediate pain and difficulty in bearing weight. Often the patient will describe a "pop," a "snap," or a sense of giving way.

Initial evaluation reveals localized tenderness over the involved ligaments. Motion may be restricted. In general, the more difficulty a person has in weight bearing, the more serious the injury.

The initial evaluation of acute injury includes the neurologic and vascular functions of the extremity. If these are intact, attention is turned to the other elements. Initially, a fracture must be differentiated from a sprain. This may be difficult with the nondisplaced spiral fracture of the fibula. Fibular pain with compression away from the area of trauma or with percussion of the heel often indicates a fracture if there is a specific referral area. Fracture at the base of the fifth metatarsal must be considered. Careful palpation of the anatomic structures generally locates the maximized area of pathology. When a physical examination suggests the need, x-ray films are acquired.

The more severe injury to the anterior talofibular ligament results in anterior

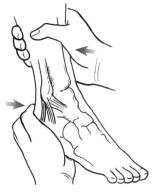

FIGURE 9-7. The anterior drawer sign. To test the stability of ankle ligaments, cup the heal in the palm of one hand and exert interiorly directed pressure while you grasp the ankle with the other hand; this exerts posteriorly directed force. With both hands cupping the ankle, it is also easy to stabilize the foot and ankle and medially and laterally rotate the foot through motion within the ankle mortise. You can palpate the ligamentous areas with your fingers or thumb at the same time and identify abnormal opening of the joint space and tenderness over the talofibular and calcaneofibular ligaments.

instability. This is demonstrated by a positive anterior drawer test (Fig. 9-7). To evaluate laxity of the anterior talofibular ligament, the patient must be relaxed and facing the examiner while seated on the examining room table with the knee flexed over the edge. Forward pressure on the heel, coupled with counter-pressure on the tibia will produce anterior lateral dimpling at the ankle and a tactile appreciation of forward motion of the foot. As the examiner grasps the patient's heel in one hand and manipulates it into inversion, there is a sense of instability or "opening" of one joint compared with the other. Ligamentous structures have a tactile end point. The talus is controlled, and the recoil slap of the unstable ankle is not appreciated when stable. Gross laxity of inversion indicates tears of both the calcaneofibular ligament and the anterior talofibular ligaments. Stress films may be obtained for documentation. They are not reliable in the acute phase unless performed under local anesthesia by the primary care provider.

The economics of medicine have forced attention on this common injury. First, the logic of the use of x-rays as a means of diagnosis by exclusion has been challenged. It is suggested that by the subjective complaints, localization of the physical findings coupled with the specificity of ligament tenderness and the findings associated with this anatomic area, there can be a 28% reduction in x-rays without missing a fracture. If examination is delayed 4 or more days, assessment between grade II and grade III injuries will be more accurate.

The Ottawa ankle rules state that if the patient has no tenderness from the tip to some 6 cm above in the posterior fibula, no tenderness from the tip 6 cm up the posterior with a history of the capacity of immediate weight bearing and walking and, certainly, this is demonstrable in the Emergency Room, the patient does not have a fracture of the ankle and does not require x-rays of the ankle. Further, if there is no medial or lateral tenderness about the navicular and base of the fifth metatarsal, x-rays of the foot are probably not needed.

One always suspects an injury to the deltoid ligament with any fracture of the fibula or any pronation mechanism of injury. Stress testing can be diagnostic by revealing widening of the medial joint space on x-ray (Fig. 9-8). Avulsion at the very tip of the lateral malleolus is diagnostic of injury to the lateral collateral ligaments. Osteochondral fractures of the dome of the talus may accompany any injury resulting in instability. Anteroposterior x-rays with the foot in equinus (ankle joint plantar flexed) and oblique views may be helpful to show this lesion. Although

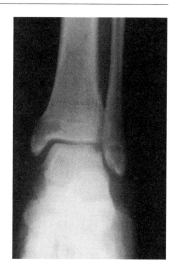

FIGURE 9-8. Widening of ankle mortise.

arthrograms of the ankle are interesting, they offer little information that impacts on treatment and prognosis. With classification based on evaluation of stability, treatment is directed toward protective support and early rehabilitation. Magnetic resonance imaging (MRI) is useful in the diagnostic evaluation of subtle articular lesion of the talus after injury. MRI is indicated in the "ankle sprain" that does not get better.

The skeletally immature person may have a different response to more severe lateral ankle sprain. The response may be the development of an ununited osteochondral fragment at the distal fibular ligament epiphyseal attachment area. Surgery for instability, in the face of failure of conservative care, is indicated.

Ankle pain in the child is a different problem. The history of trauma and its specifics may be absent. The history, on the other hand, is more detailed with an appreciation of developmental milestones, systemic or significant past medical history. Physical diagnosis includes an evaluation of the physes about the ankle as well as the calcaneal apophysis. Tarsal coalitions may become symptomatic in the child. The inflamed joint may lead to a septic arthritis. Juvenile rheumatoid arthritis, hemophilia and sickle-cell disease, as well as neurologic problems, may appear at this age. Problems such as tarsal tunnel syndrome accompanying tarsal coalitions enter into consideration.

TREATMENT. Treatment is directed toward protective support and early rehabilitation. A review of the literature suggests that, in grade I and II sprains, conservative treatment produces satisfactory results within approximately 3 weeks. The functional treatment is triphasic: (1) immediate rest, ice, cold, compression and elevation with early symptomatic-directed and ancillary-supported weight bearing and ambulation; (2) with improved symptomatology (3+ days), supportive immobilization and protection (taping, bracing, and so forth), and (3) early (10 to 21 days) active range of motion, proprioceptive training and muscle strength (emphasis on the peroneals).

The treatment of the unstable or grade III sprain of the lateral collateral ligament is still controversial. The choices are (1) short-leg plaster for 3 to 6 weeks, (2) non-cast bracing, and (3) surgical repair. Surgery is indicated in displaced interarticular fractures involving the weight-bearing surface of the joint. It may be considered in the unstable ankle joint in young, competitive athletes. There are also many people who work on extremely unstable surfaces and for whom surgery may be considered. In the very unstable ankle, where there is rupture of the anterior talofibular and calcaneofibular ligaments, the conservative versus open repair controversy continues without an absolute position established. In addition to the interarticular fractures, ankle luxation may be accompanied by peroneal tendon dislocations; this may prompt the consideration for surgery. A combination of surgical repair and cast bracing may speed the process of rehabilitation.

REHABILITATION. Rehabilitation in ankle sprains begins at the onset of treatment. Strengthening of the medial and lateral stabilizers of the ankle may begin as soon as a pain-free exercise program is made possible. Although there are arguments about full weight bearing before the pain has cleared, there are very definite benefits to progressive partial weight bearing. Exercises for dorsiflexion, plantar flexion, inversion, and eversion involve the four major muscle groups of the lower leg.

Walking is followed by jogging, running, figures of eight, and other exercises to re-establish neuromuscular integration disturbed by the injury. External support such as taping or a proprietary brace is extremely useful when a person with a second- or third-degree sprain returns to running.

Regaining proprioception should be emphasized, and this is done on tilt boards and similar apparatus. This not only aids in neuromuscular recovery but improves the subtalar motion. The rehabilitation after fractures is similar to that of sprains but is prolonged because of the injury and the required immobilization.

Subtalar Joint Sprain

Often overlooked in the ankle sprain is the frequent concomitant sprain of the subtalar joint. It is not unusual after conservative treatment of sprains in a plaster cast that the subtalar joint motion is markedly restricted. This may become a chronic problem. An "ankle sprain" that continues to be disabling beyond 6 weeks of rehabilitation should be evaluated for involvement of the subtalar joint. The joint is painful on testing of the motion. The pathology can be defined by computed tomography (CT) scan as well as a bone scan. It may not be defined with conventional x-ray. The subtalar ligamentous injuries are productive of the sinus tarsi syndrome.

The persistently painful post-sprained ankle pattern varies with the underlying disorder. There may be complaints of diffuse pain, instability, difficulty on uneven ground, swelling, stiffness and occasional locking and crepitation. The patient has a history of contemporary therapeutic failure. Physical examination may variously indicate restriction in dorsiflexion, diffuse swelling of the joint, syndesmosis tenderness, calf atrophy, skin changes, glossiness and edema suggestive of reflex dystrophy. The differential will include incomplete rehabilitation, chronic instability, subtalar sprain, fracture or instability, syndesmosis injury, fibular synostosis, medial instability, sinus tarsi syndrome, osteochondral lesions of the talus, osteochondral loose bodies and impingements (bone and soft tissue). Premature narrowing of the possibilities should be avoided.

Repetitive sprains and chronic stress can work their inroads about the ankle. Posteromedially, the differential diagnosis includes a posterior deltoid spine, osteochondritis of the talus, soleus syndrome, posterior tibial tendinitis, and posterior tarsal coalitions.

With posterolateral complaints, the differential diagnosis includes posterior impingements, fractures of the trigonal process, Achilles tendinitis, peroneal tendinitis or luxation, retrocalcaneal bursa, and pseudomeniscal syndromes.

Anterolateral considerations invoke instability patterns, osteochondral debris, pseudomeniscal syndromes with residuals of anterior tibiofibular tear, anterior osseous impacts, and sinus tarsi and subtalar instabilities. Most of these considerations are the residuals of trauma but can be certainly due to specific overuse syndromes.

Fractures

Fractures of the ankle are clinically quite different from sprains in that they will require cast immobilization and may require surgical stabilization. Rehabilitation is more difficult and prolonged due to the severity of the injury, and there is evident muscle atrophy that results from immobilization. Rigid internal fixation of these fractures may reduce the rehabilitation time and lead to a faster recovery. Presuming anatomic reduction, the ultimate prognosis in ankle fractures is related to the damage to the articular surface, which may not be evident for some period of time after the injury.

Osteochondral lesions of the ankle usually involve the superior surface of the talus, either medially or laterally, and may occasionally involve the inner surface of the fibula. Surgical removal of the bone and cartilage fragments is usually necessary to effect cure. These stress residuals may be missed if oblique views are not obtained on x-ray examination of the injured ankle. Tomograms and CT scans may prove useful in defining the condition, as well as extent and placement (Fig. 9-9). Arthroscopic techniques may be employed to treat these very specific fractures of the joint surface.

The overall principles of management of ankle fractures are concerned with the stability of the ankle joint and maintenance of the mortise. Internal fixation with screws and plates and repair of ruptured ligaments are frequently indicated to restore the integrity of the joint.

Peroneal Tendon Dislocation

These primary lateral stabilizers are the ankle's protection against an inversion injury. Injury results when the individual's foot is fixed in a position of maximal dorsiflexion, such as occurs in cross-country skiing, downhill skiing, and wrestling. Patients complain of a sudden giving-way sensation. Physical examination reveals swelling and tenderness behind the lateral malleolus that extends proximally over the peroneal tendon. Active manipulation will dislocate the tendon when the ankle is dorsiflexed. With dislocation of the peroneal tendon, there is a strong possibility of recurrence. Therefore, it is best treated initially by repair of the retinaculum, despite the fact that such treatment may lengthen the recovery phase.

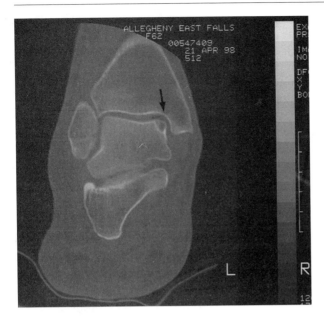

FIGURE 9-9. CT scan: Osteo-chondritis dissecans of the talus.

The Foot

Anatomy

The skeleton of the foot is composed of 26 bones, and there are as many sesamoids. The inferior surface of the talus articulates with the calcaneus, making up the subtalar joint that contributes greatly to inversion and eversion movement of the hindfoot. It may be thought of as the inferior ankle joint. The combination movement of these three articulations, talocalcaneal, talonavicular, and calcaneocuboid, results in the complex foot movement of eversion and inversion, pronation and supination. The midtarsal joints, navicular cuneiform, and cuneiform metatarsals are very stable and produce very little movement. The bone configuration conceptually is that of a stable Roman arch. Metatarsals and proximal phalanges make up the metatarsophalangeal (MP) joints. They are important for push off, particularly at the first MP joint. The individual bones are mortised together to form two arches, the longitudinal arch and the transverse arch. The ligaments of the foot and bone configuration provide intrinsic support, and the muscles provide extrinsic support (Fig. 9-10). The longitudinal arch starts at the weight-bearing surface of the calcaneus and ends at the metatarsal heads. It is supported intrinsically by the spring ligament. This ligament supports the head of the talus. The arch is also supported by the plantar fascia that runs from the calcaneal tuberosity to the proximal phalanges. The plantar fascia acts as a bowstring for the longitudinal arch and supports the muscles of the plantar surface of the foot. The extrinsic support for the medial arch comes from the anterior tibial tendon pulling on its insertion on the first cuneiform and the posterior tibial tendon and peroneus longus tendon that pass under the foot and create a dynamic sling supporting the longitudinal arch.

The three main muscle groups of the lower leg all insert on the foot and thus control the action of the foot. The deep portions of the posterior compartment contain the posterior tibial, flexor digitorum longus, and flexor hallucis longus. The

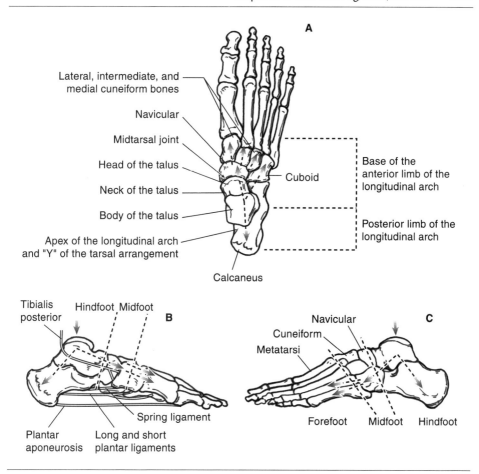

Lateral, intermediate, and medial cuneiform bones
Navicular
Midtarsal joint
Head of the talus
Neck of the talus
Body of the talus
Apex of the longitudinal arch and "Y" of the tarsal arrangement

Cuboid

Base of the anterior limb of the longitudinal arch

Posterior limb of the longitudinal arch

Calcaneus

Tibialis posterior   Hindfoot Midfoot   B

Plantar aponeurosis   Long and short plantar ligaments   Spring ligament

Navicular   C
Cuneiform
Metatarsi

Forefoot   Midfoot   Hindfoot

FIGURE 9-10. The tarsal bones and the dispersion of weight throughout the foot. (**A**) Superior view. (**B**) Medial view. (**C**) Lateral view.

posterior tibial muscle supports the longitudinal arch and inverts the foot. The flexor digitorum longus flexes the lateral four toes, and the flexor hallucis longus flexes the great toe. These three muscles enter the foot through a ligamentous tunnel behind the medial malleolus along with the posterior tibial nerve, the artery, and the vein.

The posterior tibial nerve divides into the medial and lateral plantar nerve and supplies sensation to the plantar surface of the foot while innervating the plantar muscles.

The lateral compartment is composed of two muscles, the peroneus longus and brevis. The longus crosses under the longitudinal arch from lateral to medial and inserts on the plantar surface of the first cuneiform and first metatarsal. The peroneus brevis inserts on the base of the fifth metatarsal. These muscles evert and plantar flex the foot.

The anterior compartment consists of the anterior tibial that inserts on the medial cuneiform, the extensor digitorum longus, and the extensor hallucis longus. This group dorsiflexes the foot and toes. The anterior tibial and extensor hallucis longus muscles are invertors, and extensor digitorum longus is an evertor. The intrinsic muscles of the foot are primarily related to toe function.

The plantar nerves are subjected to entrapment neuropathy as they turn around the medial edge of the foot to enter the plantar region. The posterior tibial nerve passes behind the medial malleolus where it is covered by the lanciniate ligament. This configuration has been called the tarsal tunnel. Near the tunnel, the posterior tibial nerve splits into the medial plantar, lateral plantar, and calcaneal nerves. Some of the calcaneal branches innervate the skin of the heel and pierce the ligament, but some pass completely through the tunnel. This latter group is made up of nerves that innervate the inferior aspect of the calcaneus. The medial plantar nerve carries sensation from the medial side of the sole in front of the heel and from the plantar surface of the three and one half medial toes. The nerve innervates muscles whose chief action is plantar flexion motion of the toes, particularly at the MP joint of the first toe. The flexor brevis and the abductor hallucis are very important in providing the necessary stability of the first toe phalanges for a final push-off in walking. The lateral plantar nerve carries sensation from the lateral side of the sole past the heel and from the plantar surface of the lateral one and one half toe. Motor action of this nerve helps maintain the functional conformity of the foot-innervating muscles that cause flexion at the lateral MP joints and adduction and abduction of the toes.

Entrapment of these elements may produce heel pain, or medial and lateral plantar burning pain, numbness, and changes in sweat patterns of the plantar foot. The diagnosis may be aided or established by nerve conduction and EMG studies or ninhydrin-defined sweat patterns. It has been demonstrated that forcing a foot into an overpronated position will stress the posterior tibial nerve against the fibrous-edged opening in the abductor hallucis muscle. One may suspect the involvement of the nerves in acute foot strain that presents with marked tenderness at the posteromedial plantar aspect of the foot. Although usually described as a sprained ligament, it may be due to plantar nerve trunk sensitivity. The painful heel, additionally, may be caused by involvement of the calcaneal nerves as they innervate the common origin of the muscles and fascia at the anteroinferior surface of the calcaneus.

The deep peroneal nerve is subject to an entrapment neuropathy in its terminal portions on the dorsum of the foot. Traumatic involvement of the nerve or one of its branches is a frequently unrecognized complication of a direct blow to the dorsum of the foot. As the deep peroneal nerve approaches the foot, it passes deep to the inferior extensor retinaculum. This has been designated as the anterior tarsal tunnel. In the lower portion, the nerve divides into medial and lateral branches. The lateral branch innervates the digitorum brevi. The medial branch continues on the bone plane down the dorsum of the foot to reach the junctions of the first and second metatarsal. At this point, it passes immediately under the tendon of the extensor hallucis brevis and then pierces the deep fascia to reach its final innervation of the skin of the cleft between the first and second toes.

Physical Examination

Physical examination should include complete evaluation of the lower extremity. Flat feet (or the pronated foot) is a condition in which the longitudinal arch is flattened. The hindfoot may be in valgus; this should be observed from the rear with the patient standing (Fig. 9-11). Occasionally, there is an associated accessory navicular bone. The navicular tuberosity fails to fuse to the main bone and remains as a bony prominence on the medial side of the foot. This is often locally painful (Fig. 9-12).

Flat feet are classified as flexible or rigid. The flexible flat foot (pronated foot) is the most common and is usually asymptomatic. Moderate to severe deformity may be symptomatic. Proper attention to footwear and longitudinal arch supports are helpful. The rigid flat foot is a much more difficult problem and may prohibit such activities as long, continued running. Rigid flat foot or a peroneal spastic flat foot is often due to congenital tarsal coalition, although symptoms may be delayed until adolescence or later.

Congenital deformity such as metatarsus varus or valgus may be present. Metatarsus varus (adductus) is a deformity of the forefoot in which the forefoot is angulated and rotated medially in relation to the hindfoot. Metatarsus valgus (abductus) is the opposite deformity of the forefoot. With extensive use, these deformities may place abnormal stress on the foot resulting in painful callosities. Proper footwear and orthoses may prevent problems.

The hindfoot may also be angulated either medially or laterally. Deformities are usually associated with a cavus (varus) angulated medially, or flat foot (valgus) angulated laterally. Deformities of the toes are common. Hallux valgus with or without a bunion is associated with a widened angle between the first and second metatarsals. Clawing of the toes is hyperextension of the MP joint and flexion of the interphalangeal (IP) joint. This usually results from some subtle muscle imbalance of the foot. Painful callosities can develop over the dorsum of the IP joint, as well as under the metatarsal heads. Hammertoe is a flexion deformity of the distal IP joint that puts pressure on the nail and end of the toe with contact against the sole of the shoe.

Common Problems of the Foot

Blisters

Friction produces blisters; moisture increases this effect. In sports, the premonitory sign of a blister on the sole of the foot is the appearance of redness and tenderness. If this is treated promptly with application of ice and covering with adhesive tape, the formation of the blister is prevented. Once the blister has formed on the foot, premature removal of the roof only prolongs pain and disability. One may aspirate and preserve the roof by taping. The aspiration should be performed with a fine-gauge needle through intact skin beyond the blistered area. If a blister ruptures spontaneously, the space between the roof and skin has been contaminated, and care must be exercised not to seal infection within or below the blistered skin. There should be a fairly wide area of excision. The prevention of blisters depends on minimizing the unfavorable effects of friction. Instruct the patient on the importance of properly fitting shoes and socks that fit properly, stay up and avoid wrinkles, the use of insoles, shoes that do not bind to the foot with rotary movements, and consideration of lubrication of the sole before use.

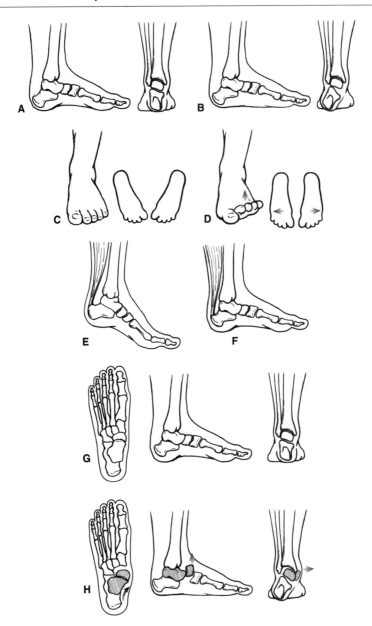

FIGURE 9-11. Pronated foot. (**A** and **B**) Hypermobile flatfoot. (**A**) Non-weightbearing. (**B**) Weight-bearing. (**C** and **D**) Correction of internal tibial torsion by intentional pronation. (**C**) Pigeon-toed stance of internal tibial torsion. (**D**) Straight stance at expense of pronation. (**E** and **F**) Adaptation to short heel cord by intentional pronation. (**E**) Non-weight-bearing. (**F**) Weightbearing. (**G** and **H**) A form of rigid flatfoot. The talus is angulated medially and plantarward. The navicular is dislocated and lies dorsal to the head of the talus. (**G**) Normal. (**H**) The rigid flatfoot.

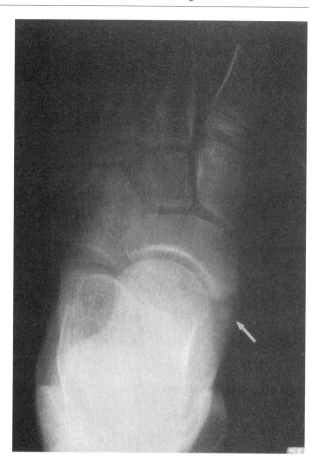

FIGURE 9-12. Accessory navicular. Note the appearance of sesamoid bone within the posterior tibial tendon.

Plantar Wart

The ubiquitous wart virus produces painful lesions on the weight-bearing surface of the foot. It must be distinguished from a foreign body and a pressure-induced corn. The surfaces may appear the same. With paring of the thickened corneum, a wart is defined by capillaries in its papillomatous surface. Ablation without a scar is the goal of treatment: chemical versus curettage.

Malignant Skin Lesions

The leg and foot are uncommon areas for malignant growth. Although uncommon compared to melanomas elsewhere in the body, malignant melanoma constitutes about 3% of all melanomas and is actually the most common malignancy of the foot. Approximately 25% of all malignant melanomas occur on the lower extremities, usually on the posterior calf, subungually and on the plantar aspect of the foot. They occur significantly more often in women younger than 40 years of age. It is to be noted that there has been an increase in the reports of Kaposi's sarcoma found in the foot related to the incidence of human immunodeficiency virus (HIV) infective states.

Soft Tissue Injuries

A bursa is a potential soft tissue space that may, with inflammation, fill with synovial fluid. External pressure from ill-fitting shoes may cause inflammation or bursitis, which is seen predominantly over the MP joint of the great toe.

The pre-Achilles bursa can suggest tendinitis. The presenting symptom is localized to the soft tissue area immediately anterior to the Achilles tendon. There may be a definitive swelling anterior to the tendon. A bursa, generally related to footwear, may develop between the Achilles tendon and the overlying skin.

A callosity is an area of thickened skin overlying a bony prominence. The presence of a callus usually indicates abnormal pressure between the shoe and the bony projection; this can be noted over the distal medial great toe. The callus can be quite bothersome over the second, third, and fourth metatarsal heads and can often be relieved by padding just proximal to the metatarsal heads. This padding may, in addition, partially correct the toe deformity that, with hyperextension of the MP joint, produces a prominence of the metatarsal head.

Neuropathy

Neuropathy of the interdigital or common digital nerve is a frequent source of foot pain. The classic Morton's neuroma is found between the third and fourth web space. Other interdigital nerves, because of a similarity in anatomic relationship, are subject to the same lesion. There are multiple causes: wearing high-heeled shoes, association with the hallux valgus or bunion formation, fixed hyperextended positions of the MP joint, and positions habitually assumed in the workplace or as a result of injury to the bones of the distal foot. The neuropathy is due to pressure and chronic irritation to the nerve with the production of a neuroma, or a nerve mass that sets in place a cycle that leads to disability. Correction of foot mechanics is sought. A modification of footwear, metatarsal pads with concomitant use of oral anti-inflammatory or injective drugs may be employed. Metacarpophalangeal joint arthritis or synovitis should not confuse the diagnosis.

Compartment Syndromes

Initially defined for the purpose of treating sequestered cavities of infection in the foot, the importance of compartments in the foot is now directed toward the consequences of trauma. Between the front of the calcaneus and the metatarsal heads, there are nine compartments within the foot. Elevated and unresolved inflammatory pressure within these compartments will produce the sequelae of intrinsic muscle and nerve loss, leading to an eventual cavus claw-toe deformity in a disabled foot. With evidence of severe injury to osseous structures or crushing injuries to the foot, attention should be directed to the possibility of compartment destructive pressures within the compartments of the foot. Pressure monitoring with multiple placement and depth changes is needed to secure a diagnosis. Clinically, beyond the subjective complaint of increasing pain, there are no other true indicators. Monitoring is based on an appreciation of the possibility of destructive swelling. If there is evidence of increased pressure, fascial compartment release is recommended.

Anterior Tarsal Syndrome

The clinical symptoms of the anterior tarsal syndromes are chiefly sensory. Numbness and paresthesias occur in the first dorsal web space. There may be aching and tightness about the ankle and dorsum of the foot. The complaints may be relieved by posturing of the foot. There may be nocturnal paresthesias that awaken the patient. Upon examination, there may be sensory loss in the web space. A Tinel's sign (reproduction of sensory symptoms by tapping with a reflex hammer over the tarsal tunnel) may be defined at the level of the ankle joint just medially to the dorsalis pedis. The extensor digitorum may be atrophic. Distal motor latency of the peroneal nerve to the extensor digitorum muscle may be useful in diagnosis.

If conservative treatment consisting of rest, night splints, and steroidal injections is unsuccessful, surgical release may be necessary.

Pain in the Hindfoot (Fig. 9-13)

Arthritis

Juvenile rheumatoid arthritis may present as a monoarticular arthritis usually seen in the lower extremity, rather than in the upper extremity. The most common site is the ankle and knee; it may occasionally arise in the subtalar joint. The painful, swollen ankle or subtalar joint in a juvenile carries a high index of suspicion for rheumatoid arthritis, especially in the absence of a history of trauma or infection. The differential diagnosis includes a screening for gonorrhea.

Flexor Hallucis Tenosynovitis

The posterior portion of the fiberosseous tunnel in which the flexor hallucis tendon passes can give rise to symptoms secondary to a stenosing vaginitis. Although most frequently found in ballet dancers, it is found definitively in less stressed feet and generally responds to conservative care.

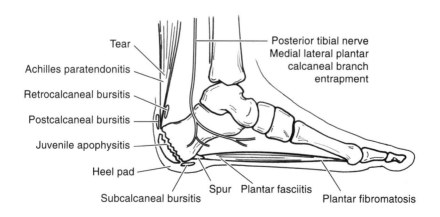

FIGURE 9-13. Sites and possible causes of heel pain.

Posterior Tibial Tendon Strain

A strain of the posterior tibial or tenosynovitis of the posterior tibial tendon may give rise to a painful flat foot. The pain may persist with swelling and definite tenderness along the course of the posterior tibial tendon as it passes beneath the medial malleolus.

TREATMENT. A valgus flat foot support or insole coupled with rest and nonsteroidal drugs will generally suffice. The condition may be associated with an accessory tarsal navicular over the medial foot. In the face of local symptoms, padding may be afforded. If the complaints continue, it may be necessary to excise the navicular prominences of the medial foot.

Posterior Tibial Tendon Rupture

The posterior tibial tendon is subject to rupture. It may be concomitant to an "ankle sprain," or it may occur during sports. Because of local swelling, it may be difficult to diagnose. Chronic "tendinitis" with fluid collection may disguise the condition. Complaints of acquired flat foot and chronic medial pain require exact definition of the condition. To aid diagnosis, obtain MRI studies of the soft tissues.

TREATMENT. With rupture, if foot support and conservative measures do not relieve the complaints, reconstruction may be necessary.

Plantar Fasciitis

Plantar fasciitis is an acute or chronic condition that is characterized by plantar heel pain. Runners with cavus feet or people who stand for long periods of time (eg, waitresses) may be particularly vulnerable. The heel is most painful, especially with the first steps after arising in the morning. Runners find that pain is severe as they begin to run. Pain is most severe at the calcaneal tuberosity but may spread along the course of the plantar fascia. Conceptually, it is a "tennis elbow equivalent" that is found anterior to the heel at the point of attachment of the long plantar fascia and the flexor brevis digitorum. The histologic pattern is the same. On physical examination, there is pain with palpation distal to the plantar surface of the heel where the plantar fascia attaches to the calcaneus. The differential includes the inflammatory arthropathies. If bilateral, the suspicion is raised. Apophysitis in the young is another osseous source. Gout may present in the heel. Neuropathy secondary to diabetes or alcohol can present in the heel. There is clinical discord between fascia and nerve as to the source of pain. The first division of the lateral plantar nerve passes just superior to the attachment of the plantar fascia. In addition, the medial calcaneal nerve has been indicted in entrapment or compressive responses.

TREATMENT. Treatment includes the introduction of an anterior heel pad, rest followed by a stretching and flexibility program. Ionotophoresis or phonophoresis with dexamethasone gel may be used as a adjunct. On occasions, injection of cortisone is necessary. Surgical release is rarely indicated.

Stress Fracture

Stress fracture of the calcaneus in adults occurs at any age and often accounts for a chronic painful heel. The calcaneus has the longest latency period in developing radiologic change. A bone scan will be positive long before the subtle radiologic change. Correct differential diagnosis avoids the overenthusiastic diagnosis of plantar fasciitis (calcaneal spur). Plantar fasciitis is sharply localized to the anterior heel. The stress fracture is much more diffuse about the heel. Heel compression is painful, and inflammation to the mediolateral leg may be present. Gout must be excluded. The treatment is reduced activity and stress-relieving pads or heel cups.

Sever's Disease

Calcaneal apophysitis, or Sever's disease, is thought to be a strain of the attachment of the tendo Achillis at the apophysis of the calcaneus or an equivalent of Osgood-Schlatter disease of the tibial tubercle. The lateral foot x-ray may demonstrate increased density of fragmentation of the apophysis. This is found on film, as opposed to the symptoms, and is almost always bilateral. There is local tenderness over the apophysis, and the patient demonstrates a limp and complains of pain with running. The condition resolves spontaneously over 3 to 6 months. Frequently, simple rest from activity will promptly reduce the symptoms, and an elevated heel pad may be useful. Occasionally, in the severe case, a short-leg walking plaster cast may be required for 3 to 6 weeks.

Pain in the Forefoot

Hallux Rigidus

Painful hallux rigidus occurs in the young and may be difficult to treat. It follows stubbing of the big toe. X-rays may show a change that suggests osteochondritis of the first metatarsal head with subsequent changes that progress to degenerative arthritis with a narrow joint line and peripheral osteophytes.

This condition is a limitation of dorsiflexion of the MP joint of the big toe. Subsequent flattening of the head and osteophyte formation produce a typical "squared-off" appearance of the metatarsal head. Repeat trauma may be the cause. Restricted motion of the fiberosseous canal of the flexor hallucis can produce this clinical finding. The flexor hallucis tendon fixed by inflammation in its sheath can produce a hallux rigidus. Treatment is directed to the tendon, not the joint.

Chronic hallux rigidus may be due to gout or rheumatoid arthritis. X-rays may reveal an erosive process at the articular margin as opposed to hypertrophy, as well as osteoporosis and joint line narrowing.

TREATMENT. Treatment consists of modification of the shoes with a rocker sole. Injections may be used but have no lasting effect. With continued disability, surgery is recommended.

Anterior Flat Foot

Diffuse callosities of the midfoot or the so-called anterior flat foot is an acquired disorder found in the obese, middle-aged person whose occupation requires standing.

TREATMENT. Treatment consists of foot supports with stress-absorbing material in the shoes, as well as soles, and exercises for the foot.

Hallux Valgus (Bunions)

Hallux valgus does occasionally develop in children and adolescents. Although 90% of the cases that come to surgery are female, the overall incidence is approximately equal for males and females. The discrepancy is probably a result of the difference in men's and women's footwear. The condition may present during adolescence from the age of 12 on, or may present at any age during adult life. Congenital hallux valgus is rare. In the adult, hallux valgus or a bunion is confused in the relevant literature. The condition may be defined by the inclusion of the following conditions: (1) rotation of the hallux, (2) metatarsus primus varus. (3) overriding of the hallux on the second toe, (4) metatarsalgia, and (5) hammer- and clawtoe deformities of the lateral toes.

The condition has multiple origins. They may be (1) hereditary, (2) secondary to metatarsus primus varus, (3) a muscular imbalance, (4) foot pronation, and (5) shoewear.

In hallux valgus, the condition is bilateral with a dominant symptomatic side. A family history is present in approximately 60% of cases. Conservative care may produce some relief or may control symptoms once they occur. The "surgical shoe" has a place, more particularly in the rheumatoid form. When all conservative measures fail, surgery becomes necessary for pain relief.

Osteochondritis

Osteochondritis of the second metatarsal (Freiberg's disease), but not limited to the second metatarsal bone, is probably an infraction of the metatarsal head. It generally occurs after 13 years of age and is more common in girls than boys. Symptoms may be treated by a metatarsal bar and inner pad; in adults, surgery may be necessary.

Stress Fractures

There is a gradual onset of pain and swelling in the foot that is aggravated by activity and relieved by rest. On palpation, a definite swelling in the dorsum of the foot may be felt. One can detect this swelling along a specific metatarsal shaft. This is particularly evident in the older person and the fracture presents with very distinct swelling, redness, and heat. It is known as a "march fracture" in military recruits. It will occur when the baseline bone activity is exceeded by imposed mechanical stress.

TREATMENT. Conservative treatment is a reduction in the general level of activity. Referral to an orthopedic surgeon may be necessary for casting. Extreme care is taken in attempting to cast the elderly osteoporotic foot, because a stress fracture, with beginning ambulation, may evolve in the contiguous metatarsals secondary to disuse osteoporosis.

Morton's Metatarsalgia (Morton's Toe)

Morton's metatarsalgia can be found from the ages of 17 to 70. The patient is usually a young or middle-aged woman. Acute neuralgic pain is felt under the middle of the forefoot, with radiation into one or more of the three central toes. In "Morton's toe," the pain is referred to the fourth toe. Pain develops with standing or walking in closed, tight-fitting footwear. The patient often takes off the shoe and manipulates the forefoot, prompting a relief of the pain. Pain is produced on physical examination by pressure upward and backward in the web space. The forefoot is alternately compressed with one hand while maintaining the pressure in the web space. If symptoms are relieved by local anesthetic injections, this is diagnostic of the condition.

Minor symptoms may be controlled by the low-heeled, open type of footwear. Occasionally, hydrocortisone injection may afford relief. When the symptoms are disabling, the treatment is surgical excision of the interdigital nerve.

Fractures of the Forefoot

Fracture-dislocations of the forefoot are probably underreported. The football interior linemen are subjected to entrapment damage to the transmetatarsal joints as well as the metatarsal shafts. The foot and toes are subject to the impact of falling objects. Because of the peroneal muscle attachment and ankle sprain patterns as well as its blood supply, the fifth metatarsal has become anatomically specific. The inability to bear weight and anatomic-specific indicators lead to confirming x-rays. Because of the confusing x-ray anatomy, oblique views as well as comparison views may be needed for definition. The goal of treatment is a stable, plantigrade, painless foot.

Sympathetic Dystrophy

As a consequence of trauma and disuse, the early "normal," nonmalignant manifestations of Sudeck's atrophy of bone will occur in the leg and foot. This condition will clear with use. Sympathetic dystrophy does occur in the lower extremity and foot. Nonsubsiding pain, intolerance to cold, and trophic changes coupled with delay in physical rehabilitation suggest the entity. Early diagnosis lessens the chance of chronicity. Treatment is trifold: sympathetic nerve blocks, drugs, and physical therapy. Care must be taken to avoid addiction.

The Diabetic Foot

The unfocused, medically transmitted anxiety surrounding the diabetic foot is changing. The tentative, minimal and intermittent conservative treatment is starting to bend in the hands of skilled interdisciplinary teams. The early identification of the diabetic condition may occur with a good physical examination of the lower extremity. Foot care starts then. The early use of a running shoe may prevent ulceration.

Subsequent progress in diabetic foot disease requires an early aggressive rather than a late response. Correction of mechanical problems in the neurotrophic foot prevents the development of deformities, secondary pressure points, and shoe-fitting problems. All wound care should be aggressive. The septic joint should be recognized early and ablated when identified. Preservation of a noninfected ambulatory extremity is the purpose of treatment.

References

Baxter, D. E., & Zingas, C. (1995). The foot in running. *Journal of the American Academy of Orthopedic Surgeons, 3,* 136.

Bennell, K. L, Malcom, S. A., Thomas, S. A., Ebeling, P. R., McCrory, P. R., Wark, J. D., & Brukner, P. D. (1995). Risk factors for stress fractures in female track-and-field athletes: a retrospective analysis. *Clinical Journal of Sports Medicine, 5*(4), 229.

Botte, M. J., Santi, M. P., Prestianni, C. A., & Reid, H. A. (1996). Ischemic contracture of the foot and ankle: principles of management and prevention. *Orthopaedics, 19,* 235.

Buckwalter, J. A., Glimcher, M. J., Cooper, R. R., & Recker, R. (1995). Bone biology: I and II. *Journal of Bone and Joint Surgery, 77A,* 1256.

Busconi, B. D., & Pappas, A. M. (1996). Chronic painful ankle instability in skeletally immature athletes. *American Journal of Sports Medicine, 24,* 647.

Churchill, J. A., & Mazur, J. M. (1995). Ankle pain in children: diagnostic evaluation and clinical decision making. *Journal of the American Academy of Orthopedic Surgeons, 3,* 183.

Climino, W. R. (1990). Tarsal tunnel syndrome: review of the literature. *Foot and Ankle, 11*(1), 47.

Dameron, T. B. (1995). Fractures of the proximal 5th metatarsal: selecting the best treatment options. *Journal of the American Academy of Orthopedic Surgeons, 3,* 110.

Dawson, D. M., Hallett, M., & Millender, L. H. (1983). *Entrapment neuropathies.* Boston: Little, Brown.

Frost, H. M. (1980). Skeletal physiology and bone remodeling. In Urist, M. R. (Ed.). *Fundamental and clinical bone physiology.* Philadelphia: J. B. Lippincott, pp. 208–241.

Gill, L. H. (1997). Plantar fasciitis: diagnosis and conservative management. *Journal of the American Academy of Orthopedic Surgeons, 5,* 109.

Gulli, B., & Templeman, D. (1994). Compartment syndrome of the lower extremity. *Orthopaedic Clinics of North America, 25*(4), 677.

Hamilton, W. G., Geppert, M. J., & Thompson, F. M. (1996). Pain in the posterior aspect of the ankle in dancers. *Journal of Bone and Joint Surgery, 78A,* 1491.

Hoppenfeld, S., Hutton, R., & Thomas, H. (1976). *Physical examination of the spine and extremities.* New York: Appleton-Century-Crofts.

Johnson, L. C. (1964). Arthrologic analysis in pathology: the kinetic of disease and general biology of bone. In Frost, H. M. (Ed.). *Bone biodynamics.* Boston: Little, Brown.

Jones, D. C., & James, S. L. (1987). Overuse injuries of the lower extremity: shin splints, iliotibial band friction syndrome, and exertional compartment syndromes. *Clinical Sports Medicine, 6*(2), 273.

Kuwada, G. T. (1995). Diagnosis and treatment of Achilles tendon. *Clinics in Podiatric Medicine and Surgery, 12*(4), 633.

Lindenfeld, T. N., Bach, B. R., & Wojtys, E. M. (1996). Reflex sympathetic dystrophy and pain dysfunction in the lower extremity. *Journal of Bone and Joint Surgery, 78A,* 1936.

Marcus, R. E., Goodfellow, D. B., & Pfister, M. E. (1995). The difficult diagnosis of posterior tibial rupture in sports injuries. *Orthopaedics, 18,* 715.

Mason, R. B., & Henderson, I. S. P. (1996). Traumatic peroneal tendon instability. *American Journal of Sports Medicine, 24,* 652.

Meyer, S. A., Saltzman. C. L., & Albright, J. P. (1993). Stress fractures of the foot and leg. *Clinical Sports Medicine, 12*(2), 395.

Mosca, V. S. (1995). Flexible flat foot. *Journal of Bone and Joint Surgery, 77A,* 1937.

Omura, E. F. (1988). Dermatological disorders. In Gould, J. S. (Ed.). *The foot book.* Baltimore: Williams & Wilkins, pp. 70–88.

Perry, J. E., Ulbrecht, J. S., Derr, J. A., & Cavanagh, P. R. (1995). The use of running shoes to reduce plantar pressures in patients who have diabetes. *Journal of Bone and Joint Surgery, 77A,* 1819.

Renström, P. A. F. H. (1994). Persistently painful sprained ankle. *Journal of the American Academy of Orthopedic Surgeons, 2,* 270.

Silas, S. I., Herzenberg, J. E., Myerson, M. S., & Sponseller, P. D. (1995). Compartment syndrome of the foot in children. *Journal of Bone and Joint Surgery, 77A,* 356.

Simonian, P. J., Vahey, S. W., Rosenbaum, D. M., Mosca, V. S., & Staheli, L. T. (1995). Fractures of the cuboid in children. *Journal of Bone and Joint Surgery, 77B,* 104.

Soma, C. A., & Mandelbaum, B. R. (1994). Achilles tendon disorders. *Clinical Sports Medicine, 13*(4), 118.

Sommer, H. M., & Vallentyne, S. W. (1995). Effect of foot posture on the incidence of medial tibial stress syndrome. *Medicine and Science in Sports and Exercise, 27,* 800.

Stiehl, I. G., McKnight, R. D., Greenberg, G. H., et al. (1994). Implementation of the Ottawa ankle rules. *Journal of the American Medical Association, 271,* 827.

Stone, J. W. (1996). Osteochondral lesions of the talar dome. *Journal of the American Academy of Orthopedic Surgeons, 4,* 63.

Stuart, J. D., Morgan, R. F., & Persing, J. A. (1989). Nerve compression syndromes of the lower extremity. *American Family Physician, 40*(4), 101.

Thompson, G. H. (1995). Bunions and deformities of the toes in children and adolescents. *Journal of Bone and Joint Surgery, 77A,* 1924.

Van Dijk, C. N., Lun, L. S. L., Bossuyt, P. M. M., & Marti, R. K. (1996). Physical examination is sufficient for the diagnosis of sprained ankles. *Journal of Bone and Joint Surgery, 78B,* 958.

Weinfeld, S. B., & Myerson, M. S. (1996). Interdigital neuritis: diagnosis and treatment. *Journal of the American Academy of Orthopedic Surgeons, 4,* 328.

Whitelaw, G. P., Wetzler, M. J., Levy, A. S., Segal, D., & Bissonette, K. (1991). A pneumatic leg brace for the treatment of tibial stress fractures. *Clinical Orthopaedics, 119,* 301.

Whitesides, T. E., & Heckman, M. M. (1996). Acute compartment syndrome: update on diagnosis and treatment. A comprehensive review. *Journal of the American Academy of Orthopedic Surgeons, 4,* 209-218.

Chapter 10

Arthritis and Rheumatic Diseases

Sally Pullman-Mooar, MD

Arthritis is the most common disabling disease in the United States, costing billions of dollars annually in lost wages and medical bills. The following discussion outlines general principles concerning the approach to a patient with arthritis and associated rheumatologic diseases so the best care plan can be formulated.

The most important step in ensuring the best treatment for the patient's condition is determining the type of arthritis present. There are more than 100 hundred types of arthritis, all associated with different pathogeneses, treatments, and outcomes. A careful history must be obtained to decide whether the problem is mechanical, degenerative or inflammatory. If indications of an inflammatory arthritis or rheumatic disease are found, the appropriate algorithm can then be followed for further diagnosis and treatment. A careful physical examination augments the history; blood work and x-rays are needed more as confirmatory tests.

Anatomy of the Joint

Knowledge of the normal anatomy of the joint is essential for understanding, diagnosing and treating different types of arthritis (Fig. 10-1). The normal joint functions as a hinge mechanism between two adjacent structures. Ideally, there will be very little friction in the joint and very little instability or laxity around the joint so that movement occurs effortlessly and painlessly. The normal diarthrodial joint is lined with smooth cartilage that provides a surface with a low-gliding coefficient of friction. A normally small membrane, called synovium, surrounds the joint cavity and attaches to the rim of bone immediately outside the gliding surface. Healthy articular cartilage is not covered by synovium. Tendons, muscles, and ligaments, which act as the mechanical "pulleys" across a joint that cause movement, also act

288

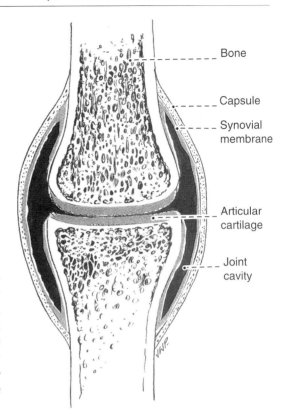

Bone

Capsule

Synovial membrane

Articular cartilage

Joint cavity

FIGURE 10-1. Diagrammatic representation of the anatomic features of a typical synovial joint seen in a section cut across the *middle* of the joint. The extent of the joint cavity is exaggerated to show the anatomic arrangement of the synovial membrane more clearly.

as stabilizing structures. Without these external structures, the joint would have excessive instability, which would cause additional biomechanical stresses to the joint. Any of the structures in and around the joint can become damaged or inflamed, which can lead to joint pain.

Data Gathering

When one approaches a patient with a painful joint, the differential diagnosis needs to be made. The history is extremely important (Tables 10-1 and 10-2). Certain key forces can cause acute or chronic swelling. When gathering information about joint pain, it is important to note many of the historical items listed in Table 10-1. The patient can usually indicate if the problem is acute or chronic, waxing and waning or constant, and whether a general sense of illness or malaise accompanies the pain. Degeneration or osteoarthritic problems and post-traumatic syndromes do not cause a sense of illness. Most of the other rheumatic diseases are accompanied by a host of systemic complaints including but not limited to morning stiffness lasting more than 45 minutes, fatigue and often polyarticular disease.

TABLE 10-1
Interview Guidelines for the Clinical History of Patients With Arthritis

Age at onset

Joints involved

Morning stiffness

Pattern of pain: constant, waxing and waning, migratory, or weight bearing

Family history of arthritis

Family history of associated illness (eg, psoriasis, colitis, iritis, sarcoidosis, gout, hypermobility, osteoporosis)

Associated systemic symptoms such as fever, rash, alopecia, weight loss, fatigue, dyspnea,
depression, sleep disturbance, Raynaud's disease, oral ulcers, photosensitivity, pleurisy,
or seizures

Sexual history

Recent changes in activities of daily living

Recent or remote trauma to affected joints

Recent changes in performance at school (children)

Osteoarthritis

The most common type of arthritis is osteoarthritis (OA), also known as wear-and-tear arthritis or degenerative arthritis. Most people over 65 years of age will have x-ray evidence of this problem, but only about 30% will have significant joint discomfort. The underlying mechanism for OA is a gradual thinning of the articular cartilage lining the joint space that leaves exposed bone in contact with bone. The underlying bone becomes thickened and sclerotic. One frequently sees bony spurs adjacent to the joint. Radiographic changes do not always parallel symptomatic severity and x-rays may markedly underestimate OA particularly in the stage of cartilaginous fibrillation, softening and ulceration. Not all radiographically abnormal joints are symptomatic, but when they are, they are characterized by joint pain, swelling, morning stiffness lasting less than 45 minutes, tenderness, limitation of movement, crepitus, and occasional joint effusion. This type of arthritis is an example of a noninflammatory arthritis that is very different from rheumatoid arthritis (RA). Joint fluids are usually noninflammatory, although commonly there may be an associated crystal disease, such as pseudogout. The involved joints are those subjected to the most mechanical stress: cervical spine, distal interphalangeal joints, lumbar spine, hips, knees and first metacarpophalangeal joints. The pain is described as an aching pain that increases with use and abates with rest. In more advanced stages, discomfort may be present in nonweight-bearing positions. It is currently thought that a family predisposition to OA exists and that several metabolic and endocrinologic disorders such as hemochromatosis and pseudogout are etiologic as well. Previous joint trauma can predispose individuals to accelerated degenerative disease because of cartilaginous injury or malalignment of the joint secondary to ligamentous instability.

Therapy or treatment of OA is aimed at decreasing the work required of a

TABLE 10-2

Assessment History and Physical Examination of the Arthritic Patient

History	
Pain	Most frequent complaint Subjective sensation Location of pain Quality (eg, sharp, radiating, or burning) Radiation Activities that worsen or improve pain
Swelling	Possible anatomic distribution: bursa, joint, or muscle
Stiffness	Duration of stiffness Time of day Differentiate from neurologic diseases, such as Parkinson's
Weakness	Secondary to painful joint Possible disuse atrophy Myopathies: inflammatory, endocrine, or other
Fatigue	Often seen with inflammatory rheumatic diseases
Physical Examination	
Swelling	Location, either intra- or extra-articular in the synovial sac, tendon sheaths, or bursae
Heat	Indicates an inflammatory process
Erythema	Usually indicates a traumatic or inflammatory process
Range of motion	Compare with normal and progression over time
Crepi-tation	Usually indicates loss of smooth gliding cartilaginous surface in joint; sometimes made from tendons slipping
Pain	During active/passive range of motion or with palpation
Instability	Loss of external ligament support or muscle strength
Deformity	Description
Strength	Normal or decreased
Flexibility	Especially important in the lumbar spine examination when considering seronegative spondyloarthropathies

joint in combination with acetaminophen or a nonsteroidal anti-inflammatory drug (NSAID) and a physical therapy program. Patients should be encouraged to lose weight, especially for painful hips, knees, and feet; wear soft-soled shoes to decrease the impact of walking; and avoid high-impact activities such as jogging and aerobics. A structured exercise program is very helpful in maximizing conservative therapy. Isometric quadriceps-strengthening exercises should be encouraged for patients with painful knees; passive and active range-of-motion exercises are also beneficial for all involved areas. Generally speaking, isometric exercises provide the greatest increase in strength without excessive stress on a joint. Swimming and water exercise therapy should be encouraged. In end-stage arthritis, particularly of the knees and hips, reconstructive surgery can provide profound pain relief and improved quality of life.

Rheumatoid Arthritis

RA is the most common inflammatory arthritis, affecting between 1% and 3% of the general population. RA has a predilection for women in their childbearing years. Typically, the disease presents with severe morning stiffness and pain in the small joints of the hands, wrists, and feet lasting more than 45 minutes. It may continue to involve joints not typically involved in OA such as elbows, shoulders, and ankles as well as the cervical spine, hips, and knees. Frequently, the patient feels ill with fatigue, and almost universally has prolonged morning stiffness. Less frequently, RA may have systemic involvement of other organ systems such as the lung, heart, skin, eye, or gastrointestinal (GI) or renal systems. Anemia, an elevated sedimentation rate, and a positive rheumatoid factor (RF) are commonly associated with RA but alone are not diagnostic of the disease. Pathologically, the synovial membrane becomes tremendously thickened and inflamed, which leads to red, hot, swollen, and tender joints and surrounding tendons. Evaluate the patient systematically (Fig. 10-2).

Many of the rheumatic illnesses affect people during the prime of their lives. Therefore, these people deserve special attention concerning adjustments in lifestyle, self-care, employment, and family planning. With the current therapies available, many people are able to live normal, productive lives. Others may need to change their lifestyles and expectations, and those expectations of a spouse or family.

Treatment is aimed at controlling the inflammation and attempting to promote an early remission. Initial therapies are aspirin or NSAIDs combined with joint conservation programs and patient education. An assessment using the Self-Report Questionnaire for Arthritis (Fig. 10-3) can lead to an individualized care plan. Patients with inflammatory arthritis benefit from referral to a rheumatologist who can help make decisions concerning interventions with potentially more toxic drugs. These medications may include sulfasalazine, hydroxychloroquine, prednisone, minocycline, gold (oral or injectable), penicillamine, methotrexate, azathioprine, cytoxan or cyclosporin. Side effects of medications and plans for monitoring drug safety such as surveillance blood counts and liver and kidney profiles need to be carefully discussed with patients. The choice of drug therapy is tailored to the person's pain tolerance and home and work responsibilities. Table 10-3 presents a comparison of OA and RA.

Psoriatic Arthritis

Psoriatic arthritis may resemble RA but has a slightly different joint distribution. Psoriatic arthritis can involve the distal interphalangeal joints of the hands and feet and also cause dactylitis, which can be described as a "sausage digit." The deformities range from mild to severe but, except for spondylitic involvement, rarely have extra-articular manifestations except the skin. Approximately 10% of patients with psoriasis may go on to develop psoriatic arthritis. About 80% of patients with psoriatic arthritis have pitted nails. Treatment is aimed at decreasing inflammation with NSAIDs, occasional use of steroids and methotrexate as the most common immunomodulator that also helps the skin disease.

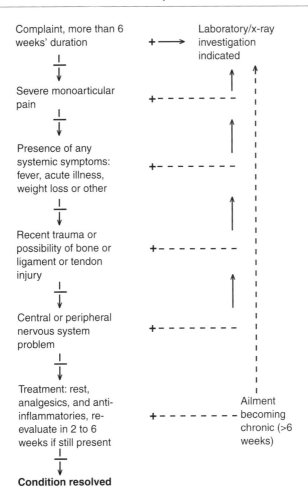

Complaint, more than 6 weeks' duration

Severe monoarticular pain

Presence of any systemic symptoms: fever, acute illness, weight loss or other

Recent trauma or possibility of bone or ligament or tendon injury

Central or peripheral nervous system problem

Treatment: rest, analgesics, and anti-inflammatories, re-evaluate in 2 to 6 weeks if still present

Condition resolved

Laboratory/x-ray investigation indicated

Ailment becoming chronic (>6 weeks)

FIGURE 10-2.   Algorithm for evaluation of the patient with rheumatic complaints. (Adapted from Kelly, W. N., Harris, E., Ruddy, S., & Sledge, C. B. [1985]. *Textbook of rheumatology,* Vol. 1 [2nd ed.]. Philadelphia: W. B. Saunders.

Infectious Arthritis

Infectious arthritis commonly presents as an acutely hot, tender, painful, and swollen joint. There are many different pathogens causing the problem, but the diagnosis needs to be made rapidly so appropriate antibiotic therapy can be instituted and joint destruction averted.

Disseminated Gonorrhea

Disseminated gonorrhea commonly affects women. It often occurs immediately after menses and may be associated with fever, a pustular rash, and tenosynovitis. A sexual history should be obtained from any sexually active person who has a

Please check (√) the ONE best answer for your abilities.

At this moment, are you able to:	Without Any Difficulty	With Some Difficulty	With Much Difficulty	Unable To Do
A. Dress yourself, including tying shoelaces and doing buttons?				
B. Get in and out of bed?				
C. Lift a full cup or glass to your mouth?				
D. Walk outdoors on flat ground?				
E. Wash and dry your entire body?				
F. Bend down to pick up clothing from the floor?				
G. Turn regular faucets (taps) on and off?				
H. Get in and out of a car?				

FIGURE 10-3. Self-report questionnaire for arthritis. (Pincus, T., Callahan, L. F., Brooks, R. H., et al. [1989]. Self-report questionnaire scores in rheumatoid arthritis compared with traditional physical, radiographs, and laboratory measures. *Annals of Internal Medicine, 100,* 259.)

new onset of an arthritis affecting only a few joints. All patients should be screened for other concurrent venereal diseases such as syphilis and *Chlamydia* and have gonorrhea cultures obtained from the urethra, cervix, rectum and pharynx. The joint fluid aspirates are usually sterile. Because of an increasing problem with penicillin-resistant organisms, patients with disseminated gonorrhea are treated with ceftriaxone, 1 g every 24 hours. Spectinomycin is an alternative. Usually improvement is noted within 48 hours. Often, the diagnosis is confirmed when the patient improves with the treatment. All sexual contacts must be notified and treatment promptly begun.

Pyogenic Arthritis

Pyogenic arthritis usually occurs as a monoarticular arthritis, most commonly caused by *Staphylococcus* or *Streptococcus*. Inquiry should be made concerning recent skin infections, dental work, surgery, or trauma. Before antibiotic therapy, joint aspiration must be performed to obtain fluid for culture to better guide prognosis and antibiotic therapy. The cell count is usually greater than 50,000 cells/mm^3 with a majority being polymorphonuclear cells. Serial daily needle aspirations are necessary to assess response to therapy and to decide if surgical drainage is necessary.

TABLE 10-3
Differential Diagnosis

	Osteoarthritis	Rheumatoid Arthritis
Pathology	Cartilage degeneration, bone regeneration (spurs)	Inflammation of synovial membrane Bone destruction Damage to ligaments, tendons, cartilage, joint capsule
Joints affected	Hands, spine, knees, hips, often asymmetric	Symmetric; wrists, PIPs, MCPs, knees, elbows, ankles
Features, symptoms	Localized pain, stiffness Heberden's nodules Usually not much swelling	Swelling, redness, warmth, pain, tenderness, nodules, fatigue, stiffness, muscle aches, fever
Other systems affected	None	Lungs, heart, skin
Prognosis: long-term	Less pain for some; more pain and disability for others Few severely disabled	
Age: onset	Age 45 to 90 Most people have some features with increasing age	Age 25 to 50 Bimodal peaks 3rd to 4th decade to 5th to 6th decade
Sex	Males and females about equal 1 : 1	Females affected more often 2.1 : 1
Heredity	One form is familial	Familial tendency
Tests	X-rays	Rheumatoid factor (80%) Blood test, x-rays, examination of joint fluid, inflammatory fluid without crystals, negative Lyme titer
Treatment	Maintain activity level, exercise, joint protection, weight control, relaxation, heat, sometimes medication and/or surgery	Reduce inflammation, balanced exercise program, joint protection, weight control, relaxation, heat, medication and/or surgery

Lyme Disease

Carried by the deer tick *Ixodes daminii,* Lyme disease is an infection caused by the spirochete *Borrelia burgdorferi.* It initially presents as an acute flulike illness but may also mimic other systemic diseases, such as pericarditis, meningitis, or Bell's palsy. About three fourths of patients will remember a typical erythema chronicum migrans (ECM) rash (an annular rash with central clearing), but only two thirds will remember a tick bite. In endemic areas, a high degree of suspicion should be entertained for Lyme disease in an oligoarticular arthritis. The blood test for Lyme disease will not become positive until 4 to 8 weeks after the exposure.

Lyme disease usually responds well to an initial course of oral antibiotics, either doxycycline 100 mg BID for 21 days, amoxicillin 500 mg QID for 21 days with probenecid or cefuroxime axetil 500 mg BID for 21 days. Some patients need intravenous (IV) therapy, but IV therapy for longer than 4 to 6 weeks is usually not indicated (Table 10-4). Approximately 10% of patients may develop a chronic inflammatory arthritis that affects only a few joints. The diagnosis of Lyme disease is made by a blood test or by history of the classic ECM rash. The arthritis may be responsive to IV or oral antibiotics. Care should be taken to ask any patient

---

TABLE 10-4

Recommendations for Antibiotic Treatment of Lyme Disease

Early Lyme Disease

Amoxicillin, 500 mg three times daily for 21 days

Doxycycline, 100 mg twice daily for 21 days

Cefuroxime axetil, 500 mg twice daily for 21 days

Azithromycin, 500 mg daily for 7 days (less effective than other regimens)

Neurologic Manifestations

Bell's palsy (no other neurologic abnormalities)
    Oral regimens for early disease suffice

Meningitis (with or without radiculoneuropathy or encephalitis)
    Ceftriaxone, 2 g daily for 14−28 days
    Penicillin G, 20 million units daily for 14−28 days
    Doxycycline, 100 mg twice daily (oral or IV) for 14−28 days
    Chloramphenicol, 1 g four times daily for 14−28 days

Arthritis

Amoxicillin and probenecid, 500 mg each, four times daily for 30 days

Doxycycline, 100 mg twice daily for 30 days

Ceftriaxone, 2 g daily for 14−28 days

Penicillin G, 20 million units daily for 14−28 days

Carditis

Ceftriaxone, 2 g daily for 14 days

Penicillin G, 20 million units daily for 14 days

Doxycycline, 100 mg twice daily for 21 days

Amoxicillin, 500 mg three times daily for 21 days

Pregnancy

Localized early disease
    Amoxicillin, 500 mg three times daily for 21 days

Any manifestation of disseminated disease
    Penicillin G, 20 million units daily for 14−28 days

Asymptomatic seropositivity
    No treatment necessary

From Malawista, S. (1996). Lyme disease. In Bennett, J. C., Plum, F. (Eds.). *Cecil's textbook of medicine*. Philadelphia, W. B. Saunders.

with a new inflammatory arthritis about exposure to ticks or whether the characteristic rash of ECM has been noticed. The highest incidence of Lyme disease is in the Northeast, Great Lake states, Pacific Northwest, and Northern California.

Parvo-19 Arthritis

A polyarticular arthritis appearing much like early RA has been recognized recently. Parvovirus, a common virus in the community that causes fifth disease in children, has been reported to cause a polyarticular inflammatory arthritis, often of the small joints of the hands and feet. Symptoms may wax and wane. RF is usually negative, but patients can be very uncomfortable for several months. Early screening with a viral titer can help to identify the IgM response, which can help prove the etiology of the arthritis.

HIV Rheumatic Syndromes

Patients with HIV infection deserve special note because of some unique problems they develop. Because of their deranged immune system, they are at risk for the more common community-acquired septic joint infections such as *Staphylococcus aureus* and streptococcal species and also myobacterial species or other less typical organisms. One also has to have a high index of suspicion with an acute monarthritis, with or without fever, to exclude unusual pathogens such as *Candida albicans.*

These patients have also been found to develop severe debilitating Reiter's syndrome as well as psoriatic arthritis and enthesopathies. Enlargement of the salivary glands can mimic Sjögren's syndrome. Blood tests are hard to interpret because of the high frequency of positive antinuclear antibodies (ANA) and other immunologic tests.

Hypermobility Syndrome (Double Jointed)

Hypermobility syndromes are a common cause of regional rheumatic pain. The features of the benign hypermobility syndrome include: (1) symmetric joint pain and stiffness, (2) sensation of joint swelling, (3) onset after prolonged inactivity, (4) joint laxity in other family members, and (5) no other contributing illnesses. The diagnosis is made when three of the five following features are found on physical examination: (1) passive apposition of thumb to forearm, (2) passive hyperextension of fingers to 90 degrees, (3) active hyperextension of the elbow greater than 10 degrees, (4) active hyperextension of the knee greater than 10 degrees, and (5) ability to flex spine and place palm on floor with knees straight.

The benign hypermobility syndrome responds well to mild anti- inflammatory drugs and strengthening and conditioning exercises. Young athletes need to be cautioned about avoiding aggravating sports. The condition may predispose the person to premature OA. Associated problems can include but are not limited to chondromalacia patella, scoliosis, low back pain, and recurrent tendinitis.

Inherited Disease of Cartilage

Certain systemic diseases have joint hyperlaxity and often are associated with internal organ pathology. Some of these diseases include Marfan's, Ehlers-Danlos syndrome, and osteogenesis imperfecta. Patients with extreme hypermobility, a heart murmur, recurrent fractures, or a family history of sudden death require primary care provider referral.

Seronegative Spondylarthropathies

As a group, these arthropathies are characterized by the absence of RF and other autoantibodies and by the predilection for inflammatory disease in the spine, peripheral joint arthritis, tendinitis with new bone formation, and extra-articular manifestations in the eyes, heart, skin, and mucous membranes. These arthropathies are found predominantly in young adult males. A strong association with the HLA-B27 antigen has been found (Tables 10-5 and 10-6).

TABLE 10-5
Laboratory Investigations for the Rheumatic Disease Patient

Disease	Minimal	Moderate	Extensive
All	CBC Creatinine Urinalysis ESR	Electrolytes Calcium Liver enzymes Albumin	CRP
RA	RF	ANA Synovial fluid WBC	HLA-DR/DW RF isotypes Serum/synovial fluid (ICs and complement) Anti-collagen Synovial biopsy
SLE	ANA Anti-DNA PTT	Anti-cardiolipin Anti-Sm, RNP, Ro, La Anti-histone Complement Coombs' VDRL	HLA-DR/DW ICs Anti-Ku Anti-neuronal
Spondylo- arthropathy		HLA-B27	HLA-B27 isotypes
Myositis	CK, ALT	Aldolase	Anti-Jo-1, RNP
Systemic sclerosis		Anti-SCL70 Anti-centromere	
Gout	Synovial fluid (crystals and WBC)	Serum uric acid	24-h urine uric acid
Vasculitis		ANCA, RF, ICs Complement HbsAg, cryoglobulin	
JRA	ANA	HLA-B27	RF, anti-DNA

From Sibley, J. (1995). Laboratory tests. *Rheumatic Disease Clinics of North America,* 21(2).

TABLE 10-6
Laboratory Tests in Polyarthritis

Test	Significance Positive	Significance Negative
Rheumatoid factor	Helpful in young persons, in whom background positivity is low	Prognostic significance only, not helpful in individual cases
Antinuclear antibody	High titer, suggestive of a rheumatic disease	Virtually rules out active systemic lupus
Uric acid	Elevated levels, indicating that gout is possible	If repeated levels are normal, gout unlikely
Antistreptolysin O	Recent streptococcal exposure	Rheumatic fever unlikely
HLA-B27	Possibly marginally useful in early-onset ankylosing spondylitis	No benefit
Anti-*Borrelia*	Only helpful if pretest probability is high	Chronic Lyme disease unlikely

From Sergent, J. S. (1997). Approach to the patient with more than one joint. In Kelley, W. N., et al. (Eds.). *Textbook of rheumatology.* Philadelphia, W. B. Saunders.

Ankylosing Spondylitis

Ankylosing spondylitis is a chronic inflammatory axial arthritis with a ratio of 3:1 male/female and an incidence of 0.1% to 0.2% in white men. Clinically, an indolent history of lower back stiffness (usually upon arising in the morning or when a static posture is maintained) is found to improve with activity. Physical examination findings may consist of lumbar spine rigidity in forward flexion, a decreased chest expansion, and pain on side-to-side compression of the pelvis. More than 90% of patients have a positive HLA-B27 marker. Fuzziness of the sacroiliac (SI) joints is a classic x-ray finding, which can be seen on anteroposterior views of the spine and SI joint. A minority of people may get cardiac, eye, or pulmonary diseases. Treatment consists of anti-inflammatories, sometimes tetracycline and disease-modifying agents, and hyperextension exercises for the neck and thoracic spine. The treatment goal, in addition to pain relief, is to prevent flexion contractures of the cervical and thoracic spine. Patients are advised to sleep without a pillow to prevent kyphosis.

Reiter's Syndrome/Reactive Arthritis

Reiter's syndrome is the presence of the clinical triad of urethritis, conjunctivitis, and an inflammatory arthritis. It may follow genitourinary infections (such as *Chlamydia*) or be associated with a diarrheal illness (also known as reactive arthritis). Rashes on the feet, fever, oral ulcers, and penile ulcers may occur. Sacroiliitis tends to be asymmetric. HLA-B27 may be positive in up to 75% of patients. Reiter's syndrome may be the most common cause of inflammatory arthritis in young men. The most common infections associated with reactive arthritis are *Chlamydia, Yer-*

sinia, Campylobacter, Salmonella, Shigella, Streptococcus, Staphylococcus, and possibly gonorrhea.

Arthritis Associated With Inflammatory Bowel Disease

Crohn's disease and ulcerative colitis may each be associated with either a peripheral arthritis or an axial (spinal) arthritis. Management is a challenge because often the NSAIDs may worsen the bowel irritability. Often, the arthritis activity parallels the disease activity in the bowel.

Polymyositis and Dermatomyositis

Polymyositis is an inflammatory disease of striated muscle most commonly affecting the proximal limb girdle, neck, and pharynx, proximal third of the esophagus, and occasionally involving the heart. The etiology is unknown, and it may occur at any age. Women are more commonly affected than men. Patients present with proximal muscle weakness and complain of being unable to comb their hair or ascend stairs. In dermatomyositis, there may be a classic violaceous rash around the eyes (heliotrope rash) or on the extensor surface of the extremities. Muscle enzymes (CPK, aldolase) and EMG are commonly abnormal, and muscle biopsies usually show inflammation.

In the patient over 40 years of age, care should be taken to exclude an underlying neoplasm. Myositis can be seen as part of other rheumatic diseases, most commonly scleroderma and systemic lupus. Other etiologies for proximal weakness should also be sought, such as hypothyroidism, steroid myopathy, and electrolyte imbalances. Polymyositis is treated with high-dose steroids or, in steroid-resistant cases, with methotrexate or azathioprine. As the inflammation subsides, care should be taken to continue passive range of motion and gradually progress to assisted active range of motion. Flexion contractures are not uncommon. Refer all patients with elevated enzymes and muscle weakness to a rheumatologist. The long-term outcome is best for the younger adult patient.

Rheumatic Fever

The prevalence of rheumatic fever has markedly decreased (compared with the pre-antibiotic era), but at least 100,000 new cases are diagnosed annually in the United States. Recently, there has been a resurgence of new cases of rheumatic fever. The illness follows infection with group A beta-hemolytic streptococcal infections, and the attack rate can be as high as 3% after epidemic streptococcal outbreaks.

The disease affects both children and adults. A febrile illness associated with a sore throat precedes the symptoms associated with acute rheumatic fever. Migrating, inflammatory arthritis, carditis, subcutaneous nodules, fevers and rashes, fatigue, malaise and a movement disorder (although rare) can all be associated with rheumatic fever. Treatment is directed toward eradication of the streptococcal infection with antibiotics and appropriate anti-inflammatories. After rheumatic fever, prophylaxis with antibiotics (penicillin or erythromycin) should be continued for at least

5 years. Antibiotics should be given 48 hours before and after tooth extraction, root canal, and certain GI and gynecologic procedures.

Raynaud's Phenomenon

Raynaud's phenomenon is a triphasic color change (blue, white, or red) of the extremities, most commonly the fingers. The etiology is unclear, and many people have no underlying connective tissue disorder. Cold exposure often provokes the symptoms, which can range from mild discomfort to intense pain in the digits. Many connective tissue diseases can have an associated Raynaud's phenomenon including scleroderma, lupus, and RA.

Treatment is aimed at preventing attacks by having the patient wear gloves or mittens, and by avoiding medications that increase vasospasm, such as pseudoephedrine in cold preparations and beta blockers for heart disease. Certain drugs have been used, with varying degrees of success, including nitropaste and nifedipine and amlodipine. The patient needs at least one initial rheumatologic evaluation for the possibility of an underlying disease.

Scleroderma

Scleroderma is a disease of unknown etiology that is characterized by the deposition of abundant collagen in the skin and, less commonly, in internal organs such as the kidney, stomach, heart, and lungs. Patients complain of puffiness and tightening of the skin of the fingers and sometimes the feet. Many people have Raynaud's disease and may have chronic recurring superficial digital ulcers that are prone to infection.

Treatment is aimed at keeping the joints mobilized to prevent flexion contractures, and palliative drugs, such as NSAIDs, are used to treat joint pains. Occasionally, additional medications for dilating blood vessels are helpful for severe Raynaud's disease. Reflux esophagitis is often symptomatic and responds well to H_2 blockers. For rapidly progressive skin involvement or in pulmonary disease, D-penicillamine is sometimes used. Patients need to be monitored for the development of hypertension, which may signal kidney involvement. If not recognized early and treated aggressively with angiotensin-converting enzyme inhibitors, this condition can lead to renal failure and death.

A subset of scleroderma patients have CREST syndrome (calcinosis, Raynaud's, esophageal motility disorders, sclerodactyly and telangiectasias). They generally have a benign outcome but sometimes develop severe pulmonary hypertension. There is no cure for scleroderma.

Systemic Lupus Erythematosus (SLE)

SLE is an autoimmune disease that most commonly affects women in their childbearing years. Fatigue and fevers are commonly present. Other symptoms are pleuritis, a facial butterfly rash, alopecia, photosensitivity, arthralgias and arthritis, anemia, and oral ulcers. Most patients have a positive ANA (>90%), and surveillance for other organ involvement needs to be done, especially the kidney. Currently, the prognosis is generally good for lupus for the majority of patients. The disease creates great psychosocial stress because it often strikes women in their reproductive years. Many symptoms, such as profound fatigue and arthralgias, may not be easily seen on casual examination. Often the treatment may include high-dose steroids, which can be disfiguring and cause secondary morbidity from osteoporosis, depression, steroid myopathy, diabetes and cataracts. The person should be counseled to rest when possible, avoid prolonged sun exposure, and use sunscreens and hats. Steroids are often used for more serious cases of lupus that are not adequately controlled by hydroxychloroquine or NSAIDs. More severe cases are treated with methotrexate, azathioprine, or cyclophosphamide.

A common orthopedic problem in lupus patients is avascular necrosis of the hips, knees and shoulders. This can present unique problems when anticipating joint reconstruction in a young patient.

Polymyalgia Rheumatica (PMR)

Polymyalgia rheumatica most commonly affects women over the age of 50 but can be seen in men also. The onset of symptoms occurs suddenly. Symptoms are best characterized by profound morning stiffness lasting more than 45 minutes of the proximal shoulder girdle and hip girdle musculature. Often, there are systemic symptoms such as fatigue, anemia and weight loss. Over 90% of patients have sedimentation rates over 45 mm Hg. Etiology of the syndrome is unknown. Because other conditions mimic PMR, these should be excluded, such as postviral arthralgias, hypothyroidism, and early RA and systemic lupus. Symptoms respond beautifully and rapidly to low-dose oral prednisone.

Conditions Associated with ANAs

Lupus erythematosus
Sjögren's syndrome
Rheumatoid arthritis
Juvenile arthritis
Leprosy
Infectious mononucleosis
Scleroderma
Liver disease
Primary pulmonary fibrosis
Vasculitis
Dermatomyositis/polymyositis
Mixed connective tissue disease
Mixed cryoglobulinemia
Aging
Medications

From Shur, P. (1996). Systemic lupus erythematosus. In Bennett, J. C., Plum, F. (Eds.). *Cecil's textbook of medicine.* Philadelphia, W. B. Saunders.

Temporal Arteritis

Temporal arteritis is a vasculitis characterized by inflammation in medium-sized blood vessels. Patients are usually elderly women who present with headaches, tender temporal arteries, weight loss, and occasionally fever. Fifty percent of patients with temporal arteritis will have symptoms of polymyalgia rheumatica as well.

Evaluate for jaw claudication, anorexia, and systemic illness. Because there is a risk of blindness if the arteritis is left untreated, a high index of suspicion should be maintained with patients with severe headaches, visual disturbances, scalp tenderness, and tender temporal arteries. A temporal artery biopsy should be obtained if the sedimentation rate is elevated in combination with these symptoms.

Treatment is moderate- to high-dose steroids for several months. The elderly are very sensitive to this high-steroid dose and may have secondary psychosis, insomnia, depression, myopathy, new diabetes, and hypertension and osteoporosis. Education about osteoporosis prevention is important for patients on these medications, and consideration should be given to starting antiresorptive drugs.

Classification of Rheumatic Disease

Category	Prototypes	Useful Tests	Treatments
Synovitis	Rheumatoid arthritis Autoimmune collagen diseases	Latex, erythrocyte sedimentation rate ANA test	Methotrexate Prednisone
Enthesopathy	Ankylosing spondylitis B27 spondylarthropathies	Sacroiliac radiographs	Indomethacin
Crystal-induced synovitis	Gout Pseudogout	Joint fluid crystal examination Radiographic chondrocalcinosis Joint fluid crystal examination	Indomethacin Indomethacin
Joint space	Septic arthritis	Joint fluid culture	Antibiotics
Cartilage degeneration	Osteoarthritis	Radiographs of affected area	Physical therapy Analgesics
Osteoarticular	Avascular necrosis bone	Radiographs, magnetic resonance imaging	Prosthetic joint replacement
Polymyositis	Dermatomyositis Inclusion body myositis	Muscle enzymes, EMG, muscle biopsy	Corticosteroids
Local conditions	Tendinitis	None, radiographs of affected area	Local
General conditions	Fibromyalgia	Erythrocyte sedimentation rate, TSH, ANA	Fitness exercises

Modified from Gordon, E. (1996). Approach to the patient with musculoskeletal disease. In Bennett, J. C., Plum, F. (Eds.). *Cecil's Textbook of Medicine*. Philadelphia, W. B. Saunders.

Crystal Diseases

Gout

Gout is a common disorder of middle-aged and older males and postmenopausal women. The characteristic pattern of the arthritis includes development of an acutely painful joint, most often the first metatarsophalangeal joint. The pain is excruciating. Gout is a consequence of hyperuricemia (elevated serum uric acid levels). This may be due to a variety of etiologies including overproduction of urate as with psoriasis, reduced renal excretion of urate, adverse reaction to certain drugs such as diuretics, chronic renal failure, or certain genetic defects in purine metabolism.

Uric acid is soluble in serum up to levels of 8.0 mg/dL. In patients with hyperuricemia (uric acid levels greater than 8.0 mg/dL), small crystals of uric acid in the form of monosodium urate become deposited in joints, bursa, tendons, and in nodular skin deposits called tophi. Renal calculi are found in 10% of patients with gout. All joints may be affected, although by far the most common joint is the first metatarsophalangeal joint, followed by the hips, knees, and hands. Chronic hyperuricemia with gout can lead to an erosive destructive arthritis. The diagnosis can only be made by examination of the joint fluid for intracellular monosodium urate crystals.

Treatment is aimed at rapid relief of the acute attack, usually by NSAIDs followed by long-term prevention of repetitive episodes. Patients with normal renal function and no history of kidney stones may be placed on probenecid to increase renal clearance of urate. Colchicine has been found useful for both acute treatment (although in high doses it may cause GI side effects) and prophylaxis. Allopurinol, which inhibits purine degradation to uric acid, is often the drug of choice, and subsequent attacks can be prevented and the tophi gradually resorbed. Patients should be screened for renal disease because abnormal renal function is a relative contraindication for the use of NSAIDs, colchicine and allopurinol. Doses may have to be adjusted for those with renal disease. For patients with renal disease, other options include tapered oral steroids or intramuscular long-acting steroids. ACTH may be used in the treatment of gout, but it is less potent.

Pseudogout: Calcium Pyrophosphate Deposition Disease (CPPD)

The attack of CPPD arthritis may mimic gout or septic arthritis. The diagnosis is made by examination of joint fluid for the typical crystals. An associated x-ray finding is calcification of the articular cartilage known as chondrocalcinosis. The disease may be associated with other conditions such as hyperparathyroidism, hemochromatosis, hypothyroidism, gout, and OA. Treatment with NSAIDs is usually successful.

Juvenile Rheumatoid Arthritis (JRA)

JRA affects approximately 60,000 to 200,000 children in the United States. The disease is characterized by synovial inflammation and is divided into subgroups; prognosis is based on mode of onset, seropositivity, and related systemic symptoms.

The systemic symptoms include fever, rash, splenomegaly, and adenopathy. Certain types of JRA have a predisposition for eye involvement.

Treatment is aimed at relief of painful joints and presenting systemic symptoms. Anti-inflammatories such as aspirin and NSAIDs are the first-line drugs of choice. Adolescents should be monitored closely for adverse drug reactions. These drugs should be withheld if the child develops an acute febrile illness, because the combination of the drugs and the acute illness may predispose the child to Reye's syndrome. Recognition should be made also of possible limb length discrepancy, which may occur after a chronic inflammatory process that is adjacent to a growth plate. Family counseling is important.

Osteoporosis

Over 20 million people in the United States have osteoporosis leading to 1.3 million fractures yearly. By the ninth decade, one third of elderly women and one sixth of elderly men will have sustained a hip fracture.

By definition, osteoporosis is a decrease in total bone calcium/unit volume, which, in turn, leads to a more brittle bone. Plain radiographs may not reveal a decrease in the density until approximately 30% to 40% of the normal calcium is gone. Often, the first indication of underlying osteoporosis becomes evident at the time of a fracture in the postmenopausal female. The most common fractures with osteoporosis are seen in the thoracic and lumbar spine, the distal radius, humerus, hips, and ribs (Fig. 10-4).

Normal bone is constantly remodeling with osteoclastic and osteoblastic activity. The rate of remodeling depends on a balance between osteoclastic and osteoblastic activity and is regulated by many different factors including hormones, dietary calcium, phosphorus and vitamin D, exercise, gender, genetic predispositions, and environmental influences. At any given age, men have more body calcium than women. After menopause, whether naturally or by oophorectomy, bone loss in women accelerates and may range from 0.5% to 2% per year. This negative balance occurs because bone formation remains relatively constant, but resorption increases. The skeleton acts as the major calcium reservoir in the body; therefore, blood levels of calcium will remain constant despite large changes in total body calcium.

Replacing the calcium content of osteoporotic bone is almost impossible; therefore, the two most important interventions for improvement in the condition are identifying premenopausal women who are at risk and working with postmenopausal women to lessen the rate at which calcium is lost.

Premenopausal women, especially those with a strong family history of osteoporosis, should be instructed in a preventive program to decrease the rate at which calcium leaves the bones. Adequate dietary calcium is important; 1000 mg to 1500 mg/day can be taken as a supplemental vitamin as long as there is no history of renal calculi. Calcium carbonate and calcium citrate are the best absorbed calcium preparations. A diet high in calcium can supplement these as well. Vitamin D should also be taken daily in doses between 400 and 800 IU. An average multivitamin has 400 IU/tablet. Daily weight-bearing exercise has been found to be helpful in maintaining good bone stock. Patients should be encouraged to walk 20 minutes daily when possible. Elimination of environmental factors such as excessive alcohol

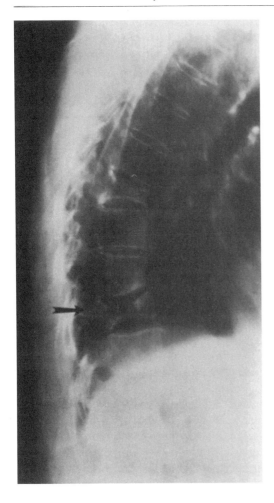

FIGURE 10-4. Severe osteoporosis with multiple thoracic and lumbar vertebral body compression fractures.

consumption and cigarette smoking is also important. Women undergoing oophorectomy should discuss the risks of supplemental estrogens/progesterone compared with the risks of premature osteoporosis. Patients at risk for fractures, or in whom fractures have occurred, should be evaluated and counseled concerning the risks and benefits of additional antiresorptive therapy. The approved agents are estrogen therapy, calcitonin, bisphosphonates, and raloxifene (selective estrogen receptor modulator; SERM).

The postmenopausal woman who sustains a fracture should have at least one evaluation for other causes of pathologic fractures. Radiographs should be obtained; they are often helpful for excluding a neoplastic process. A bone scan may need to be performed to identify a new fracture that may not be visible on x-ray. A complete blood count, sedimentation rate, alkaline phosphatase, and serum calcium test should be obtained and, if there is any evidence of an underlying pathologic process, a serum protein electrophoresis is needed to evaluate the patient for multiple myeloma. Occasionally vitamin D_3 levels and PTH levels may be indicated. Osteoporotic fractures, as a rule, do not occur in men, and, if a male develops a nontraumatic fracture, he should always be evaluated for an underlying malignancy, infection, or metabolic bone disease.

Controversy exists about which populations to screen, but those women who have multiple risk factors for osteoporosis, with or without a previous fracture, should probably undergo bone density scanning. This is a simple radiographic test with low x-ray exposures. The best, more sensitive and reproducible scans are the standard DEXA scans. Falsely elevated densities can occur with scoliosis and osteophytes as well as a calcified aorta. Scanners that also do a lateral view of the lumbar spine have less problem with false negatives. Other less expensive scans called P-DEXAs (peripheral DEXAs) are not nearly as sensitive and may be difficult to reproduce because of positioning problems of the wrist or calcaneus. Newer means such as ultrasound techniques are also being studied for screening purposes.

In the identified high-risk perimenopausal woman, the primary care provider should consider the addition of estrogens, which have been found to decelerate bone loss. Ideally, hormone replacement therapy should begin within 3 years after menopause (the time of most rapid bone loss). Good evidence exists for starting estrogen therapy even into the eighth decade with studies showing up to a 50% decrease in hip fracture rate. When estrogen therapy is withdrawn, the risk of fracture returns to near peer-group level. Careful gynecologic and breast examinations should be done throughout therapy. In addition, as previously discussed, less controversial interventions should be undertaken.

Calcitonin has been in use for more than 3 decades and was initially used to treat Paget's disease of bone. It is a potent disrupter of osteoclast activity and hence slows down bone loss and has been shown to have promoted modest bone gain. Calcitonin can be administered either subcutaneously or intranasally. The most bothersome problems tend to be flushing and diarrhea. The nasal spray, although generally better tolerated, is associated with nasal irritation and headache. Skin testing before subcutaneous administration is encouraged to screen for patients sensitive to calcitonin.

The bisphosphonate family of chemicals was introduced almost 100 years ago as water softeners. Bisphosphonates also inhibit osteoclasts. The first drug used for osteoporosis in this class was etidronate. This product has fallen out of favor because of its weaker bone avidity and the osteomalacia caused by long-term use, but studies are supporting its use for steroid-induced osteoporosis. Alendronate, an amino-bisphosphonate, is one hundred times more potent than etidronate. Alendronate has been shown to decrease the rate of spinal and hip fractures. Because of the poor bioavailability of the drug, it has to be administered on an empty stomach or at least 30 minutes before eating. GI problems, particularly esophagitis, are the biggest side effects, and special caution should be taken when administered simultaneously with an NSAID.

Enthusiasm for fluoride treatment has waxed and waned. Initial studies showing an increase in bone density did not show any change in fracture rate but had increase in stress fractures. A more recent study by Pak (Pak et al, 1995) using a 25 mg BID slow-release fluoride with calcium supplement suggested an increase in bone density and a decrease in fracture rate.

New agents under investigation include SERMs. Recently approved for use is raloxifene, which acts as an estrogen agonist in bone and increases bone density.

In a report by the National Osteoporosis Foundation, patients receiving raloxifene 30 to 150 mg/day and calcium 500 mg/day demonstrated a 2% to 4% increase in bone mass. Its action as an estrogen agonist in the liver resulted in a 10% decrease in low-density lipoprotein (LDL) cholesterol.

Treatment of vertebral fractures usually is conservative. The sharp pain subsides after 2 to 3 weeks, and most discomfort should be gone in 6 weeks. Calcitonin can be used for acute fracture pain because it has an analgesic component. Lumbar braces and thoracic posture supports can minimize the chronic pain felt secondary to irreversible deformities in the spine. Gradual progressive ambulation should be encouraged, but frequent rest in the supine position often is the best treatment for the aching, kyphotic back. Neurologic complications rarely occur secondary to osteoporotic spinal fractures. Fractures in the limbs are managed by the orthopedist, either through casting or appropriate surgical intervention. After the acute pain starts to subside, one should encourage the patient to increase gradually the number of minutes he or she can sit and then to resume normal activities when comfortable. The home environment should be screened for scatter rugs or slippery floors where falls may be likely (see Chapter 1). Spinal hyperextension exercises should be done, and walking should be encouraged (see Appendix E for exercises).

Interventions with osteoporotic patients should be directed toward minimizing loss of bone and prevention of fractures and related injuries. The osteoporosis intervention model proves suitable for designing an inclusive patient care framework.

Nonorthopedic problems encountered in the osteoporotic patient include chronic intractable pain, loss of self-esteem and poor self-image, loss of ability to wear one's clothing secondary to increasing girth, fear of previously enjoyed activities, restrictive lung disease, and exacerbation of cervical neck pain secondary to exaggerated cervical lordosis as compensation for thoracic kyphosis.

Paget's Disease of Bone

In Paget's disease, osteoclasts are excessively destroyed and the resorption of bone is followed by uncontrolled osteoblastic new bone formation. The result is a bone that is mechanically defective, enlarged, and deformed. Paget's disease affects people after 40 years of age; the peak incidence is between 50 and 70 years of age. The etiology of Paget's disease is unknown.

Although most people are asymptomatic, the following symptoms may be present: Pain in the hip, sacrum, spine, pelvis, skull, femur, and tibia (worse with weight bearing and cold weather). Patients may experience difficulty with walking, increasing head size, hearing loss, a compromise of spinal cord and nerve roots (radiculopathy) and possible high-output cardiac failure. The cardinal clinical finding is an elevated alkaline phosphatase. The alkaline phosphatase can be as high as ten times the upper limits of normal. Audiograms may reveal a hearing loss. Pain on palpation over affected areas may be appreciated on physical examination. Diagnostic studies will help differentiate between ankylosing spondylitis and other rheumatic, metastatic, and metabolic diseases. The bone scan is the most sensitive screen and will pick up skeletal changes before the standard x-ray. X-ray examination reveals osteolytic areas with new bone formation (Fig. 10-5).

Interventions for Osteoporosis

Primary prevention

(before the disease is present)
Goal: Reducing risk factors

Risk factors
Female sex
Small frame
Caucasian or Asian ethnicity
Positive family history
Lifelong low calcium intake (particularly in
  adolescents)
Early menopause or oophorectomy
Sedentary lifestyle
Nulliparity
Alcoholism
High sodium intake
Cigarette smoking
High caffeine intake
High phosphate intake
High protein intake
Steroids, heparin, anticonvulsants
Hyperthyroidism, hyperparathyroidism
Multiple myeloma
Rheumatoid arthritis
Height loss >1.5 inches
Low trauma fracture
Secondary osteoporosis (thyrotoxicosis,
  postgastrectomy, malabsorption
  syndrome)
Prolonged immobilization
Organ transplantation
Chronic renal failure

Health education
Adequate calcium carbonate intake
  1000 mg qd before menopause
  1200 mg qd during menopause
  1500 mg qd after menopause
Adequate vitamin D intake
  200 units qd before menopause
  400 units during and after menopause
Exercise regimen
  Muscle-building exercise (weightlifting)
  Weight-bearing exercise (walking 30
  minutes/day)
Nutritional intake (48-hour diet recall)
  Referral to nutritionist when appropriate

Secondary prevention

Goal: (1) To detect problem at an early
          stage
      (2) To prevent fractures and to limit
          disability once the diagnosis is
          made

Screening
DEXA scan
Thyroid functions
ESR, calcium, alkaline phosphatase

Therapeutic regimen (*health education*)

Dietary
Ongoing nutritional support
(1) Avoid bone meal as a calcium
    supplement; it may contain lead
(2) Drink at least 8 oz of water with each
    1 g of calcium to decrease the risk of
    developing renal stones
(3) Increase calcium absorption by taking
    calcium supplement with the meal/
    snack that contains the least amount of
    fiber (fiber can reduce absorption)
(4) Take Lactaid as a supplement to aid
    absorption if there is a history of lactose
    intolerance
(5) Take up to 600 mg calcium at one
    time—maximal absorption/

Hormones
Patient education regarding estrogen/
  progesterone replacement therapies
Estrogen replacement in conjunction with
  physician consultation
Perimenopausal high-risk female
Postmenopausal female with radiographic
  evidence of osteopenia

Exercise
Walking, swimming, and social dancing
Loading exercises for the upper extremities
  (lifting 1-lb weights to build the strength
  of the radius for 15 min 3 times/week).
Referral to a physical therapist for
  individualized exercise regimen

Tertiary prevention (symptomatic osteoporosis)

Goals: (1) To promote patient adaptation to
           orthopedic intervention
       (2) To restore the individual to
           optimal level of functioning

Expected Outcome

Fx	Healing time	Recovery
Wrist	6–12 weeks	3–6 months
Spine	4–8 weeks	1–2 years
Hip	6–12 weeks	1 year

Treatment regimen: may consist of
Estrogen therapy, bisphosphonates
Calcitonin (SQ or nasal spray).
Selective estrogen receptor modulator
  (SERM)
Exercise (eg, walking [30 min 5 times/
  week]
Loading exercises of the upper extremities
  (15 min 3 times/week)

Health teaching regarding:
Fall prevention
Back strain
  Keep commonly used items in reach
  Use proper body machanics
  Maintain a safe home environment
  Proper usage of canes and crutches

Adapted from Lindsay, R. (1987). Estrogens in prevention and treatment of osteoporosis. In
  The osteoporotic syndrome: Detection, prevention, and treatment. Orlando, FL: Grune & Stratton, p 101.

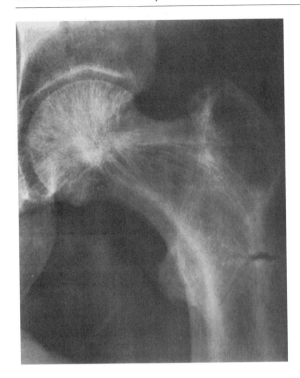

FIGURE 10-5. Osteolytic areas with new bone formation.

The treatment of Paget's disease depends on the severity of the disease. Mild bone pain is treated with NSAIDs. The first line of treatment is alendronate (Fosamax). If this is not effective or is contraindicated, bisphosphonates (Skelid) or etidronate (Didronel) may be tried. IV pamidronate is currently being evaluated. Some patients will have complete remission with drug therapy.

Patients with Paget's may be referred to a rheumatologist, orthopedist, endocrinologist, cardiologist or neurosurgeon for further evaluation. Patients with mild disease will need annual follow-up visits. Those with severe disease should be seen routinely.

Drug-Associated Musculoskeletal Syndromes

Drug reactions or allergies are common and can present as acute febrile illnesses with rash, myalgia and arthritis, oral ulcers, and renal findings. This is also known as serum-sickness. The most common offending agents are antibiotics, but many drugs have a similar effect. Certain medications (eg, procaine, pronestyl, hydralazine, beta blockers, aldomet, and hydrochlorothiazide) may induce a picture much like lupus. Any patient with rheumatic complaints needs to have a careful drug history taken.

Drug Therapy for Arthritis

Before initiating either a prescription or nonprescription drug program for a rheumatic disease, the exact diagnosis needs to be established. When this is done, the drug with the fewest side effects for the greatest possible benefit is administered.

In conditions such as OA, an NSAID or acetaminophen is often beneficial in conjunction with joint preservation advice. The inflammatory arthropathies often require additional medications known as disease-modifying agents or immunosuppressants. All patients need baseline hematologic liver and kidney function tests, with periodic testing at 6 weeks, 3 months, and at regular intervals afterward while on NSAIDs. Changes in normal function warrant discontinuation of the drug and consultation with a primary care provider. High-risk patients such as diabetics and hypertensives and patients with underlying renal disease should be screened more frequently.

Analgesics

Nonsteroidal Anti-inflammatory Drugs

This family of products, including salicylates as well as nonsteroidals, shares similar toxicity profiles. They are usually used to decrease pain, swelling and stiffness and improve function. There is no evidence that they change the course of the disease. Because of the mechanisms of action of inhibiting prostaglandins, the anti-inflammatory class of drugs may cause gastritis as well as renal insufficiency and hypertension. Routine surveillance of side effects, particularly in high-risk patients such as diabetics or hypertension patients, is important.

Acetaminophen

Patients can take acetaminophen in conjunction with other drugs for arthritis. Acetaminophen is a good analgesic for mild to moderate pain but has no anti-inflammatory properties. Patients should take no more than 4000 mg/day. With higher doses (near 7000 mg/day), liver toxicity and kidney failure are possible. In doses under 4000/mg, side effects are uncommon.

Disease-Modifying Antirheumatic Drugs

Antimalarials (Hydroxychloroquine, Chloroquine)

The antimalarials are beneficial in the treatment of RA and systemic lupus. These drugs, especially hydroxychloroquine, have relatively low toxicity but may cause retinal damage. Ophthalmologic examinations are recommended every 6 months.

Gold Therapy (Oral and Injectable)

Gold is one of the "remittive" drugs in RA. Side effects are common and include a decreased leukocyte count and thrombocytopenia, rash, proteinuria, and diarrhea (more common with the oral preparation). The mechanism of action is unknown, and any beneficial effect does not occur for 3 months. Surveillance for bone marrow suppression, rash, and proteinuria should be done on a regular basis.

D-Penicillamine

This drug is used primarily in RA and scleroderma and may work by inhibiting collagen deposition. Many patients respond well to D-penicillamine after 6 months of treatment. Unfortunately, a large number need to discontinue the drug because of the side effects, including loss of taste, leukopenia, rash, proteinuria, and drug-induced lupus.

Corticosteroids

ORAL PREPARATION. The most commonly administered steroid is prednisone, but many other preparations are also available. Topically applied steroid creams, when applied to large areas of the body, can also have the effect of systemic steroids. Steroids are given for refractory inflammatory conditions and severe allergic reactions. If used over a long period of time, they can have severe consequences.

Some of the more common and important side effects include adrenal insufficiency, diabetes, hypertension, accelerated atherosclerosis, accelerated osteoporosis, truncal obesity, striae, cataracts, gastritis, decreased immunity to infections, edema, myopathy, aseptic necrosis of bone, psychosis, and headaches. Discontinuation of steroids, especially after prolonged use, requires a gradual withdrawal with a tapered dose schedule. Because of the possibility of sudden adrenal insufficiency, *steroids should never be withdrawn abruptly.*

Patients should be taught the dangers of abrupt discontinuation and the necessity of strict adherence to the prescribed dosing schedule. Because of the associated osteoporosis seen with steroid use, patients should have bone density scans performed and be evaluated for use of antiresorptive drugs.

STEROID INJECTIONS. Injections can be made into the joints or the soft tissues (for treatment of carpal tunnel syndrome or bursitis). Intra-articular injections should be used judiciously. The risk of infection is low, but repeated injections may soften the cartilage or ligaments. Intra-articular steroid injections have some systemic effects, particularly in transient elevation of blood sugars in diabetics.

Immunomodulators (Cytoxan, Imuran, Methotrexate, Cyclosporin)

Immunomodulators are drugs reserved for advanced refractory diseases where conventional (less toxic) therapy has been inadequate. GI symptoms, mucosal ulcers, and decreased blood counts are the most common side effects. All patients on immunosuppressants are at an increased risk for infections so any fever or even superficial skin infection should be reported to a primary care provider.

Methotrexate is the most commonly used medication in this class with extraordinary usefulness particularly for RA. Careful surveillance for leukopenia and liver function abnormalities should be done, and other environmental factors that can also contribute to cirrhosis (such as alcohol) should be evaluated. Certain drugs such as trimethoprim should be avoided because of the synergism with methotrexate to cause bone marrow suppression. Patients at higher risk for side effects are those with diabetes, renal disease and alcohol use.

Cytoxan has a high-toxicity problem when administered as a daily oral dose particularly from interstitial cystitis. Patients should keep themselves well hydrated. Another common mode of administering the cytoxan is with monthly bolus IV doses. These are given for potentially life-threatening problems, and the patients receiving it usually have systemic lupus or vasculitis.

Azathioprine shares some of the side effects of methotrexate. Monitoring for hematologic and liver toxicity is recommended. The drug has been useful for treatment of refractory cases of RA, systemic lupus, polymyositis, vasculitis and other less common diseases.

Cyclosporin has been used successfully for organ transplantation and has gained favor for resistant cases of RA and other diseases. Abnormalities in renal function and new hypertension are the two most ominous side effects, but others include hirsutism, tremor and the immunocompromised state.

Diagnostic Tests for Arthritis Patients

Laboratory Tests

Complete Blood Count (CBC)

The CBC is a very helpful test to determine if there are concurrent abnormalities indicating an underlying inflammatory condition. Leukocytosis can be seen with an infectious process or an inflammatory etiology. Leukopenia (WBC <4000) may suggest a disease such as SLE or may be a side effect of an immunosuppressant. Anemia is not found in a normal healthy patient, even in the elderly, and thus can also be a marker of an underlying systemic disease. Patients should be screened for anemia after prolonged use of NSAIDs because of associated gastritis and occult GI bleeding.

Westergren Erythrocyte Sedimentation Rate (ESR)

This is a very sensitive but nonspecific test for inflammation. The ESR may be elevated with infections, inflammatory autoimmune diseases and malignancy. It is usually normal in people with noninflammatory conditions, such as OA or a traumatic joint injury.

Renal and Liver Functions

Chemistry profiles should be obtained before starting elderly patients on aspirin or NSAIDs. The kidney function should also be checked intermittently while the patient is taking these medications, because occasionally they may cause renal insufficiency and elevated blood pressure. These hazards are especially common in a patient with preexisting hypertension or a mild degree of creatinine elevation.

Rheumatoid Factor

An aggregation of immune complexes found in the sera of the majority of people with RA has been labeled a rheumatoid factor (RF). It is not necessary to have a positive RF to be diagnosed with RA. RF can be seen in other diseases such as endocarditis, sarcoid, and systemic lupus and leprosy as well as aging.

Antinuclear Antibody (ANA)

A positive ANA is found in more than 90% of persons who are diagnosed as having SLE. ANA may also be present in patients with RA, progressive systemic sclerosis, and poorly differentiated connective tissue diseases, polymyositis, and sarcoidosis. Usually, low-titer ANA appears in the elderly and may not indicate the presence of an associated connective tissue disease. Several medications have been linked with the syndrome of drug-induced lupus. Two of the most common ones are procainamide and hydralazine.

Tine or PPD

All patients to be treated with steroids should first be tested for tuberculosis. Patients with a positive result should be treated with INH concomitantly with the steroid therapy.

Arthrocentesis–Synovial Fluid Analysis

Joint fluid analysis is used for differentiating inflammatory from noninflammatory processes. Cell counts less than 1500 cells/mm3 indicate a noninflammatory process such as OA. RA classically will give you counts from 3000 cells/mm^3 to 50,000/mm^3. Septic arthritis and gout will yield counts often greater than 100,000/mm^3. The joint fluid should be placed in a green top (heparinized) tube to prevent clotting and to minimize crystal artifact. Inflammatory fluids, in general, should be sent for culture and sensitivity and polarized light examination to look for crystals.

Imaging Techniques

Radiographs

Radiographs are very helpful in evaluating a patient with arthritis. Diagnostic changes are seen with certain types of arthritis, and the stage and prognosis can also be determined by x-rays. For example, typical changes seen in OA include asymmetric loss of the joint space from the narrowing of cartilage with osteophyte or bony spur production and subchondral sclerosis. An inflammatory arthritis will give a picture of symmetric joint space narrowing and possible juxta-articular erosions. Changes with acute infectious arthritis are swelling of the soft tissues with bony changes seen with chronic infection (osteomyelitis). These changes include osteopenia and loss of the bony cortex. Certain crystal diseases have pathognomonic calcification seen in cartilage. Often after an injury, only soft tissue swelling will be visualized, but fractures and foreign bodies need to be excluded, especially if the skin integrity has been broken.

Magnetic Resonance Imaging

MRI is very helpful especially when looking for avascular necrosis and herniated discs in the spine and will also help when assessing for a hairline fracture or tumor. Bone scans are also sensitive for avascular necrosis, certain tumors, and fractures, and are less expensive but also less specific.

Therapeutic Modalities

Physical Therapy

Physical therapy is often recommended to treat the sore, stiff joints and muscles of people with arthritis and to teach patients adaptive, appropriate skills for home therapy and prevention of disability.

Treatment consists of various modalities including hot packs, ultrasound, whirlpool, paraffin wax and massage to decrease muscle spasm and pain. The therapist uses gentle, passive range of motion to stretch tightened muscles and prevent flexion contractures. "Hot" joints are handled carefully, limiting movement to passive range of motion. As symptoms subside, exercise can continue to include a strengthening exercise program emphasizing isometric techniques and mild resistance exercises using elastic bands and light weights. The daily routine includes use of massage, use of hot/cold therapy for 20 minutes three times a day, and the proper sequencing of anti-inflammatory and mild pain-relieving medications before showers that are then followed by range-of-motion exercise and relaxation techniques.

Despite small gains, the physical therapist has the opportunity to soothe and encourage the patient through the use of techniques in touch, helpful modalities, and constant encouragement. Most importantly, the therapist teaches patients how to pace themselves and how to modify the home environment for improved activities of daily living.

Exercise

Patients are instructed to do range-of-motion exercises 3 to 4 times a day, gradually increasing strengthening exercises daily. Finally, an endurance exercise program can be included after careful evaluation of the patient's major joint dysfunctions and overall conditioning. Again, gradual progression is important from the beginning. Activities such as freestyle swimming (the water temperature should be at least 82°) or swimming with flotation devices, fast walking (treadmill or street), and bike riding (stationary or mobile), light racquet games (badminton and ping-pong), croquet, dancing, and light weight resistance exercises (<20 lb) are most often recommended.

Patients are advised to avoid the following activities unless suitable adaptation can be made: Activities that impact or jar the joints (jogging, jumping, running, and aerobics), activities that require heavy racquets (tennis), highly competitive team sports and contact sports (Banwell, 1984).

Occupational Therapy

The occupational therapist contributes to the rehabilitation process of the patients by teaching activities of daily living, joint protection, energy conservation techniques, and splinting.

The arthritic patient is taught coping skills for everyday living. Patients learn to put on stockings, open jars, and adapt to their chronic illness in a manner that preserves their self-esteem. The occupational therapist uses self-help aids and teaches the importance of balancing rest with work activities to avoid fatigue.

Patients usually need special help in alternating their work and rest periods. Teach them to rest when they feel tired or in pain; doing a little each day rather than overdoing exertion on one day is essential. The learned techniques in joint protection and energy conservation allow patients to continue with a more normal daily life at home and at work.

Making splints for patients to provide proper alignment of joints and adequate rest of inflamed joints has also become a major responsibility of the occupational therapist. Proper alignment helps prevent joint contractures, tendon ruptures, and deformities. Rest for joints, alternating with gentle range-of-motion exercise, helps to reduce inflammation and pain while maintaining joint function.

Nontraditional Treatments

Nontraditional treatments or remedies used for rheumatic diseases are common. A patient who has been told that there is no cure for the chronic, painful condition will naturally try almost anything to obtain relief of pain and (hopefully) a cure. In addition to the feelings of desperation, well-meaning friends and relatives continue to bombard the patient with suggestions and recommendations. Some suggestions are as easy as purchasing and wearing a simple copper bracelet or as strange as drinking a gallon of carrot juice daily. Others include more expensive fare such as mail-order high-potency vitamins or a trip to a Mexican clinic.

The Arthritis Foundation publishes an excellent pamphlet on this subject. Patients often need the reassurance of a health professional that most people do experiment sometimes but that it is good to investigate each possible remedy through the Foundation or primary care provider.

Help the patient learn to evaluate nontraditional treatments by asking the following questions:

1. Does it help or cure all kinds of arthritis?
2. Was a control group used in the study?
3. Is it based on a secret formula?
4. Is it promoted only in the media (books or by mail order)?
5. Does it use case histories and testimonials in promotion?
6. Does it eliminate any basic foods or nutrients?

Psychosocial Considerations

Psychosocial aspects must always be addressed when caring for the person who has arthritis. The lack of cure and chronicity of the disease make adjustment difficult. The patient who deals with pain and disability on a daily basis experiences fears: of increasing disability, harmful medications, guilt about being ill or burdensome to the family, and depression from decreased social opportunities.

Most people with arthritis are amazingly resourceful and determined to be independent. Life for people with arthritis is in constant flux. It is through excellent medical care and comprehensive patient education that this roller coaster existence can be modified and normal goals and plans for day-to-day living can be developed.

Education on self-help techniques, involvement in support groups, and interaction with others in the same or similar circumstances seem to be particularly helpful in resolving and promoting a healthy psychological outlook. Counseling for the patient and family may be necessary for overwhelming or chronic depression that results from the loss of health. Once different, but realistic goals, projects and social interactions can be reinstituted, psychosocial adjustment is usually accomplished more easily. If the patients and their families master appropriate and helpful interventions for depression, situational stress, and flare-ups, these reactions appear less frequently and are more easily controllable. Most important is that the health professionals to whom the person with arthritis is directed are knowledgeable about the diseases, community resources, and chronic illness adjustment methods.

The adolescent with arthritis presents an additional challenge. The adolescent is normally maturing and becoming increasingly independent; the parent must allow the normal growth process to continue despite concerns about health issues, such as getting enough rest and joint protection. The adolescent must be encouraged to develop activities, hobbies, and interests that will not do damage to their joints; overprotection is not helpful. The young person needs to be as active as the disease process will allow. Career planning should take into consideration the physical limitations imposed by the disease. Physical appearance is of special concern to the adolescent. When disability, even slight, does exist, the teenager may choose to avoid activities. Teenagers, by nature, want to conform; yet treatment for arthritis often excludes the patient from gym classes. The patient may also experience drug-related cosmetic problems (weight gain and acne). Even the use of a splint can cause loss of self-esteem and make the adolescent feel even further removed from peers. Again, encouragement to participate in activities is important in and out of school so that friendships can be built. Parents should encourage normal activities within the limits set by the primary care provider that promote normal development. Warm baths and splinting are useful in promoting and maintaining range of motion. Physical or occupational therapy and swimming are additional measures suggested for adolescents with more active inflammation. Counseling may be necessary for both teens and their parents so the normal process of growing and maturing will not be hindered more than necessary.

Diffuse Pain Syndromes

Fibromyalgia (FM) is a chronic diffuse musculoskeletal pain syndrome. Myofascial pain syndromes (MPS) are chronic regional or localized pain syndromes. FM and myofascial pain are common conditions that still often evade diagnosis. Careful diagnosis avoids unnecessary and expensive testing. Helpful general management issues in treating patient with soft tissue pain include the following:

Exclude systemic disease such as malignancy or inflammatory arthritis. Often a thorough physical examination and basic laboratory studies such as a CBC, sedimentation rate, calcium, alkaline phosphatase, serum protein electrophoresis (where indicated), liver profile and thyroid studies are adequate.

Spend time getting to know the patient carefully in terms of the social network, workplace, and activity level.

Reassure the patient that this is not a life-threatening illness, although it might be chronic.

Give the patient literature or other resources such as support group information.

Eliminate factors in the patient's work and home life that seem to aggravate the symptoms.

Provide an extensive and graded exercise plan often with a physical therapist.

Provide pain relief with non-narcotic analgesics or anti-inflammatory medications.

Treat a sleep disturbance appropriately with relaxation techniques and tricyclic antidepressants.

Listen carefully to the patient's complaints.

Fibromyalgia

FM is an increasingly recognized syndrome of musculoskeletal pain and fatigue, often associated with an array of other musculoskeletal and neurologic symptoms. Most studies suggest a female-to-male predominance of approximately 9:1. The overall prevalence in the population is 2% (3.4% of all women and 0.5% of men).

Historically, there has been great variability in the criteria used to diagnose FM. In 1990, the American College of Rheumatology published criteria to discriminate FM from other musculoskeletal disorders. These criteria include widespread pain and tenderness in at least 11 of 18 specified locations. These tender points are broadly distributed throughout the musculoskeletal system and are typically found over tendinous insertions, bony prominences, and muscle bellies (Fig. 10-6). In addition to these areas of reproducible pain, patients with FM invariably complain of disabling fatigue and sleep disturbances. Nonrestorative, disturbed sleep is believed to be important in the pathogenesis of FM. Other common symptoms include unexplained headache and abdominal symptoms suggesting irritable bowel syndrome. Affective symptoms (ie, depression, anxiety) are common in patients with FM, although it is unclear if they are primary or secondary.

The etiology of FM is unknown and has been debated for many years; it is probably multifactorial. Most patients with FM cannot identify a precipitating factor, but some identify a triggering flulike or viral illness. Minor or substantial physical trauma such as a motor vehicle accident is also cited, and emotional trauma, prolonged use of corticosteroids and other chronic illnesses have been associated with FM. Patients with chronic infections such as HIV, Epstein-Barr virus and Lyme disease have an increased incidence of FM. Before making the diagnosis of FM, care should be given to search for other underlying causes for the complaints such as polymyalgia rheumatica, lupus, and endocrine problems such as hypothyroidism, osteoporosis, and cervical OA.

There is no specific treatment for FM, but individual patients may be considerably helped with a number of diverse available therapies. The single most important intervention is patient education and reassurance. Patients readily understand an explanation based on poor sleep and reduced fitness. Interventions to restore sleep are important as is a program of cardiovascular exercise. Low-impact activities such as fast walking, biking, swimming or water aerobics are the most helpful. The type and intensity of the exercise program should be individualized.

American College of Rheumatology 1990 Criteria for Classification of Fibromyalgia*

History of widespead pain

Pain is considered widespread when all of these are present:
Pain in left side of body
Pain in right side of body
Pain above waist
Pain below waist

In addition, axial skeletal pain must be present in at least one of the following areas:
Cervical spine
Anterior chest
Thoracic spine
Low back

Shoulder and buttock pain is considered as pain for each involved side

Low back pain is considered lower segment pain

Pain in 11 of 18 tender point sites on digital palpation†

Tender point sites are defined as follows (all are bilateral):
Occiput: at suboccipital muscle insertions
Low cervical: at anterior aspects of intertransverse spaces at C5-C7
Trapezius: at midpoint of upper border
Supraspinatus: at origins, above scapular spine near medial border
Second rib: at second costochondral junctions, just lateral to junctions on upper surfaces
Lateral epicondyle: 2 cm distal to epicondyles
Gluteal: in upper outer quadrants of buttocks in anterior fold of muscle
Greater trochanter: posterior to trochanteric prominence
Knee: at medial fat pad proximal to joint line

*Patients have fibromyalgia if both criteria are satisfied. Widespread pain must have been present for at least 3 months. Presence of a second clinical disorder does not exclude diagnosis of fibromyalgia.

†Digital palpation should be performed with an approximate force of 4 kg. For a tender point to be considered "positive," subject must state that palpation was painful; "tender" is not to be equated with "painful."

Adapted from Wolfe, F., Smythe, H. A., Yunnus, M. B., et al. (1990). *Arthritis and Rheumatism, 33,* 160–172. With permission, American College of Rheumatology.

Approximately 50% of patients with FM will have a striking response to tricyclic antidepressants; others will get a partial response. Anxiety and depression need to be addressed as well. Improving the patient's coping mechanisms, possibly with the use of yoga, meditation or biofeedback, support groups and counseling is an important adjunct to treatment. Patients with FM should be closely monitored and given encouragement, reassurance and education.

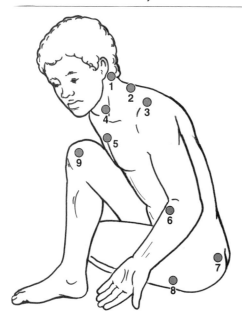

FIGURE 10-6. Fibromyalgia trigger points.

Myofascial Pain

MPS are usually regional in nature and overlap with other common regional pain disorders such as idiopathic low back and cervical strain syndrome, chest wall pain syndromes, and temporomandibular joint syndrome. According to Simons and Travell (1995), the syndrome is defined by the presence of trigger points. These localized trigger points, when palpated, create a local twitch response that then causes a characteristic pain pattern (Fig. 10-7). They are thought to be brought on by continual straining of the muscle, often from the repetition of a certain posture or task.

Contributing and associated factors in MPS include (1) neurologic pain syndromes such as cervical radiculopathy and entrapment neuropathies that can mimic myofascial pain syndrome, (2) tension and vascular headaches that can create trigger points in the temporalis, posterior cervical and sternocleidomastoid muscles, and (3) physical and mechanical factors such as poor posture or leg length discrepancies. Repetitive motion, awkward postures, and poor workspace design predispose to specific MPS.

FM and myofascial pain can be differentiated by the presence of trigger points and the localized or regional pain of MPS versus the widespread or generalized pain of FM. Furthermore, MPS can often be permanently relieved by local measures such as massage, stretch and spray manipulation and local injections. Such treatment is not successful in FM. As symptoms improve, prevention of recurrence through exercise and work modification becomes essential.

Temporomandibular Pain Syndrome

Temporomandibular pain syndrome is an acute or chronic musculoskeletal condition involving jaw motion. The syndrome is most common in young women. Pain with motion of the jaw is the most common symptom. The pain is usually dull and worse with chewing hard foods; sometimes it is poorly localized. Patients often describe spasm of the muscles of mastication, clicking and grinding of the jaw, and locking or limited motion of the jaw. Temporomandibular pain syndrome is often associated with other syndromes, including tension headache, neck and back pain, and chronic GI and pelvic discomfort. Dizziness, earaches, sinus pain, and arm and shoulder pain are also associated with temporomandibular pain syndrome. Other etiologic factors include malocclusion, which causes overstretching of the lateral pterygoid and the mastication muscles; sports or motor vehicle trauma that results in overstretching; and stress manifested by clenching or grinding of the teeth.

A thorough physical examination of the temporomandibular joint is important. Rule out other causes of facial pain, including trigeminal neuralgia, salivary gland abnormalities, sinusitis, and dental disease. Elderly patients should be evaluated for giant cell arteritis or temporal arteritis. Tomography, magnetic resonance imaging (MRI), or computed tomography (CT) scanning may be indicated.

Treatment includes patient reassurance and avoiding eating hard foods that can cause jaw clenching. Bite plates help reduce joint pressure and muscle activity. Relaxation techniques may also be helpful. Tricyclic antidepressant medications are the mainstay of medical management. Doxepin 25 mg or nortriptyline 25 mg have been shown to be successful in several studies. Other treatment options to be performed by either an otolaryngologist or an oral surgeon include repositioning and surgical meniscectomy of the joint. Treatment alleviates discomfort and in some instances provides a cure.

Chest Wall Pain Syndromes

Musculoskeletal problems involving the chest wall are common causes of chest pain. Up to 10% of patients presenting with chest pain have musculoskeletal chest pain syndromes. Lack of familiarity with these disorders can often lead to errors in diagnosis, unnecessary testing such as stress tests, and delays in appropriate treatment. However, angina pectoris, pericarditis, pneumonia, pleurisy and other more serious disorders need to be ruled out in equivocal cases. Obtain an electrocardiogram (ECG) if there is a suspicion of angina pectoris, other cardiac disease, or if the patient is in a high-risk group for early cardiac death. Obtain a chest x-ray if there is a suspicion of pulmonary disease such as a pulmonary tumor.

Musculoskeletal chest wall pain is usually insidious in onset. The pain is often well localized, nagging and exacerbated by movement. There may be a history of prior minor or repetitive trauma, or a history of increased physical activity. Patients may have trouble falling asleep due to the pain, and it is not uncommon for the pain to be associated with chest tightness and shortness of breath. These symptoms make it difficult to distinguish musculoskeletal chest wall pain from other causes of chest pain. Physical signs on examination include local chest wall tenderness and possibly swelling. A thorough physical examination of the heart and lungs is necessary. Of extreme importance is evaluation of the ribs, costochondral and

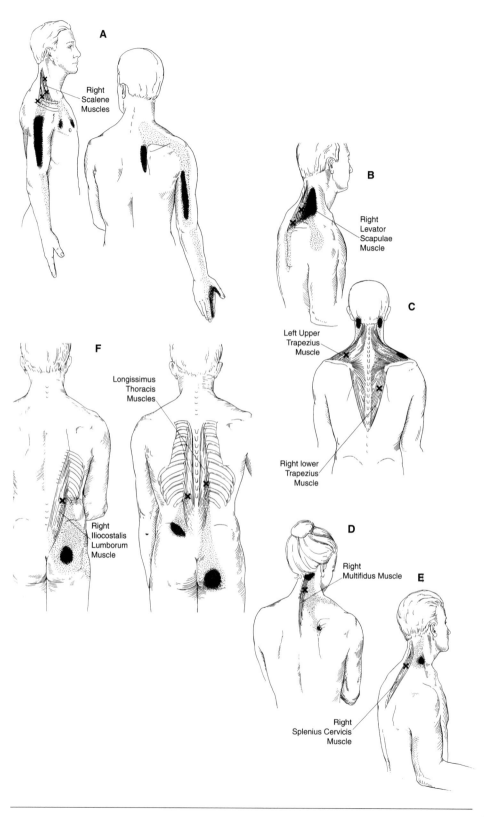

A

Right
Scalene
Muscles

B

Right
Levator
Scapulae
Muscle

C

Left Upper
Trapezius
Muscle

Right lower
Trapezius
Muscle

F

Longissimus
Thoracis
Muscles

Right
Iliocostalis
Lumborum
Muscle

D

Right
Multifidus Muscle

E

Right
Splenius Cervicis
Muscle

FIGURE 10-7.

costosternal articulations, intercostal musculature, sternum, sternoclavicular and acromioclavicular joint, and cervical and thoracic spines. Laboratory evaluations should include a complete blood count, ESR, chest x-ray and ECG.

Costochondritis, or anterior chest wall syndrome, is a common cause of anterior chest pain. Often there is a prior history of cough or congestion due to an upper respiratory infection. Patients are typically over 40 years of age. Pain is elicited at numerous costochondral junctions. Swelling is typically absent. *Tietze's syndrome* is an inflammation of the costocartilage typically occurring in the young and mid-adult years. Tietze's syndrome is a less common cause of chest pain. There is tenderness and often swelling present at the cartilaginous articulations of the anterior chest wall. It can be distinguished from costochondritis by numerous features—younger age at onset, predilection for the second and third costochondral articulations, unilateral distribution and single lesions in most patients.

Costochondritis, Tietze's syndrome, and most musculoskeletal chest wall syndromes usually resolve in 2 to 3 days. In some cases the symptoms may persist for 6 to 8 weeks or may be refractory and last months or years. If symptoms persist beyond 6 weeks, a bone scan may be helpful in determining the diagnosis, which can include systemic inflammation, insufficiency fracture, infection and tumor.

Local treatment with ice or heat and NSAIDs is usually sufficient. Carefully explain the disease process, reassure the patient, allow him or her time to express fears and concerns, and stress elimination of causative activities. Occasionally, patients require local corticosteroid and lidocaine injections of the involved costochondral site. Intercostal nerve blocks have been used in refractory cases. Physiotherapy is of limited benefit.

Pharmacologic Agents and Symptom Control

Tricyclic Antidepressants (TCA)

TCAs have been found to be effective in the treatment of FM and other soft tissue musculoskeletal pain syndromes. Care must be taken in using this group of medications, because none is currently approved for this purpose. One should be

---

FIGURE 10-7. Referred pain from trigger points (Xs) in right scalene muscles (**A**) extends down front and back of the arm (over the biceps and triceps). Pain skips the elbow and reappears in the radial side of the forearm, the thumb, and the index finger. Other reference zones are in the back and chest. Trigger points in right levator scapulae muscle (**B**) produce consolidated pain pattern shown. Trigger points in left upper trapezius and right lower trapezius refer pain ipsilaterally (**C**). (**D**) Trigger point (X) above the base of the neck (left) is the most common posterior cervical location and often leads to entrapment of the greater occipital nerve. Pain and tenderness are referred upward to the suboccipital region and sometimes downward to the upper vertebral border of the scapula. (**E**) Lower splenius cervicis trigger point (right) refers pain to the angle of the neck. (**F**) Referred pain patterns associated with trigger points (Xs) at different levels of the superficial paraspinal muscles are shown. The essential reference zones are depicted in *solid black* and the spillover areas in *stippled black.*

familiar with several more commonly used TCAs in varying dosage ranges. Although TCAs have been available for use for nearly 40 years, their exact mechanism of action is still not known. At low doses, they do not seem to affect depression, but have sleep, regulatory and pain-modulating properties. Suggested dosing strategies for TCAs are as follows:

Start with amitriptyline 10 mg 1 to 2 hours before bedtime. There is a 1- to 3-week delay in achieving effective analgesic and sleep modification. Symptoms of dryness of the eyes and mouth (anticholinergic properties) should abate in several weeks.

If the patient has no benefit, increase the dose after 3 to 4 weeks to 25 mg of amitriptyline. If there is still no effect, consider switching to another TCA such as doxepin.

Doxepin has less anticholinergic and other undesirable side effects. Recommend starting at 10 mg 1 hour before bed. Doxepin is also available in a liquid form such that extremely low doses (less than 5 mg hs) could also be tried.

If neither amitriptyline nor doxepin is effective, or if either causes intolerable side effects, nortriptyline or desipramine may be tried. Trazodone (Deseryl), a drug with strong sedating but minimal anticholinergic properties, can be used in doses of 50 to 100 mg at bedtime.

Nonsteroidal Anti-inflammatory Drugs

Used alone, NSAIDs have not proven effective in reducing the pain of FM. However, the efficacy of tricyclic antidepressants is increased when used in combination with nonsteroidals. NSAIDs should be used in low analgesic doses as adjunctive therapy for patients with FM. Because of the great variation in dosing and frequency of administration of NSAIDs, care should be given to choosing the appropriate agent. Under no circumstance should the recommended maximum dose be exceeded. Assess the patient's renal and hepatic status before starting the NSAID. Prolonged and regular use of acetaminophen while commonly prescribed is not advisable. Again, hepatic and renal toxicity when taken on a regular basis need to be of a major concern. A new non-narcotic analgesic, tramodol (Ultram) has been approved for use in patients with chronic pain. Anecdotal experience with this analgesic has been favorable in patients with FM and myofascial pain. It is preferable to start at the lowest dosing range (ie, 50 mg every 4 to 6 hours on a prn basis).

Patients who are taking narcotic analgesics must be weaned off them. If withdrawal is not possible by the primary health care provider alone, a carefully selected pain center or clinic is often helpful. The same is true for sedatives or hypnotics.

Muscle Relaxants

Muscle relaxants, particularly cyclobenzapine (Flexeril), may be an adjunct in the management of diffuse pain syndromes. The exact mechanism of action is unknown; it does not directly relax muscles but appears to act in the spinal cord or at the brain stem.

Arthritis Foundation

The Arthritis Foundation was established as a national organization in 1947. It was begun by a group of primary care providers who wanted to pursue funds to support research to find the cause and cure for arthritis.

The organization has its national headquarters in Atlanta, Georgia and 76 local chapters throughout the United States. The goals of the Foundation are public education and information, patient services, professional education, and research.

The programs of the Arthritis Foundation that are particularly noteworthy include (1) the Arthritis Self-Help Course, (2) the Arthritis Joint Venture Dry Exercise Program and (3) the Arthritis Foundation YMCA Aquatic Program. The national address is Arthritis Foundation, 1314 Spring Street, NW, Atlanta, Georgia 30309, (404) 872-7100.

The author acknowledges Hal Dinerman, MD, Department of Medicine, Beth Israel Deaconess Medical Center, Harvard Medical School, for his contribution of Diffuse Pain Syndromes.

References and Recommended Readings

Aloia, J. F., Vaswani, A., Yeh, J. K., et al. (1994). Calcium supplementation with and without hormone replacement therapy to prevent postmenopausal bone loss. *Annals of Internal Medicine, 120,* 97.

Arnett, F. (1987). Seronegative spondylarthropathies. *Bulletin on the Rheumatic Diseases, 37*(1), 1.

Banwell, B. F. (1984). Exercise and mobility in arthritis. *Nursing Clinics of North America, 19*(4), 605.

Black, D. M., Cummings, S. R., Karpf, D. B., et al. (1996). Randomized trial of effect of alendronate on risk of fracture in women with existing vertebral fractures. *Lancet, 348,* 1535.

Calabrese, L. (1993). Human immunodeficiency virus (HIV) infection and arthritis. *Rheumatic Diseases Clinics of North America, 19*(2), 477.

Deal, C. L. (1997). Osteoporosis: prevention, diagnosis and management. *American Journal of Medicine, 102*(suppl 1A), 35S.

Felson, D. T., Zhang, Y., Hannan, M. T., Kiel, D. P., Wilson, P. W., & Anderson, J. J. (1993). The effect of postmenopausal estrogen therapy on bone density in elderly women. *New England Journal of Medicine, 329,* 1141.

Fries, J. F. (1997). General approach to the rheumatic disease patient. In Kelley, W. N., et al. (Eds.). *Textbook of rheumatology.* Philadelphia: W. B. Saunders.

Goldberg, V., & Kuettner, K. (Eds.). (1995). Osteoarthritic disorders: workshop, Monterey, California, April 1994. *American Academy of Orthopedic Surgeons,* pp. xxii–xxiii.

Goldenberg, D. L. (1994). Fibromyalgia. In Klippel, J. H., & Dieppe, P. A. (Eds.). *Rheumatology.* St. Louis: Mosby.

Gordon, E. (1996). Approach to the patient with musculoskeletal disease. In Bennett, J. C., Plum, F. (Eds.) *Cecil's textbook of medicine* (20th ed.). Philadelphia: W. B. Saunders.

Huch, K., Kuettner, K., & Dieppe, P. (1997). Osteoarthritis in ankle and knee joints. *Seminars in Arthritis and Rheumatism, 26,* 667.

Kelley, W. N., Harris, E. D., Ruddy, S., & Sledge, C. B. (1997). *Textbook of rheumatology* (5th ed.). Philadelphia: W. B. Saunders.

Liberman, V. A., Weiss, S. R., Broll, J., et al. (1995). Effect of oral alendronate on bone mineral density and the incidence of fractures in postmenopausal osteoporosis. *New England Journal of Medicine, 333,* 1437.

Malawista, S. (1996). Lyme disease. In Bennett, J. C., Plum, F. (Eds.). *Cecil's textbook of medicine* (20th ed.). Philadelphia: W. B. Saunders.

Naides, S. (1993). Parvovirus B19 infection. *Rheumatic Diseases Clinics of North America, 19*(2), 457.

Pak, C., Khashayar, S., Damas-Huet, B., Piziak, V., Peterson, R., & Poindexxer, J. (1995). Treatment of postmenopausal osteoporosis with slow release sodium fluoride. *Annals of Internal Medicine, 123,* 401.

Schumacher, H. R., Klippel, J., & Koopman, W. (Eds.). (1993). *Primer on the rheumatic diseases* (10th ed.). Atlanta, GA: Arthritis Foundation.

Sergent, J. S. (1997). Approach to the patient with more than one joint. In Kelley, W. N., et al. (Eds.). *Textbook of rheumatology.* Philadelphia: W. B. Saunders.

Shur, P. (1996). Systemic lupus erythematosus. In Bennett, J., C., Plum, F. (Eds.). *Cecil's textbook of medicine* (20th ed.). Philadelphia: W. B. Saunders.

Sibley, J. (1995). Laboratory tests. *Rheumatic Diseases Clinics of North America, 21*(2), 407.

Simons, D. G., & Traveil, J. G. (1995). *Myofascial pain and dysfunction trigger point manual.* Baltimore: Williams and Wilkins.

Sparling, P. F. (1996). Gonococcal infections. In Bennett, J. C., Plum, F. (Eds.). *Cecil's textbook of medicine.* Philadelphia: W. B. Saunders.

Wolf, F., & Hawley, D. F. (1993). Fibromyalgia. In Kelly, W. N., Harris, E. D., Ruddy, S., & Sledge, C. G. (Eds.). *Textbook of rheumatology.* Philadelphia: W. B. Saunders.

Wolf, F., Simons, D. G., Fricton, J. et al. (1992). The fibromyalgia and myofascial pain syndrome: A preliminary study of tender points and trigger points in persons with fibromyalgia, myofascial pain syndrome and no disease. *Journal of Rheumatology, 19,* 944–951.

● ●

Drug Therapy for Musculoskeletal Conditions

This appendix provides a brief overview of the classes of drugs used in orthopedic drug therapy. The prudent practitioner will consult the pharmacologic references cited at the end of the appendices for more details.

Analgesics and Antiinflammatory Drugs

Acetaminophen

Acetaminophen is a mild analgesic and antipyretic. It is not an antiinflammatory and may be less effective when inflammation is contributing to pain. Acetaminophen is less irritating to the GI tract than NSAIDs.

PRACTITIONER AND PATIENT CONSIDERATIONS. Severe liver damage may result from overdosage or interaction with alcohol. Advise patients to avoid alcohol and other OTC drugs that contain acetaminophen during treatment. Adult doses should not exceed 4 g/day or 2.6 g/day if taken on a long-term basis. Long-term therapy is contraindicated in patients with hepatic or renal disease or anemia.

Tramadol Hydrochloride

Tramadol binds to mu-opioid receptors and inhibits the reuptake of norepinephrine and serotonin. Tramadol causes CNS effects similar to opioids—dizziness, somnolence—but does not cause respiratory depression.

PRACTITIONER AND PATIENT CONSIDERATIONS. Adverse effects include seizures; tramadol should be used with caution in patients with seizure disorders, on MAOIs, or on medication that lowers the seizure threshold. Limit the use of tramadol in patients with a history of substance abuse. Use with caution in patients with renal or hepatic impairment.

Nonsteroidal Antiinflammatory Drugs/Analgesics

Nonsteroidal antiinflammatory drugs (NSAIDs) are indicated for mild to moderate pain relief and/or for subduing inflammation. They are often recommended after surgery or injury or on an acute or chronic basis for rheumatoid arthritis and degenerative joint disease. They have analgesic, antiinflammatory, and antipyretic properties.

NSAIDs are classified as salicylates (e.g., aspirin), non-acetylated salicylates (e.g., choline magnesium salicylate), indoles (e.g., indomethacin), propionic acid derivatives (e.g., ibuprofen), pyrroles (e.g., tolemetin sodium), fenemates (e.g., meclofenamate), and pyrazolones (e.g., phenylbutazone). Pyrazolones are very potent drugs used selectively for short terms because of their potential for renal and bone marrow toxicity. NSAIDs work by inhibiting prostaglandin formation. The GI tract rapidly absorbs them and they are frequently irritating to it. Toxic levels of NSAIDs may cause tinnitus and eighth cranial nerve damage. In addition, they cause sodium and fluid retention and decrease the ability of platelets to aggregate. Other adverse effects include peptic and duodenal ulcers, gastritis, hemolytic anemia, nephrotoxicity, and elevated liver enzymes.

PRACTITIONER AND PATIENT CONSIDERATIONS. The patient should be instructed to take NSAIDs with food and/or antacids and at least 8 ounces of fluid to prevent GI irritation or erosion. Patient teaching includes observing for bleeding tenancies such as bruisablity, bleeding gums, smoke-colored urine, and dark, tarry stools. Hemoccult testing of the stool should be done at least once a month for those on long-term therapy. It is recommended that renal and hepatic function be tested every 1 to 2 months in patients on long-term NSAIDs whether or not they display symptoms. Patients must be questioned about tinnitus. If tinnitus occurs the dosage is lowered; if it persists, the drug should be discontinued. Patients who are taking these drugs for long-term antiinflammatory effects need to be advised that therapeutic effect may not be noticeable for 2 to 4 weeks. Because sodium and fluid retention are common side effects of NSAIDs, they should be used cautiously in the elderly and in those with cardiac or renal disease.

Warn patients that many OTC drugs contain NSAIDs, and teach the importance of reading the labels. Patients should be encouraged to tell their pharmacist or practitioners about any OTC drugs they may be taking and to ask about possible drug interactions or adverse effects.

Corticosteroids

Corticosteroids are frequently used in rheumatic disorders and collagen diseases for their antiinflammatory properties when remittive agents have not been effective. Although the precise mechanisms of action are unknown, corticosteroids non-specifically inhibit inflammatory effects of many microorganisms, chemical or thermal irritants, allergens, and trauma. Steroids suppress symptoms but do not treat the underlying cause of the problem. Continuous daily therapy is usually reserved for acute conditions (e.g., trauma, SLE). For chronic disorders enough steroid should be administered to allow function, but usually not enough to provide complete symptomatic relief since this would require much higher doses.

The use of alternate-day therapy should be considered in chronic disease. Patients receive a 2-day dosage in a single administration every other morning. This mode of administration may reduce side effects, particularly adrenal suppression. Theoretically, the patient has lower steroid bloods levels on the "off" days, which allows a day of reactivation of the adrenal glands by the normal mechanism of CRF-ACTH and recovery of other tissues from the metabolic effects of exogenous steroids. Steroids that are inactivated in less than 30 to 36 hours must be used to allow the body's own secretory mechanisms to prevail on non-treatment days. The dose should be given in the morning to simulate the normal diurnal rhythm and to achieve maximum benefit with minimum dose.

PRACTITIONER AND PATIENT CONSIDERATIONS. Corticosteroids may increase susceptibility to infection, suppress skin sensitivity tests, and elevate serum amylase and blood glucose levels. When glucocorticoids are administered over a long period the patient may display sodium and water retention, potassium depletion, and symptoms similar to Cushing's syndrome, including hirsutism, cervicothoracic hump, moon face, edema, amenorrhea, striae and thinning of the skin, hyperglycemia, hypokalemia, hypochloremia, metabolic alkalosis, mental disturbances, and hyperglycemia. In addition, increased appetite, weight gain, peptic ulcer, puerpera, headache, and dizziness have been reported. Osteoporosis and vertebral compression are well-recognized complications of long-term (over 2 months) therapy.

Antirheumatics

Anti-malarials: Hydoxycholooquine Sulphate, Chloroquine Phosphate

These drugs were originally used to treat malaria and were subsequently found to have antiinflammatory properties, which are useful in the treatment of RA and both systemic and discoid lupus erythematosus. Their mechanism of action is unknown. The most common side effects are GI disturbances, especially gastric burning. Other adverse reactions include headaches, visual disturbances, tinnitus, vertigo, blood dyscrasias, and dermatitis.

PRACTITIONER AND PATIENT CONSIDERATIONS. Visual acuity and a slit lamp ophthalmologic examination should proceed administration of these drugs and should be repeated every 3 to 6 months, as retinopathy is a rare side effect. For this reason the drugs are contraindicated in patients with retinal or visual field changes and are not recommended for diabetics. Because the drugs concentrate in the liver, extreme caution is urged in using these medications in patients with hepatic problems or in alcoholics. CBC and liver function tests should be obtained routinely in those on long-term therapy. Toxic symptoms include headache, drowsiness, and visual disturbances and can proceed to cardiovascular collapse, seizures, and respiratory and cardiac arrest. Since children are especially susceptible to toxicity, avoid long-term treatment. Patients should be cautioned to avoid sun exposure as drug-induced dermatosis may result.

Gold Sodium Thiomalate

Gold salts have been shown to be effective against RA. Seventy-five percent of patients started on the therapy have a favorable response. However, numerous and serious side effects, which are frequently a dose-related problem, may require the discontinuation of the drug. Owing to the frequency and severity of these adverse reactions, gold salts are indicated only in patients in whom NSAIDs and D-penicillamine have not been helpful.

Intramuscular injection should be into large muscles. Patients should lie down for 10 to 20 minutes after injection and be observed for 30 minutes after injection for acute reactions. Gold sodium thiomalate is a suspension. It requires warming and agitation in order to resuspend and to obtain an accurate dose. It is pale yellow in color and should not be used if the solution has darkened.

PRACTITIONER AND PATIENT CONSIDERATIONS. Gold salts are contraindicated in the presence of many medical conditions but show no significant drug interactions. Advise patients that benefits of the therapy may not be observed for 6 to 12 weeks. Patients may remain on gold therapy for years.

Dermatitis, including rash and/or pruritus, is the most common adverse reaction. Pruritic skin reactions will often progress to more serious skin problems; therefore, it is necessary to discontinue the drug until the reaction clears. Concomitant stomatitis often occurs. Nephrotoxicity with initial proteinuria and albuminuria may occur; therefore, frequent urine dipstick urinalysis is crucial. Blood dyscrasias, most notably thrombocytopenia (with or without purpura), aplastic anemia, and granulocytosis, are well-known side effects. A CBC and platelet count must be obtained at least biweekly routinely. Other adverse reactions include nausea, vomiting, diarrhea, metallic taste, hepatitis, and jaundice. Since thrombocytopenia, aplastic anemia, granulocytosis, proteinuria, and nephritic syndrome are common and potentially life-threatening side effects, authorities recommend that a urinalysis or dipstick for urine protein and a hematocrit precede every gold injection. Caution patients to report any adverse reactions promptly to their practitioner. Dimercaprol is used to treat acute gold toxicity.

D-Penicillamine

The precise mechanism of action of D-penicillamine is not known; however, it lowers IgM rheumatoid factor and reduces the excessive excretion of cystine. Many patients respond well to D-penicillamine after 6 to 8 weeks of treatment. Unfortunately, a large number need to discontinue the drug due to side effects, including renal and hepatoxicity, leukopenia, thrombocytopenia, rash, drug-induced lupus, and loss of taste.

PRACTITIONER AND PATIENT CONSIDERATIONS. Urinalysis and CBC with differential and platelet count must be obtained every 2 weeks; if abnormalities are seen, D-penicillamine usually is discontinued. Proteinuria of greater than 2 to 5 g/day calls for discontinuation to preserve renal function. Taking D-penicillamine on an empty stomach prevents binding with dietary metals, which can cause the loss of essential minerals as well as decrease drug efficacy.

Immunomodulators

Azathioprine and Cyclophosphamide

Azathioprine and cyclophosphamide are highly effective against arthritis and provide complete or partial remission in up to 75% of patients. However, they are reserved for advanced refractory conditions due to their hepatotoxicity and the frequency of secondary infections from the immunosuppression. Giving immunosuppressives in conjunction with steroids reduces the dose of steroids needed.

PATIENT AND PRACTITIONER CONSIDERATIONS. Response may take up to 6 weeks. Leukopenia, bone marrow depression, hepatotoxicity, and other blood dyscrasias necessitate monitoring of CBC and liver enzymes. Therapy must be stopped if WBC is less than 3000/mm3 to prevent irreversible bone marrow depression. GI complaints are frequent, including, nausea, vomiting, diarrhea, and stomatitis. Taking the drug with meals and antiemetics may lessen nausea and vomiting, and scrupulous oral hygiene may help stomatitis. Patients on cyclophosphamide are at risk for hemorrhagic cystitis and bladder cancer and, therefore, should drink copious amounts of fluid to minimize the concentration in the bladder. Taking the drug earlier in the morning helps prevent retention of the metabolites overnight in the bladder. Advise patients to observe for opportunistic infections—thrush, herpes zoster, colds—and to consult their practitioner promptly when even mild fever or symptoms occur.

Anti-gout

Allopurinol

Allopurinol acts as a hypouricemic agent and is used for long-term treatment of gout. It is especially beneficial for those with elevated uric acid, renal insufficiency, or for those who cannot use uricosuric drugs. Side effects are generally rare and mild. Side effects indicative of hypersensitivity include rash, hepatotoxicity, and/or blood dyscrasias. These usually occur 1 to 6 weeks into treatment but may occur at any time during therapy; the drug must be discontinued if they occur. Allopurinol is contraindicated in patients with idiopathic hemochromatosis and should not be given to those on iron therapy.

PRACTITIONER AND PATIENT CONSIDERATIONS. Liver function tests and CBC are indicated on a weekly basis during the first few months of therapy to screen for hepatic and/or blood problems. Advise patients that a rash can lead to serious complications (exfoliative dermatitis, toxic epidermal neurolysis) and that their practitioner should be notified promptly so that the drug can be discontinued. Encourage patients to drink large amounts of fluid. Urine output should be at least 2 L/day.

Colchicine

Colchicine has been used to treat gout for centuries; it is the drug of choice for acute gout and can also be used on a long-term basis. Colchicine is believed to act by inhibiting the migration of granulocytes to an area of inflammation. It has mild antiinflammatory effects but no analgesic properties. Nausea, vomiting, and diarrhea are common side effects and reasons for discontinuation. Chronic administration infrequently may result in bone marrow depression.

PRACTITIONER AND PATIENT CONSIDERATIONS. A baseline CBC should be obtained and monitored as leukopenia, aplastic anemia, and/or agranulocytosis may occur with chronic use. If administering intravenously, use undiluted or diluted in 0.9% Sodium Chloride Injection. Do not use 5% glucose and water. Infuse over 2 to 5 minutes. Do not give subcutaneously or intramuscularly.

Probenecid, Sulfinpyrazone

These medications are indicated for hyperuricemia and chronic gout. They should not be started for an acute gouty attack. They work by blocking tubular reabsorption of urate, thereby causing a marked increase in the excretion of uric acid.

PRACTITIONER AND PATIENT CONSIDERATIONS. Treatment should begin with small doses to decrease the probability of renal stones. Instruct patients to drink enough fluid to maintain a urine output of 2 to 3 L/day (also to prevent renal stones). Alkalinization of the urine increases the solubility of urates, reducing the possibility of renal stone formation. A dietician can provide information on foods that will alkalize the urine. Because GI irritation is a frequent complaint, these medications should be given with food to decrease GI irritation. Antacids may also be given with probenecid to decrease GI irritation. Avoid prescibing to patients with BUN greater than 40 or creatine clearance of less than 40 mL/minute and in those with blood dyscrasias. Advise patients that this drug may take up to 6 to 12 months to become effective and that gouty attacks may increase in the first 6 to 12 months of therapy. Despite this, treatment should continue in conjunction with colchicine or other antiinflammatory agents. Salicylates inhibit the uricosuric activities of the drug and therefore should be avoided.

●●

Comparative Costs of Commonly Used NSAIDs

Drug	Rating
Ibuprofen (Motrin, Rufen, Ibu-tab)	$
Indomethacin (Indocin)	$
Piroxicam (Feldene)	$
Naproxen (Naprosyn)	$$
Sulindac (Clinoril)	$$
Meclofenamate (Meclomen)	$$
Fenoprofen (Nalfon)	$$$
Trilisate (Tricosal)	$$$
Flurbiprofen (Ansaid)	$$$$
Diclofenac (Voltarin)	$$$$$
Etodolac (Lodine)	$$$$$
Ketoprofen (Oruvail)	$$$$$
Nabumetone (Relafen)	$$$$$
Oxaproxin (Daypro)	$$$$$

Rating based on 30-day supply of generic drug. *Brand names cost one and a half to three times more.*

....

Care of Casts and Back Braces

Synthetic (Fiberglass and Plastic) Casts

The fiberglass cast obtains maximum hardness immediately after application; therefore, molding (unwanted shaping, dents, or depressions) during the drying process is not a problem. The patient need not avoid resting the cast on hard surfaces after application. Weight bearing may begin immediately. The fiberglass cast may be cleaned with mild soap and a damp cloth. Water on the outside of the cast will not harm it; however, water on the inside of the cast may lead to moldiness and/or skin irritation. To avert any possible skin irritation or infection, advise the patient that the cast should stay dry. If the cast becomes wet, a blow dryer set on low may be used to expedite the drying process.

Plaster Casts

A plaster cast dries in 24 to 72 hours. Smaller casts, such as a child's arm cast, will dry in 24 hours; larger casts, such as an adult body cast, may take up to 72 hours. During the drying process the cast must be positioned to prevent unwanted molding or depressions. Weight bearing must be avoided. Warn the patient that the cast will feel warm when "setting." Until the cast is completely dry, avoid placing it on plastic or other waterproof pillows, as these materials trap heat and condensation may occur. The resulting damp cast will not "set" properly.

After the cast is dry, the rough edges may be petaled to prevent skin irritation. To petal a cast, cut 4-inch lengths of 2-inch-wide moleskin, adhesive, or silk tape, rounding the cut edges. Place one-half of the strip under the cast, firmly sticking it to the inside of the cast. Bring the remaining end over the edge to the outside of the cast (keeping the tape smooth and taut to avoid wrinkles). Continue to apply petals around the edge of the cast, overlapping each piece over the previous one.

The cast may be "cleaned" by using a large eraser to remove marks; white shoe polish may be used to cover marks. Avoid covering the entire cast with polish as it needs to "breathe."

General Cast Care and Patient Teaching

Prior to cast application, baseline neurovascular status and skin integrity should be assessed and documented. Following application of the cast, neurovascular status is reassessed. The patient should be instructed how to assess neurovascular status. Instruct the patient to report any adverse change in this status and to report if the cast is rubbing or otherwise uncomfortable. Following cast application, an x-ray is required to verify proper positioning. Additional patient instructions include:

1. Elevate the injured extremity whenever possible (ideally above the heart).

2. Call the practitioner if the cast is damaged and needs repair, if it has become too loose or rubs, if the cast develops an odor, if a fever develops, or if there is an increase in pain.

3. Avoid inserting anything into the cast, including lotion, powders, backscratchers, or liquids.

4. Maintain the integrity of the cast. Do not chip, break, crush, or otherwise mutilate the cast.

5. Keep the skin near the plaster cast's edges clean by using rubbing alcohol.

6. Immediately report any sign of new bleeding inside the cast or seepage to the outside.

The patient should be provided with a written record of exercises, weight bearing limits, instructions for cleaning the cast, a list of cast do's and don'ts, and the phone number of a resource person to call with questions or problems.

Brace Care

Patients who wear back braces must be taught about preventing skin breakdown. Instruct the patient to take the following measures:

- Bathe or shower daily.
- Apply rubbing alcohol to all parts of the skin that the brace covers, especially in areas of increased pressure. Explain that the alcohol and friction toughen the skin.
- Avoid creams, lotions, or powders under the brace.
- Wear a 100% cotton undershirt that does not have side seams.
- Wear the brace as tightly as possible to avoid chafing the skin by brace movement.
- Inspect the skin daily for signs of pressure and skin breakdown.
- Do not wear the brace and contact the practitioner if skin breakdown occurs.

●●●

Ambulatory Assistive Devices

Most people whose mobility is restricted because of lower-extremity impairment require some type of ambulatory assistive device. The selection of one type of device over another depends primarily on the injury, the patient's physical strengths and limitations, the degree of weight bearing allowed, and the patient's coordination. Patient education and instruction are necessary to prevent patient mobility problems associated with the use of ambulatory assistive devices.

Axillary Crutches

Proper Measurement

When checking a pair of crutches for proper fit, it is crucial that there be a handsbreadth between the top pad on the crutch and the patient's axilla. Encourage patients to avoid leaning or placing their body weight on the top of the crutches. Sustained pressure on the radial, ulnar, and median nerves can lead to crutch paralysis. The patient should be able to flex his elbows comfortably at approximately 20 degrees while bearing weight on the padded hand bars of the crutches. Adjustment of the hand bars should allow for this flexion.

Standing From a Seated Position

To rise from a seated position using axillary crutches, have the patient slide forward in the chair. The leg on the unaffected side should be placed firmly on the floor slightly underneath the chair. Instruct the patient to hold onto the chair's armrest on the unaffected side and the hand bars of both crutches with the other hand, and push himself or herself up into a standing position. Once erect, one crutch may be shifted to the other arm.

Sitting Down

Have the patient stand with his or her back to the chair (perferably a chair with two armrests). The patient should be close enough to the chair so that the back of the *un*affected leg touches the chair. Both crutches are then placed under the arm on the *un*affected side. Holding onto the hand bars of the crutches with one hand, have the patient reach back and grasp the armrest on the affected side and slowly lower himself or herself into a sitting position.

Ambulating

When ambulating with crutches, two types of gaits should be considered: the swing-to and the swing-through gaits. For the non–weight-bearing patient, the swing-to gait is the gait of choice, at least until the patient is able to balance well.

335

SWING-TO GAIT. The patient who is able to bear weight should be instructed to place both crutches securely on the floor approximately 1 foot in front. With elbows slightly bent and bearing weight on the hand bars (not the axilla), have the patient propel or swing both feet up to but not beyond the location of the crutches. Repaet this cycle by placing both crutches approximately 1 foot ahead, then propelling both feet to a point up to but not beyond the placement of the crutches. The non–weight-bearing patient should place weight on the unaffected limb only.

SWING-THROUGH GAIT. Once adept at the swing-to gait, the patient may be progressed to the swing-through gait. The swing-through gait is the most vigorous in terms of energy expenditure, and it also provides the most rapid means of ambulation.

The swing-through gait is similar to the swing-to gait, but it requires that the patient propel his or her feet *beyond* the placement of the crutches. Have the non–weight-bearing patient move both crutches approximately 1 foot forward. While bearing weight on the hand bars of the crutch (not the axilla), have the patient step through or swing through with the legs to a point approximately 8 to 12 inches *beyond* the previously positioned crutches. The non–weight-bearing patient should place weight only on the *un*affected limb.

Neogotiating Stairs

ASCENDING STAIRS. To ascend stairs with hand railings, have the patient position both crutches on the *un*affected side opposite the railing. With the hand on the affected side, have him or her grasp the railing. Using the crutches on the *un*affected side and the hand railing for support, tell the patient to swing the *un*affected leg up to the next stair, followed by the affected leg and crutches. For stairs without hand railings, both crutches are used for support; the good leg is brought up to the next stair, followed by the affected leg and crutches. The patient who is able to partially bear weight should follow the same sequence.

DESCENDING STAIRS. Have the patient place both crutches into position on the *un*affected side opposite the railing on the stairs. Grasping the railing on the affected side, have him or her lower the crutches and the affected leg to the stair below, followed by the *un*affected leg. For stairs without railings, both crutches are used for support, one on each side. The sequence is the same for the patient who is able to partially bear weight. A good rule of thumb to tell patients is *"Up* with the *good...down* with the *bad."*

Walkers

A walker may be used for either the full or partial weight bearing patient. It is considered a stable walking device. To ensure optimal efficiency of the device with the least amount of strain on the patient, it is necessary to assess proper fit.

PROPER MEASUREMENT. To adjust the walker size for each patient, have the patient stand "inside" the walker. The hand grips should be at the level of the greater trochanter of the hip, allowing for a 15- to 20-degree flexion at the elbow. If the height is not accurate, adjust the walker accordingly.

STANDING FROM A SEATED POSITION. To rise from a seated position, place the walker directly in front of the seated patient. Have the patient slide to the chair's edge. The *un*affected leg should be flexed and slightly under the chair. Instruct him or her to rise by grasping both armrests of the chair, pushing up using arm strength and the *un*affected leg. With the hand on the *un*affected side first, have the patient grasp the walker. Next, instruct the patient to release his or her grip on the chair's armrest with the other hand, and grasp the walker with this hand as well. The patient should shift the body weight forward to the strong or *un*affected limb, into an erect position. Do not allow patients to use the walker to pull themselves up.

SITTING DOWN. To assist the patient into a sitting position, encourage them to use chairs of average height, preferably with armrests. Have the patient stand with his or her back to the chair, making sure the *un*affected leg touches the chair before beginning to lower himself or herself into the chair. The patient should reach back for the chair's armrest with the hand on the affected side. Instruct the patient to release the other hand from the walker, grasp the chair's remaining armrest, and lean forward and slowly lower himself or herself into the chair.

AMBULATING. To begin ambulation, instruct the patient to advance the walker approximately 8 to 10 inches. Placing the weight on his or her hands, have the patient step into the walker with the affected leg and then follow through with the *un*affected leg. The cycle continues as the patient advances the walker, bears weight using the hands and *un*affected extremity, steps into the walker first with the affected leg, and then with the *un*affected leg.

DESCENDING STAIRS. To descend the stairs, have the patient grasp the railing with one or both hands. Have him lower himself one stair at a time beginning with the affected limb first, then the *un*affected limb. If the patient must cary the walker while descending the stairs, have him or her grasp the stair railing with one hand and place the folded walker on the next stair down. While grasping the top of the walker, the patient can then descend the stairs slowly, beginning with the affected foot and followed by the *un*affected foot.

ASCENDING STAIRS. To ascend the stairs, the patient should first grasp the railing with one or both hands. Using the railing for leverage, he or she should ascend the stairs, *un*affected leg first, followed by the affected leg. If the patient must carry the walker, have him or her fold the walker. Grasping the hand railing with one hand and placing the folded walker on the next stair up, the patient can grasp the top of the walker with the free hand and advance to the next stair, *un*affected foot first, followed by the affected foot. The sequence is then repeated.

Canes

Canes are another ambulatory assistive device often used for balance, security, and support. Additionally, canes function to help absorb the body weight for those who are partial weight bearers. Canes may be used unilaterally or bilaterally, depending on the patient's needs. They may be triangular- or quadrangular-based to provide greater support.

Proper Measurement
Metallic canes are adjustable. Wood canes may be cut to size. The proper length should allow the patient approximately 20 to 30 degrees of flexion at the elbow.

Ambulating
The cane is held in the hand on the *un*affected side. When ambulating, the patient should move the cane in conjunction with the affected leg. The *un*affected leg is then brought forward. The patient's body weight and level of balance are maintained with the cane.

Negotiating Stairs
Negotiating stairs using a cane is accomplished by applying the "*up* with the *good...down* with the *bad*" rule.

Descending Stairs

To descend stairs, the cane is placed in the hand on the *un*affected or uninvolved side. Grasping the stair railing on the affected side, the patient should move the cane down one stair. He or she then steps down with the affected limb, followed by the *un*affected limb. Remember, "*up* with the *good...down* with the *bad.*"

Ascending Stairs

To ascend stairs, the cane is placed in the hand on the *un*affected side. Grasping the stair railing on the affected side, the patient should move the *un*affected leg up the stair, followed by the affected leg.

Safety Tips

SHOES. Have the patient wear flat shoes, with approximately a 1/2-inch heel. The sole of the shoes should be a non-skid surface. Shoes that strap on are safer than loafers or slip-ons, which are apt to slip off.

DEVICE. The rubber suction tip(s) on the bottom of the ambulatory assistive devices, as well as the hand grips, should be checked for secure fit, cracks, and uneven wearing.

ENVIRONMENT. All potential obstructions should be removed from the floor to ensure safe passage. Throw rugs, electrical cords, and telephone cords are especially hazardous. Optimal lighting, without excessive glare, should be provided. The room should be arranged so that frequently used items are placed in close proximity to the patient.

STAIRS. Have someone stand behind the patient when he or she is first learning to ascend stairs, and beside or in front as he or she descends stairs for the first time.

●●

Beginning Exercise
for Rehabilitation

This appendix should be used as a guide to provide beginning exercise for rehabilitation of various regional musculoskeletal problems. The exercise recommendations are not intended to take the place of a comprehensive rehabilitation program. The prudent practitioner should always consult a rehabilitation specialist for more individualized treatment plans. The exercises follow the text chapters.

Keep in mind to start *slowly:* advise the patient to hold each exercise for 5 to 10 seconds. Suggest that the patient count out loud to avoid breath holding. Initially each exercise should consist of 5 to 10 repetitions and should be done twice each day. Always instruct the patient in the exercise, and supervise the patient for correct performance in order to ensure that directions and techniques are understood. Warming up the area to be exercised before starting is as important as cooling the area following exercise. Either can be accomplished by stretching or by application of a warm pack to the area for warm up or a cold pack for cool down.

Stretching and range-of-motion exercises should be performed before strengthening exercises.

Cervical Spine

Isometric (Strengthening)

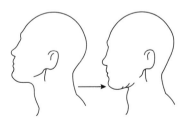

Neck Glide (Axial Extension)
- Begin sitting or standing naturally.

- Tuck your chin in and pull your head slowly and gently back.

- Hold for 10–30 seconds.

- _____ repetitions, _____ times per day.

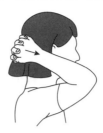

Neck Extension

- Sit or stand.

- Place hands behind head over large bony prominence as shown.

- Press head backwards into hands, without letting either head or hands move.

- Hold _____ seconds.

- _____ repetitions, _____ times per day.

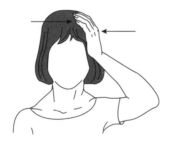

Neck Side-to-Side Bend (Lateral Flexion)

- Sit or stand.

- Place hand on _____ side of head as shown (heel of hand just above the ear).

- Press head sideways into hand.

- Hold _____ seconds.

- _____ repetitions, _____ times per day.

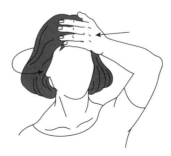

Neck Side-to-Side Rotation

- Sit or stand.

- Place hand on left side of head as shown.

- Slowly rotate your head toward your hand (as if looking over your shoulder). Stop at the point of pain. Repeat on the right.

- Hold _____ seconds.

- _____ repetitions, _____ times per day.

Range of Motion (Flexibility)

- Sit or stand.

- Shrug shoulders in all directions both together and alternately to begin.

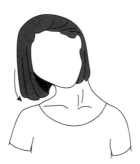

Neck Side Bending

- Sit or stand.

- Keeping face forward, tip right ear toward shoulder.

- Hold _____ seconds and relax by returning to starting position. Repeat on left.

- _____ repetitions, _____ times per day.

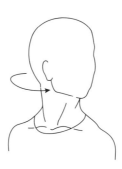

Side-to-Side Neck Rotation

- Sit or stand.

- Slowly turn head and chin to the _____.

- Hold _____ seconds. Relax and repeat on the _____.
- _____ repetitions, _____ times per day.

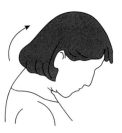

Neck Flexion

- Sit or stand.

- Bend head forward as shown.

- Hold _____ seconds, relax.

- _____ repetitions, _____ times per day.

Lumbar Spine

Strengthening (to be done on a protected, firm surface, such as a carpeted floor or exercise mat)

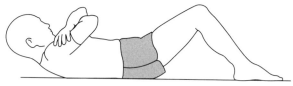

Abdominal Curl/Back Flexion

- Lie on back with knees bent.

- Cross arms over chest.

- Raise head and shoulders, curl trunk upward no more than 6 inches, as shown. Keep small of back pressed against the mat. Exhale during the curl up.

- Hold _____ seconds.

- _____ repetitions, _____ times per day.

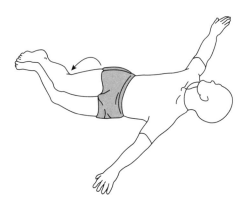

Back Rotation
- Lie on back with knees bent and feet together, arms out to the side.

- Rotate knees to the left as you turn head in the opposite direction, until you feel a stretch.

- Hold _____ seconds. Relax and repeat on the right.

- _____ repetitions, _____ times per day.

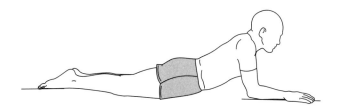

Back Extension (Beginning Extension Exercise)
- Lie on stomach and place hands as shown.

- Hold 30–60 seconds.

- _____ repetitions, _____ times per day.

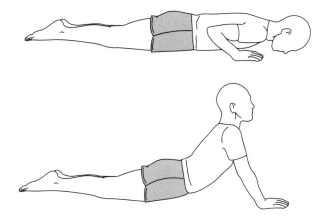

Back Extension (Prone Push-Up)
- Lie on stomach and place hands on floor, as shown.

- Slowly straighten arms to press upper body off floor, keeping pelvis against the floor.

- Hold 30–60 seconds.

- _____ repetitions, _____ times per day.

Stretching

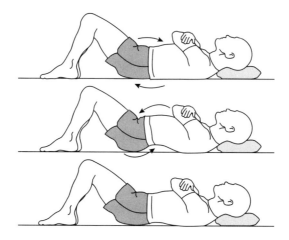

Pelvic Posterior (Tilt)

- Lie on back with knees bent.
- Tighten your abdominal muscles, squeeze buttocks muscles, and flatten your back as shown.
- Hold _____ seconds.
- _____ repetitions, _____ times per day.

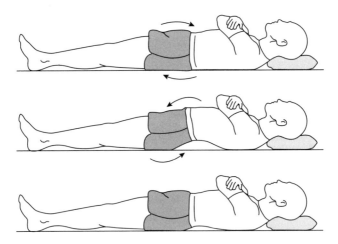

Pelvic Rotation (Tilt)

- Lie on back with legs straight.
- Tighten your abdominal muscles, squeeze buttocks muscles, and flatten your back as shown.
- Then, rotate tailbone backward/upward and arch back as shown.
- Hold _____ seconds.
- _____ repetitions, _____ times per day.

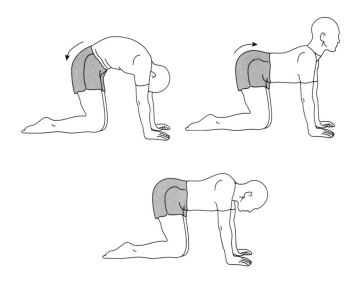

Pelvic Rotation (Cat and Camel)

• Assume hands and knees position.

• Tuck chin to chest. Tighten your abdominal muscles, squeeze buttocks muscles, and tuck tailbone under, arch back upward as shown. Keep the elbows straight.

• Then raise head, let low back sag toward floor. Keep the elbows straight.

• Hold _____ seconds.

• _____ repetitions, _____ times per day.

Shoulder

Range of Motion

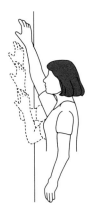

Shoulder Flexion/(Wall Climb)

- Stand 1–2 feet from a wall as shown.

- Slowly "walk" your fingers up the wall so that you feel a stretch.

- Increase distance walked up wall as motion improves.

- _____ repetitions, _____ times per day.

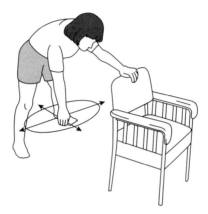

Shoulder Pendulum (Codman Exercises)

- Lean forward as shown, letting _____ arm hang down (elbow may be bent 90 degrees).

- Keep knees slightly bent; let arm swing forward and backward, then side to side ("elephant's trunk").

- Increase length of swing as motion improves.

- Repeat, with the arm moving in small circles, clockwise and counterclockwise; gradually make larger circles.

- _____ repetitions, _____ times per day.

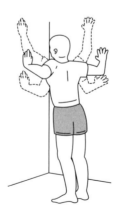

Shoulder Abduction

- Stand in a corner about 1 to 2 feet from the wall with hands on wall as shown; or stand in a door frame (see p. 144).

- Lean into corner so that you feel a stretch.
- Vary the stretch by moving arms higher or lower or by standing away from wall.
- Hold _____ seconds.
- _____ repetitions, _____ times per day.

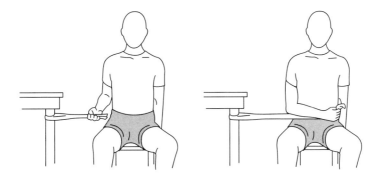

Strengthening (see p. 144)

Shoulder Internal Rotation
- Anchor rubber tubing to solid object (table leg or doorknob).
- Sit or stand with arm at side, elbow bent as shown.
- Slowly rotate arm inward toward body.
- Hold _____ seconds.
- _____ repetitions, _____ times per day.
- Repeat sequence in opposite direction for external rotation conditioning.

Elbow, Wrist, and Hand

Strengthening
Elbow Flexion and Extension With and Against Gravity

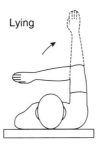

Lying

- Lie flat with _____ arm extended.
- Flex elbow to 90 degrees.

- Extend to straight position.

- Hold _____ seconds/minutes.

- _____ repetitions, _____ times per day.

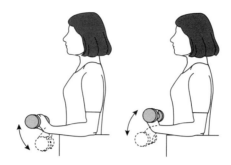

Wrist Curls and Reverse Wrist Curls (start when you are pain free)
- Support arm on flat surface.

- With palm up, flex and extend wrist fully; with palm down, flex and extend wrist fully (can be done up fast, down slow).

- Hold _____ seconds/minutes.

- _____ repetitions, _____ times per day.

- May be done with light weights or rubber tubing.

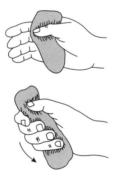

Hand Flexion and Extension
- Hold putty (Play-Doh) or soft rubber ball with your _____ hand.

- Squeeze as firmly as you can.

- Hold _____ seconds/minutes.

- _____ times a day.

Elbow Stretch
- Hold _____ arm at shoulder level, as shown.

- With hand clenched, flex the wrist as far as possible.

- Hold _____ seconds/minutes, relax.

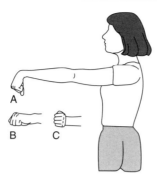

* Return the wrist to neutral position; alternately turn the arm inward with a flexed wrist and then outward with an extended wrist.

* _____ times a day.

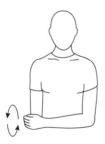

Forearm Rotation

* With elbow flexed at ninety degrees, hold arm in front of you as shown.

* Rotate wrist so that your palm is facing the floor.

* Hold _____ seconds.

* Rotate wrist so that palm is facing up.

* Hold _____ seconds.

* _____ repetitions, _____ times a day.

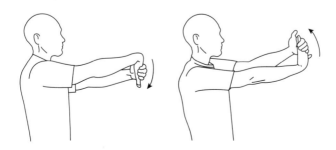

Forearm Extensor and Flexor Stretch

- Extend _____ arm as shown.

- Firmly hold wrist as shown.

- Hold _____ seconds.

- _____ times a day.

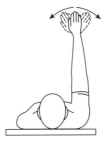

Range of Motion of the Wrist

- Lie flat with _____ arm as shown.

- With palm facing up, move wrist from side to side.

- Move wrist in circles. Gradually increase circles, alternating with wrist facing up and wrist facing down.

- _____ repetitions, _____ times per day.

Hip

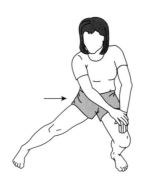

Hip Abduction

- Assume a half-squat position as shown, with _____ leg out to the side. (Never let your knee come over your foot.)

- Press inside of thigh downward by shifting weight toward the bent leg.

- Hold _____ seconds, relax.

- _____ repetitions, _____ times per day.

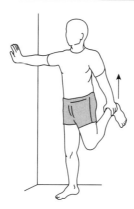

Hip Flexor Stretch
• Stand grasping right ankle as shown.

• Bend knee further by pulling ankle towards buttocks with hand.

• Maintain good erect posture. Do not arch your back or lean forward during the stretch.

• Hold _____ seconds, relax; repeat grasping left ankle.

• _____ repetitions, _____ times per day.

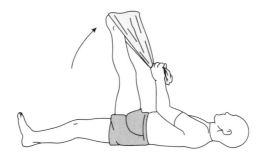

Hamstring Stretch (beginners may try without the towel)
• Lie on back, holding right leg as shown.

• Straighten the knee as far as you can to feel a stretch, keeping your other leg straight on the floor.

• Hold _____ seconds, relax; repeat holding left leg.

• _____ repetitions, _____ times per day.

Illiotibial Band Stretching
• While standing, place the affected hip toward the wall as shown.

• Lean hip toward wall while keeping trunk away from wall.

• Hold _____ seconds.

• _____ repetitions, _____ times per day.

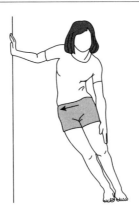

Knee

Strengthening

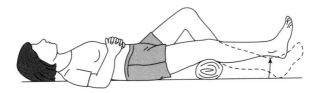

Short Arc Quadriceps Strengthening

- Lie on your back with knee supported and bent 30–45 degrees.

- Lift heel off floor until knee is straight.

- Hold 10 seconds and slowly allow knee to bend; relax (see p. 241).

- _____ repetitions, _____ times per day.

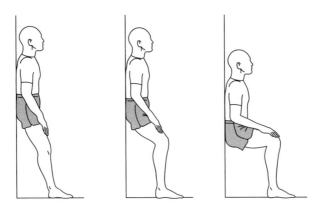

Quadriceps—Slide

- Stand with back against wall, feet shoulder width apart and 18 inches from wall.

- Slowly slide down wall until you are in a "chair position."

- Hold 10 seconds, relax.

- _____ repetitions, _____ times per day.

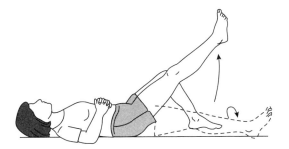

Straight Leg Raise

- Lie on back with _____ knee straight and the other knee bent as shown.

- Keep the leg straight, with toes pointed outward, then raise it 10 inches. (Do not let your back arch.)

- Hold _____ seconds.

- _____ repetitions, _____ times per day.

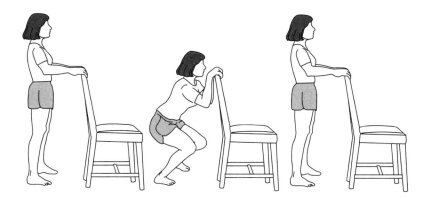

Quadriceps—Squats

- Hold onto chair back or table.

- Keep feet flat on the floor spaced shoulderwidth apart.

- Keeping heels on the floor, squat as far as you can, then stand up using as little help from arms as possible.

- _____ repetitions, _____ times per day.

Lower Leg

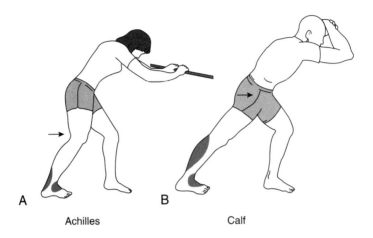

A   Achilles   B   Calf

Lower Leg Stretches (Calf/Achilles Tendon)

- Hold foot against wall with knee flexed, as shown.

- Bend knee and push body toward wall (**A**); straighten knee (**B**).

- Hold _____ seconds.

- _____ repetitions, _____ times a day.

Ankle and Foot

Strengthening

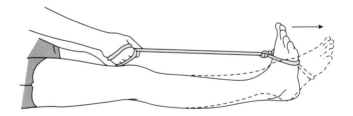

Resisted Plantar Flexion

- Wrap tubing or towel around _____ foot, sitting with knee extended.

- Press foot away from knee as shown.

- Hold 10–30 seconds, relax.

- 5 repetitions, _____ times per day.

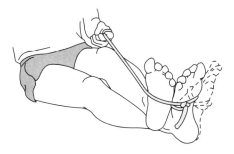

Resisted Inversion
- Cross legs with affected ankle underneath.
- With tubing anchored around foot as shown, slowly turn affected foot inward.
- Hold _____ seconds, relax.
- _____ repetitions, _____ times per day.

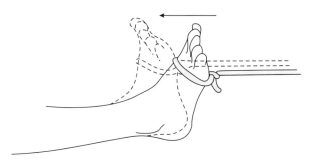

Resisted Dorsiflexion
- Wrap tubing around _____ foot; anchor tubing around solid object (eg, table leg).
- Sit with knee extended; pull forefoot toward knee.
- Hold 10–30 seconds, relax.
- 5 repetitions, 2 times per day.

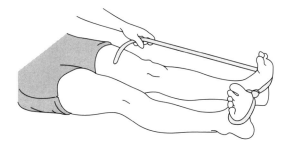

Resisted Eversion
- Wrap tubing around uninvolved foot and behind involved foot as shown.
- Slowly turn involved foot outward.

- Hold _____ seconds, relax.

- _____ repetitions, _____ times per day.

Stretching
Ankle Alphabet

- Move your ankle around slowly to trace the letters of the alphabet.

- Start slowly with six letters; gradually increase by adding a letter each day.

- Repeat _____ times per day.

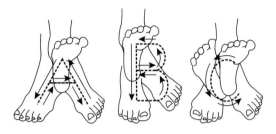

Forefoot

Range of Motion

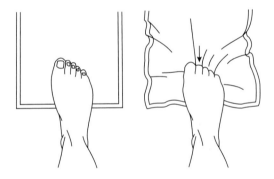

Toe Towel Curls

- Sit comfortably.

- Place towel on floor as shown.

- Grasp the towel with the toes.

- Start slowly, 1–2 minutes, 2 times a day.

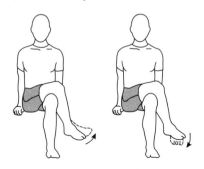

Toe Flexion and Extension
- Sit comfortably.

- Straighten and spread the toes.

- Curl the toes up and down.

- Start slowly, 1–2 minutes daily.

Osteoporosis

Weight Bearing or Impact Exercises
Walking, 3 to 4 times each week for 1 hour.

Modest Weight Training
Add 1- to 3-lb weights to the wrists when walking.

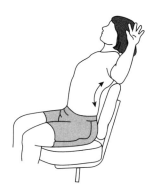

Back Bends (Extension)
- Sit with back against chair as shown.

- Slowly reach upward and lean backward until you feel a stretch.

- Hold _____ seconds.

- _____ repetitions, _____ times per day.

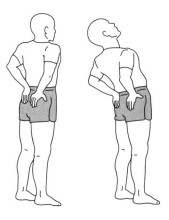

Back Bends (Extension)

- Firmly place hands against lower back as shown.

- Slowly bend backward until you feel a stretch.

- Hold _____ seconds.

- _____ repetitions, _____ times per day.

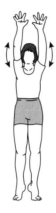

Back Extension (Thoracic Stretch)

- Stand on tiptoes, arms overhead as shown.

- Slowly reach toward the ceiling.

- Hold _____ seconds.

- _____ repetitions, _____ times per day.

The authors wish to acknowledge the following dedicated rehabilitation specialists: Doreen Robinson, RPT; Julie Jacobs, RPT; Kathy Baker, RPT; and Robin Masuda, RPT.

Intraarticular Aspiration and Injection

Intraarticular aspiration is frequently used to diagnose rheumatic conditions such as crystal disease (gout, pseudogout). Arthrocentesis of a joint can aid in distinguishing betweeen inflammatory, non-inflammatory, and septic joint conditions. Synovial fluid analysis must be completed in order to effect a diagnosis for the patient with a joint effusion. Therapeutic aspiration can reduce pain by relieving pressure within the joint capsule.

Corticosteroid injection therapy may be used to treat inflammation of soft tissues, bursae, tendon sheaths, and joints. Commonly used preparations are shown in Table F-1.

Sodium hyaluronate injections are used to treat osteoarthritic knee joints. Since the patient will not obtain relief unless the medication is injected precisely within the synovial space of the articulating joint surfaces, these new and costly injections should be done only by a specialist (orthopedic surgeon or rheumatologist).

Indications

Joint aspiration with or without injection is indicated for the temporary relief of inflammation and pain associated with rheumatic and rheumatic soft tissue conditions.

Contraindications

Joint diagnostic aspiration and therapeutic corticosteroid injection are contraindicated in the following:

Diagnostic Aspiration
- Soft tissue sepsis in the area of aspiration (cellulitis)

- Bacteremia

- Coagulopathy

Therapeutic Injection
- All of the above

- Avascular necrosis

- Charcot joints

- Trauma

- Septic arthritis

TABLE F-1
Corticosteroids in Current Use

Corticosteroid	Concentrations Available	Dose Range
Prednisolone tebutate (Hydetra TBA)	20 mg/mL	5–15 mg
Betamethasone acetate and betamethasone sodium phosphate (Celestone Soluspan)	6 mg/mL	1.5–3 mg
Methylprednisolone acetate Depo-Medrol)	20–40–80 mg/mL	10–20 mg
Triamcinolone acetonide or diacetate (Aristocort)	10–25–40 mg/mL	5–15 mg
Triamcinolone hexaacetonide (Aristospan)	5–20 mg/mL	5–20 mg
Dexamethasone acetate suspension (Decadron-LA)	8 mg/mL	0.8–3.2 mg

(From Schoen, R. P., Moskowitz, R. W., & Goldberg, V. M. [1996]. *Soft tissue rheumatic pain* [3rd ed.]. Baltimore: Williams and Wilkins)

Precautions

• Patients who require injection of the hip, spine, hand, and foot/ankle should be referred to a specialist due to the technical difficulties associated with injection and aspiration of these joints.

• Frequent injection of weight-bearing joints of patients with osteoarthritis should be avoided. Frequent use of corticosteroids in these joints can hasten joint destruction.

Potential Complications

• Steroid arthropathy

• Soft tissue atrophy

• Tendon rupture

• Infection

• Needle trauma

• Allergic reaction

• Nerve damage

• Post-injection flare (most common)

- Cushing's syndrome
- Exacerbation of diabetes
- Uterine bleeding
- Intraarticular bleeding

Frequency of Injection

- Weight bearing joints—no more than every 4 months.
- Soft tissue and other joint injections—no more than every 6 weeks (no more than three injections a year)

Patient Preparation

Explain the risks and benefits of the procedure and obtain the patient's informed consent.

Technique

The following is suggested as one approach to joint aspiration and injection. Refer to specific chapters for additional information.

1. Use aseptic technique and standard precautions.
2. Palpate the joint and mark the insertion site with a pen with the point retracted. This will create an impression that will last 5 to 15 minutes.
3. Clean the skin with an antiseptic solution.

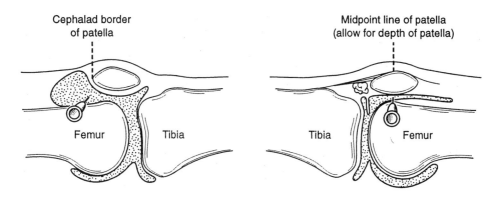

FIGURE F-1. Aspiration of the knee: (**A**) lateral approach; (**B**) medial approach. (From Gatter, R.A. [1993]. Arthrocentesis technique and intralesional therapy. In McCarty, D.J., & Koopman, W.J. [Eds.]. *Arthritis and allied conditions* (12th ed., p. 712). Philadelphia: Lea and Febiger.)

4. Spray with ethylchloride.

5. Stretch the skin and insert the needle through the impression mark; aspirate gently as the needle is advanced into the joint space.

6. If aspiration will be followed by injection, leave the needle in the joint, change syringes, and inject the steroid preparation. *Never* inject against resistance.

7. If aspiration will not be followed by injection, or after injection is complete, remove the syringe and needle and apply pressure to the puncture site.

Specific Technique: The Knee (Fig. F-1)

• Use a 1½-inch, 18-gauge needle.

• Enter laterally just below the patella and advance toward the superior pole for a large effusion (*A*).

• Enter medially under the midpoint of the patella for a small effusion (*B*). Allow an extra 1 to 2 cm posterior to the medial edge of the patella to avoid hitting the V-shaped gliding surface.

• Aspirate continuously while advancing the needle.

Discharge Instructions

Advise the patient to observe the following measures:

• Rest the joint and apply ice packs to the site for 15 minutes four times a day for 2 days. This helps to prevent a post-injection flare.

• Avoid ballistic stress, such as throwing a ball or swinging a golf club, for several weeks if the injection was near a tendon.

• Continue previous therapy such as medications and thermotherapy.

• If there is increased pain following the injection beyond 24 hours, patient evaluation is indicated to rule out infection.

Recommended Readings

Anderson, B.C. (1994). *Office orthopedics for primary care*. Philadelphia: Saunders.
Gatter, R.A. (1993). Arthrocentesis technique and intralesional therapy. In McCarty D.J., & Koopman, W.J. (Eds.). *Arthritis and allied conditions* (12th ed., p. 712). Philadelphia: Lea and Febiger.
Owen, D.S. (1997). Aspiration and injection of joints and soft tissues. In Kelley, W.N., Harris, E.D., Ruddy, S., & Sledge, C.B. (Eds.) *Textbook of rheumatology* (5th ed., p. 591). Philadelphia: Saunders.
Shoen, R.P., Moskowitz, R.W., & Goldby, V.M. (Eds). (1996). *Soft tissue rheumatic pain* (3rd ed.). Baltimore: Williams and Wilkins.

Index

Page numbers followed by *f* refer to figures; page numbers followed by *t* refer to tables.

A

Abductor pollicis tendons, anatomy of, 168
Abscess, epidural, and low back pain, 113
Acetaminophen, 327
  for arthritis, 312
Achilles tendinitis, 263–264
Achilles tendon, rupture of, 264, 265f
Acromioclavicular joint
  anatomy of, 119f
  separation of, 131, 131f–132f
Acromion, anatomy of, 117
Activities of daily living (ADLs), 28
ADLs (activities of daily living), 28
Adolescents. *See also* specific disorders
  adaptation to illness by, 5
  chronic conditions in, 14–15
  developmental tasks of, 4
  exercise in, 15t, 15–16
  fractures in, 8
  musculoskeletal system of, 5
  overuse injuries in, prevention of, 3t
  psychosocial issues of, 4–5
  sports preparticipation examination of, 5, 6f, 7
  trauma in, 7–8
Adson maneuver, in cervical spine assessment, 56
Adults
  developmental tasks of, 16
  psychosocial issues of, 16
Aging, demographics of, 27–29
Alcohol abuse, in older adults, 32
Alendronate, for prevention of osteoporosis, 308
Allen test, 175
Allopurinol, for gout, 305, 330–331
Ambulation, assistive devices for, 335–338
Amoxicillin, for Lyme disease, 296, 296t
ANA (antinuclear antibody), in arthritis, 314
Analgesics, 327–328
  for arthritis, 311–312
Animal bites, on hand, treatment of, 181
Ankle
  anatomy of, 266–268, 267f
  exercise for, 355–357
  fractures of, 273–274
  sprains of, 268–272, 269f–271f
    mechanism of injury in, 268, 269f
    physical examination in, 268–272, 270f
    rehabilitation after, 272
    treatment of, 272

Ankylosing spondylitis, 202–203, 298t–299t, 299
Anterior drawer sign, 231, 270f
Antidepressants, tricyclic, for diffuse pain syndromes, 324
Antimalarials, for rheumatoid arthritis, 311
Antinuclear antibody (ANA), in arthritis, 313
Antirheumatic drugs, disease-modifying, 312–313, 329–330
Apley compression test, 232
Apophyseal avulsion fractures, 211–212, 212t
Apophysitis, of tibial tubercle, 10–11
Arteritis, temporal, 303
Arthritis, 38–39, 40t
  in adolescents, 317–318
  crystalline, hip pain from, 205
  degenerative, of cervical spine, 61–64
  diagnosis of, 313–315
  differential diagnosis of, 292f, 294t
  in elbow, 159–160
  history in, 289, 290t–291t, 293f
  in human immunodeficiency virus infection, 297
  infectious, 295–297, 296t
  inflammatory, hip pain from, 204–205
  inflammatory bowel disease and, 300
  from parvovirus-19, 297
  physical examination in, 291t
  psoriatic, 294–295
  psychosocial issues in, 317–318
  reactive, 299–300
  in rearfoot, 281
  rehabilitation in, 40t
  rheumatoid, 39, 292–293, 293f
    differential diagnosis of, 294t
    of hand, 191
    juvenile, 305
    of wrist, 190–191
  treatment of
    analgesics in, 311–312
    exercise in, 315
    nontraditional, 316
    occupational therapy in, 315
    physical therapy in, 314–315
Arthritis Foundation, 324
Arthrocentesis, 314
Aspiration. *See* Joint aspiration
Assistive devices, ambulatory, 335–338
Ataxic gait, 254–255
Athletes, recreational, injuries in, 21–22

363

The following figures and tables were borrowed from Lippincott Williams & Wilkins sources:

Figure 1-1 Weinstein, S., and Buckwalter, J. (1994). *Turek's Orthopaedics, 5/e.* Philadelphia: Lippincott-Raven Publishers. *Figure 13-2, page 451*

Figure 2-1 Rosse, C., and Rosse, P. G. (1997). *Hollinshead's Textbook of Anatomy, 5/e.* Philadelphia: Lippincott-Raven Publishers. *Figure 12-1, page 110*

Table 2-2 Rosse, C., and Rosse, P. G. (1997). *Hollinshead's Textbook of Anatomy, 5/e.* Philadelphia: Lippincott-Raven Publishers. *Table 9-3, page 347*

Figure 2-2 Rosse, C., and Rosse, P. G. (1997). *Hollinshead's Textbook of Anatomy, 5/e.* Philadelphia: Lippincott-Raven Publishers. *Figure 12-11, page 119*

Figure 2-3 Porth, C. M. (1998). *Pathophysiology: Concepts of Altered Health States, 5/e.* Philadelphia: Lippincott-Raven Publishers. *Figure 50-13A, page 1051*

Figure 2-4 Weinstein, S., and Buckwalter, J. (1994). *Turek's Orthopaedics, 5/e.* Philadelphia: Lippincott-Raven Publishers. *Figure 13-33, page 480*

First unnumbered table in Chapter 3 Weinstein, S., and Buckwalter, J. (1994). *Turek's Orthopaedics, 5/e.* Philadelphia: Lippincott-Raven Publishers. *Table 13-4, page 466*

Second unnumbered table in Chapter 3 Hardy, R. (1993). *Lumbar Disc Disease, 2/e.* Philadelphia: J.B. Lippincott Company. *Table 1, page 26*

Figure 3-2A Rosse, C., and Rosse, P. G. (1997). *Hollinshead's Textbook of Anatomy, 5/e.* Philadelphia: Lippincott-Raven Publishers. *Figure 12-12, page 119*

Figure 3-3A Unni, K. K. (1996). *Dahlin's Bone Tumors.* Philadelphia: J.B. Lippincott Company. *Figure 22-3, page 309*

Figure 3-3B Porth, C. M. (1998). *Pathophysiology: Concepts of Altered Health States, 5/e.* Philadelphia: Lippincott-Raven Publishers. *Figure 50-13B, page 1051*

Figure 3-4 Rosse, C., and Rosse, P. G. (1997). *Hollinshead's Textbook of Anatomy, 5/e.* Philadelphia: Lippincott-Raven Publishers. *Figure 12-3, page 113*

Figure 3-6 Burnside, J. W., and McGlynne, T. J. (1987). *Physical diagnosis, 17/e.* Baltimore: Williams & Wilkins. *Page 262*

Figure 3-8 Burnside, J. W., and McGlynne, T. J. (1987). *Physical diagnosis, 17/e.* Baltimore: Williams & Wilkins. Page 262

Figure 4-1 Rosse, C., and Rosse, P. G. (1997). *Hollinshead's Textbook of Anatomy, 5/e.* Philadelphia: Lippincott-Raven Publishers. *Figure 15-6, page 201*

Figure 4-2 Rosse, C., and Rosse, P. G. (1997). *Hollinshead's Textbook of Anatomy, 5/e.* Philadelphia: Lippincott-Raven Publishers. *Figure 15-28, page 226*

Figure 4-3 Rosse, C., and Rosse, P. G. (1997). *Hollinshead's Textbook of Anatomy, 5/e.* Philadelphia: Lippincott-Raven Publishers. *Figure 15-32, page 230*

Figure 4-4 Rosse, C., and Rosse, P. G. (1997). *Hollinshead's Textbook of Anatomy, 5/e.* Philadelphia: Lippincott-Raven Publishers. *Figure 15-33, page 232*

Figure 4-5 Rosse, C., and Rosse, P. G. (1997). *Hollinshead's Textbook of Anatomy, 5/e.* Philadelphia: Lippincott-Raven Publishers. *Figure 15-21, page 219*

Figure 4-6 Burnside, J. W., & McGlynne, T. J. (1987). *Physical Diagnosis, 17/e.* Baltimore: Williams & Wilkins.

Figure 4-7 DePalma, A. F. (1973). *Surgery of the Shoulder.* Philadelphia: J.B. Lippincott. *Figure 9-73, page 349*

Figure 4-12 Weinstein, S., and Buckwalter, J. (1994). *Turek's Orthopaedics, 5/e.* Philadelphia: Lippincott-Raven Publishers. *Figure 10-30, page 384*

Figure 4-14 Weinstein, S., and Buckwalter, J. (1994). *Turek's Orthopaedics, 5/e.* Philadelphia: Lippincott-Raven Publishers. *Figure 10-38 and 10-39, page 388*

Figure 4-15 Hertling, D., and Kessler, R. M. (1996). *Management of Common Musculoskeletal Disorders: Physical Therapy Principles and Methods, 3/e.* Philadelphia: Lippincott-Raven Publishers. *Page 183*

Figure 4-17 Weinstein, S., and Buckwalter, J. (1994). *Turek's Orthopaedics, 5/e.* Philadelphia: Lippincott-Raven Publishers. *Figure 10-25, page 379*

Figure 4-18 Weinstein, S., and Buckwalter, J. (1994). *Turek's Orthopaedics, 5/e.* Philadelphia: Lippincott-Raven Publishers. *Figure 10-26, page 379*

Figure 4-19   Weinstein, S., and Buckwalter, J. (1994). *Turek's Orthopaedics, 5/e.* Philadelphia: Lippincott-Raven Publishers. *Figure 10-7, page 368*

Table 5-1   Steinberg, G. C, Akins, C., and Baran, D. T. (1992). *Ramamurti's orthopedics in primary care, 2/e.* Baltimore: Williams & Wilkins.

Figure 5-1   Steinberg, G. C., Akins, C., and Baran, D. T. (1992). *Ramamurti's orthopedics in primary care, 2/e.* Baltimore: Williams & Wilkins. *Figure 3-1, page 63*

Figure 5-2   Rosse, C., and Rosse, P. G. (1997). *Hollinshead's Textbook of Anatomy, 5/e.* Philadelphia: Lippincott-Raven Publishers. *Figure 16-61, page 296*

Figure 5-3   Steinberg, G. C., Akins, C., and Baran, D. T. (1992). *Ramamurti's orthopedics in primary care, 2/e.* Baltimore: Williams & Wilkins. *Figure 3-6, page 65*

Figure 5-4   Rosse, C., and Rosse, P. G. (1997). *Hollinshead's Textbook of Anatomy, 5/e.* Philadelphia: Lippincott-Raven Publishers. *Figure 16-22, page 265*

Figure 5-5A   Rosse, C., and Rosse, P. G. (1997). *Hollinshead's Textbook of Anatomy, 5/e.* Philadelphia: Lippincott-Raven Publishers. *Figure 16-27, page 269*

Figure 5-5B   Rosse, C., and Rosse, P. G. (1997). *Hollinshead's Textbook of Anatomy, 5/e.* Philadelphia: Lippincott-Raven Publishers. *Figure 16-28, page 270*

Figure 5-8   Burnside, J. W., and McGlynne, T. J. (1987). *Physical diagnosis, 17/e.* Baltimore: Williams & Wilkins.

Figure 5-12   Morrey, B. F. (1993). *The Elbow and Its Disorders.* Philadelphia: J.B. Lippincott Company. *Figure 18-1, page 283*

Figure 5-13   Morrey, B. F. (1993). *The Elbow and Its Disorders.* Philadelphia: J.B. Lippincott Company. *Figure 18-4, page 286*

Figure 6-1   Rosse, C., and Rosse, P. G. (1997). *Hollinshead's Textbook of Anatomy, 5/e.* Philadelphia: Lippincott-Raven Publishers. *Figure 16-5, page 245*

Figure 6-4   Rosse, C., and Rosse, P. G. (1997). *Hollinshead's Textbook of Anatomy, 5/e.* Philadelphia: Lippincott-Raven Publishers. *Figure 16-30, page 273*

Figure 6-5   Rosse, C., and Rosse, P. G. (1997). *Hollinshead's Textbook of Anatomy, 5/e.* Philadelphia: Lippincott-Raven Publishers. *Figure 16-47, page 285*

Figure 6-6   Bates, B. (1995). *A Guide to Physical Examination and History Taking.* Philadelphia: Lippincott-Raven Publishers. *Page 325*

Figure 6-14   Weinstein, S., and Buckwalter, J. (1994). *Turek's Orthopaedics, 5/e.* Philadelphia: Lippincott-Raven Publishers. *Figure 12-12A, page 434*

Figure 6-15   Weinstein, S., and Buckwalter, J. (1994). *Turek's Orthopaedics, 5/e.* Philadelphia: Lippincott-Raven Publishers. *Figure 12-13, page 435*

Figure 7-1   Rosse, C., and Rosse, P. G. (1997). *Hollinshead's Textbook of Anatomy, 5/e.* Philadelphia: Lippincott-Raven Publishers. *Figure 17-1, page 308*

Figure 7-2   Rosse, C., and Rosse, P. G. (1997). *Hollinshead's Textbook of Anatomy, 5/e.* Philadelphia: Lippincott-Raven Publishers. *Figure 17-3A, page 310*

Figure 7-3   Burnside, J. W., and McGlynne, T. J. (1987). *Physical diagnosis, 17/e.* Baltimore: Williams & Wilkins.

Figure 7-4   Drave, D. J. (1986). *Anatomy of the lower extremity.* Baltimore: Williams & Wilkins. *Figure 3-33, page 63*

Figure 7-5   McNab, I. (1977). *Backache.* Baltimore: Williams & Wilkins.

Figure 7-6   Rosse, C., and Rosse, P. G. (1997). *Hollinshead's Textbook of Anatomy, 5/e.* Philadelphia: Lippincott-Raven Publishers. *Figure 17-20, page 330*

Figure 7-7   Steinberg, G. C., Akins, C., and Baran, D. T. (1992). *Ramamurti's orthopedics in primary care, 2/e.* Baltimore: Williams & Wilkins.

Figure 7-8   Steinberg, G. C., Akins, C., and Baran, D. T. (1992). *Ramamurti's orthopedics in primary care, 2/e.* Baltimore: Williams & Wilkins. *Figure 6-27, page 187*

Figure 8-1   Rosse, C., and Rosse, P. G. (1997). *Hollinshead's Textbook of Anatomy, 5/e.* Philadelphia: Lippincott-Raven Publishers. *Figure 18-34, page 381*

Figure 8-2   Rosse, C., and Rosse, P. G. (1997). *Hollinshead's Textbook of Anatomy, 5/e.* Philadelphia: Lippincott-Raven Publishers. *Figure 18-36, page 382*

Figure 8-3   Rosse, C., and Rosse, P. G. (1997). *Hollinshead's Textbook of Anatomy, 5/e.* Philadelphia: Lippincott-Raven Publishers. *Figure 18-39, page 385*

Figure 8-4   Rosse, C., and Rosse, P. G. (1997). *Hollinshead's Textbook of Anatomy, 5/e.* Philadelphia: Lippincott-Raven Publishers. *Figure 18-11, page 356*

Figure 8-5   Weinstein, S., and Buckwalter, J. (1994). *Turek's Orthopaedics, 5/e.* Philadelphia: Lippincott-Raven Publishers. *Figure 17-1, page 586*

Figure 8-10   Scott, W. N. (1984). *Principles of sports medicine.* Baltimore: Williams & Wilkins. *Page 302*

Figure 8-12   Steinberg, G. C., Akins, C., and Baran, D. T. (1992). *Ramamurti's orthopedics in primary care, 2/e.* Baltimore: Williams & Wilkins. *Figures 7-21, 7-22, 7-23, and 7-24, pages 208–209*

Figure 8-13   Steinberg, G. C., Akins, C., and Baran, D. T. (1992). *Ramamurti's orthopedics in primary care, 2/e.* Baltimore: Williams & Wilkins.

Figure 9-1   Rosse, C., and Rosse, P. G. (1997). *Hollinshead's Textbook of Anatomy, 5/e.* Philadelphia: Lippincott-Raven Publishers. *Figure 18-19, page 377*

Figure 9-2   Steinberg, G. C., Akins, C., and Baran, D. T. (1992). *Ramamurti's orthopedics in primary care, 2/e.* Baltimore: Williams & Wilkins. *Figure 8-8, page 236*

Figure 9-3   Steinberg, G. C., Akins, C., and Baran, D. T. (1992). *Ramamurti's orthopedics in primary care, 2/e.* Baltimore: Williams & Wilkins. *Figure 8-14, page 246*

Figure 9-6   Gorroll, A. H., May, L. A., and Mulley, A. G. (1995). *Primary Care Medicine.* Philadelphia: J.B. Lippincott. *Figure 154-2, page 777*

Figure 9-7   Burnside, J. W., and McGlyne, T. J. (1987). *Physical diagnosis, 17/e.* Baltimore: Williams & Wilkins.

Figure 9-10   Steinberg, G. C., Akins, C., and Baran, D. T. (1992). *Ramamurti's orthopedics in primary care, 2/e.* Baltimore: Williams & Wilkins. *Figure 9-1, page 259*

Figure 9-11   Steinberg, G. C., Akins, C., and Baran, D. T. (1992). *Ramamurti's orthopedics in primary care, 2/e.* Baltimore: Williams & Wilkins.

Figure 9-12   Weinstein, S., and Buckwalter, J. (1994). *Turek's Orthopaedics, 5/e.* Philadelphia: Lippincott-Raven Publishers. *Figure 18-10, page 623*

Figure 10-1   Rosse, C., and Rosse, P. G. (1997). *Hollinshead's Textbook of Anatomy, 5/e.* Philadelphia: Lippincott-Raven Publishers. *Figure 5-8, page 37*

Figure 10-4   Hardy, R. (1993). *Lumbar Disc Disease, 2/e.* Philadelphia: J.B. Lippincott Company. *Figure 3, page 27*

Figure 10-5   Unni, K. K. (1996). *Dahlin's Bone Tumors.* Philadelphia: J.B. Lippincott Company. *Figure 27-113, page 416*

Figure 10-6   Weinstein, S., and Buckwalter, J. (1994). *Turek's Orthopaedics, 5/e.* Philadelphia: Lippincott-Raven Publishers. *Figure 5-16, page 206*

Figure 10-7   Warfield, C. (1990). *Manual of Pain Management.* Philadelphia: J.B. Lippincott Company. *Figures 28-1 and 28-2, pages 168 and 169*

Appendix E, Forefoot exercises   Steinberg, G. C., Akins, C., and Baran, D. T. (1992). *Ramamurti's Orthopedics in Primary Care,* 2/e. Baltimore: Williams & Wilkins